A Sketch of the Life and Writings of
Robert Knox
the Anatomist

HENRY LONSDALE

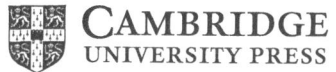

CAMBRIDGE
UNIVERSITY PRESS

CAMBRIDGE
UNIVERSITY PRESS

University Printing House, Cambridge, CB2 8BS, United Kingdom

Published in the United States of America by Cambridge University Press, New York

Cambridge University Press is part of the University of Cambridge.
It furthers the University's mission by disseminating knowledge in the pursuit of
education, learning and research at the highest international levels of excellence.

www.cambridge.org
Information on this title: www.cambridge.org/9781108065290

© in this compilation Cambridge University Press 2013

This edition first published 1870
This digitally printed version 2013

ISBN 978-1-108-06529-0 Paperback

CAMBRIDGE LIBRARY COLLECTION

Books of enduring scholarly value

History of Medicine

It is sobering to realise that as recently as the year in which On the Origin of Species was published, learned opinion was that diseases such as typhus and cholera were spread by a 'miasma', and suggestions that doctors should wash their hands before examining patients were greeted with mockery by the profession. The Cambridge Library Collection reissues milestone publications in the history of Western medicine as well as studies of other medical traditions. Its coverage ranges from Galen on anatomical procedures to Florence Nightingale's common-sense advice to nurses, and includes early research into genetics and mental health, colonial reports on tropical diseases, documents on public health and military medicine, and publications on spa culture and medicinal plants.

A Sketch of the Life and Writings of Robert Knox, the Anatomist

Among the ablest anatomical teachers of his day, Robert Knox (1791–1862) also busied himself with the study of zoology and ethnology. Prepared by his pupil and colleague Henry Lonsdale (1816–76), this 1870 biography explores the scope of Knox's scientific research and the nature of his character. It describes how Knox developed at Edinburgh one of the most significant anatomical schools in Britain, playing a dominant role in expanding the comparative anatomy collection held by the city's Royal College of Surgeons. Despite his eminence and popularity as a lecturer, his reputation was deeply tarnished by his association with the notorious murderers Hare and Burke, who had provided Knox with bodies for dissection. Drawing on surviving correspondence and information gathered from friends and colleagues, Lonsdale's work stands as a robust defence and sympathetic portrait of a prominent yet controversial figure in the history of nineteenth-century medicine.

Cambridge University Press has long been a pioneer in the reissuing of out-of-print titles from its own backlist, producing digital reprints of books that are still sought after by scholars and students but could not be reprinted economically using traditional technology. The Cambridge Library Collection extends this activity to a wider range of books which are still of importance to researchers and professionals, either for the source material they contain, or as landmarks in the history of their academic discipline.

Drawing from the world-renowned collections in the Cambridge University Library and other partner libraries, and guided by the advice of experts in each subject area, Cambridge University Press is using state-of-the-art scanning machines in its own Printing House to capture the content of each book selected for inclusion. The files are processed to give a consistently clear, crisp image, and the books finished to the high quality standard for which the Press is recognised around the world. The latest print-on-demand technology ensures that the books will remain available indefinitely, and that orders for single or multiple copies can quickly be supplied.

The Cambridge Library Collection brings back to life books of enduring scholarly value (including out-of-copyright works originally issued by other publishers) across a wide range of disciplines in the humanities and social sciences and in science and technology.

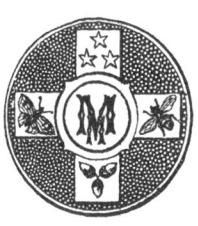

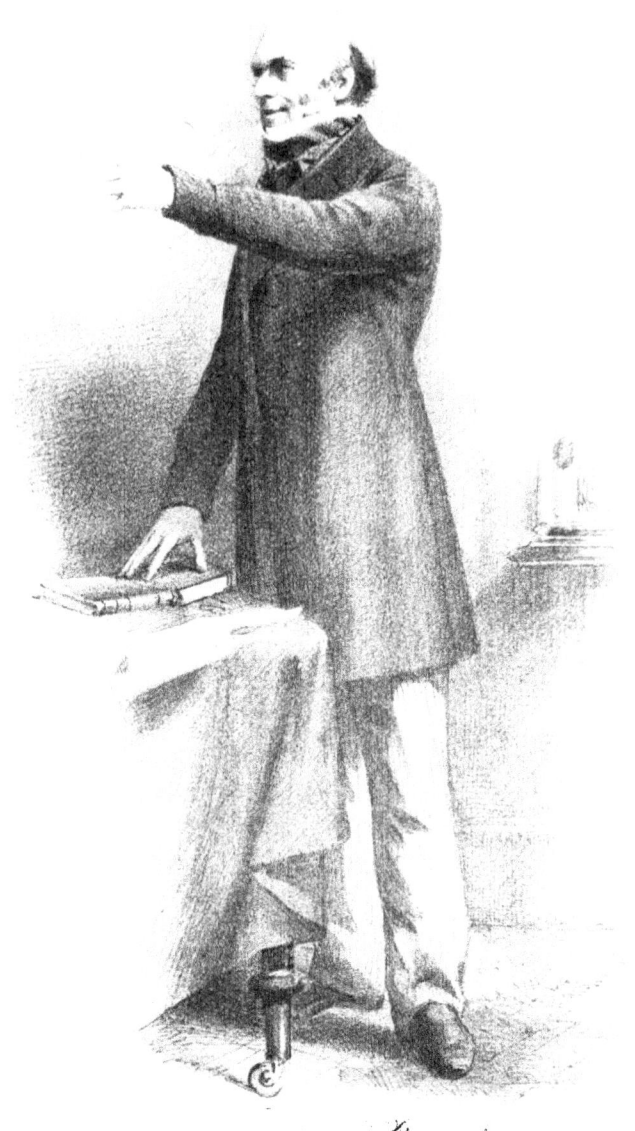

Believe me the
very faithfully yours
R Knox

A SKETCH

OF THE

LIFE AND WRITINGS

OF

ROBERT KNOX

THE ANATOMIST.

BY

His Pupil and Colleague,

HENRY LONSDALE.

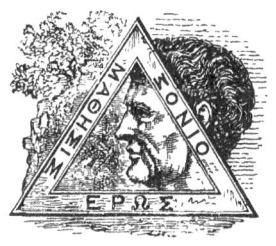

London:

MACMILLAN AND CO.

1870.

LONDON:
R CLAY, SONS, AND TAYLOR, PRINTERS,
BREAD STREET HILL.

TO

SIR WILLIAM FERGUSSON, Bart.

F.R.S.,

SERJEANT-SURGEON TO THE QUEEN, AND PRESIDENT OF THE ROYAL
COLLEGE OF SURGEONS OF ENGLAND.

MY DEAR FERGUSSON,

I have very sincere pleasure in dedicating this volume to
you, the favoured pupil, the zealous colleague, and attached friend
of Dr. ROBERT KNOX.   In associating your excellent name with this
Biography, I do honour to the memory of our Anatomical Teacher.
I also gladly avail myself of this opportunity of paying a grateful
tribute to our long and cordial friendship.

Heartily rejoicing in your well-merited position as one of the
leading representatives of British Surgery,

I am,

Ever yours faithfully,

HENRY LONSDALE.

ROSE HILL, CARLISLE,
September 15, 1870.

PREFACE.

SHORTLY after the decease of Dr. Robert Knox (Dec.
1862), several friends solicited me to write his Life, but
I respectfully declined, on the grounds that I had no
literary experience, and that there were other pupils
and associates of the Anatomist senior to myself, and
much more competent to undertake his biography:
moreover, I was borne down at the time by a domestic
sorrow so trying that the seven years since elapsing
have not entirely effaced its influence. My hopes of
seeing an historical record of Knox lay chiefly with
his distinguished pupil Professor John Goodsir, with
whom I had conversed on this subject in 1864, and
whose remark at the time was pretty much as follows.
"Well, Lonsdale, it (the biography) should be done by
one or both of us: you knew Knox's character and

thoughts better than any one; I'll gather his science, and show the import of his teachings." Unfortunately, the amiable Professor made no progress in the work; and, greatly to the loss of the science which he adorned, he followed his master to the grave in March 1867. Towards Christmas of the same year, the Rev. Joseph Goodsir, an eminent scholar and divine, honoured me with the trust of writing his brother John's biography. In sketching the history of my friend and companion Goodsir, Knox's presence oft came visibly before me, and with it arose the wish to do justice to his character and memory. In January 1868, an advertisement appeared in the *Anthropological Review*, announcing that a Life of Dr. Knox was in preparation, and information was solicited to render that Life more complete. On inquiry, Dr. James Hunt disclosed himself as the writer, and with great courtesy not only offered to give way to what he was kind enough to designate my superior claims, but furnished me with Knox's correspondence for the years 1860-62, excerpts from which will be found in Chapter XIX.

In 1868 my pen was occupied with the memoir of Professor Goodsir, and in completing the Life of Sir James Graham. Wishing to see a better known name than my own attached to Knox's history, I would gladly, as late as October of that year, have persuaded my friend Sir William Fergusson, Bart. to become the biographer of his great teacher : his engagements, however, were too important to permit of such an undertaking; so that the work declined in 1863 eventually comes to be done by me in 1870.

Dr. Knox only a short time before his death destroyed numerous letters and manuscripts ; what was left, though of much less avail than had been anticipated, was kindly placed at my disposal by the only surviving member of his family, his son, Mr. Edward Knox. The gist of the information thus furnished me is contained in the first chapter.

Whilst courteously acknowledging words of encouragement received from various quarters, I regret to say that the direct aid afforded me has been comparatively small. My cordial thanks are due, however, to

my friends Sir W. Fergusson, Bart., Dr. David Skae, of
the Morningside Asylum, Edinburgh, and Dr. James
Adams, of Glasgow, for both anecdote and narrative.
Many friends, like the late Dr. Adams, sen., of Edinburgh, from whom I learned something of Dr. Knox's
career previous to 1834, have passed beyond my
grateful acknowledgments.

Some historical record, however imperfect, was due to
a man of Dr. Knox's eminence, the great notability of
the Edinburgh Medical School during the third and
fourth decades of this century.   He was without dispute
the ablest anatomical teacher of his day.   The character
of a man so scholarly and many-sided, so original and
versatile in thought, so broad and comprehensive in
views, is not easily portrayed; and all that can be
said of the present effort is, that an honest wish not
to extenuate, nor set aught down in malice, has been
the guiding principle.   A more popular cast might
have been given to his biography by saying less about
his scientific career, and more about his personal traits;
on the other hand, to have passed over his zoological

labours with too light a hand would have been unjust to his professional status. It was imperative to notice, however briefly, his varied march over the vast domain of art and literature, as well as science.

A chapter has been devoted to the early history of the Anatomical School of Edinburgh, to enable the reader to comprehend the injustice of the stigma cast upon Dr. Knox by the West Port atrocities, which *happened* to culminate in the rooms of his anatomical establishment. I would gladly have kept the Resurrectionists out of sight, and all remarks bearing upon the history of transactions both painful and harrowing to the general sentiment; but to have written Knox's Life without a clue to the events which damaged his name and destroyed his prospects, would have been as incongruous as playing the Shakesperian Hamlet and omitting altogether the part of the Ghost. The fault of the Resurrectionist system—a terrible blot upon our social status as a Christian nation —lay with the Executive Government of the country, who for half a century proved deaf to all remonstrance, and evinced not the slightest regard for the science of medicine till the anatomical affairs of the kingdom fell into a state of fearful chaos.

As an English boy on the Scottish borders, I was nurtured in the anatomical prejudices of the day, and these prejudices were still fresh in my mind in 1834 when I joined Dr. Knox's class. It was from this cause probably that, during many years' intercourse with the Anatomist, I used to find myself instinctively studying his character in the hope of obtaining a clue to the shadows of his public career; and those who knew our friendly relations will at once concede my claim to be considered fairly conversant with his inner life and opinions. Throughout my medical probation the mode of conducting anatomical establishments previous to and after the passing of the legislative Act of 1832 oft engaged my attention. Now my opportunities were ample, and it may be said unusual, for knowing what has been so unhesitatingly advanced in this volume on all matters pertaining to the operations of the Resurrectionists and their employers. Nor was I less cognizant

of the character of the proletariat population of the
Old Town of Edinburgh.   On my becoming Dr. Knox's
partner in 1840, the anatomical affairs of the city were
in a state of confusion ; and before the winter session
commenced, the Associated Professors and Teachers of
Anatomy and Surgery (Professors Monro, Sir C. Bell,
Sir Geo. Ballingall, Drs. Knox, Handyside, Duncan, and
others) did me the honour of appointing me their
Secretary and Treasurer.   This onerous and anomalous
position gave me large insight over a period of five
years ; at the same time I acted as Physician to the
Royal Public Dispensary, and had charge of the
largest and worst district of Edinburgh (including a
great portion of the High Street and Cowgate, the
whole of the Grassmarket, West Port, &c.).   The re-
lapsing fever which prevailed as an epidemic in 1843
brought me daily in contact with the filthiest dens of
the city, and a population indescribably brutal and
debased.   Indeed in my walks through the worst parts
of Paris, Rome, Naples, Stamboul, Cairo, and Jerusalem, I do not remember seeing anything so shocking

in the relations of humanity as was presented to me in the capital of Christian Scotland during the summer of 1843.

This explanation seemed necessary, as some persons may be disposed to view the picture of Edinburgh "low life" as a little overcharged; whilst others, and those possibly nearer the mark, will opine that the curtain is only partially drawn up, and that some of the more tragical shadows are not presented on the canvas.

The work has been a labour of love, or it would never have been done. It will constitute a reward for the pains bestowed upon this volume, the greater part of which has been written whilst suffering from impaired health and sorely-tried vision, if the reader can be induced to rely on the data it contains, and accept the sentiments based thereon—it may be a little bluntly, but not less honestly expressed.

The headings of each chapter, along with the Index, should suffice for every reference. Whilst thanking my publisher for the excellent getting-up of the work, I ought to add that the portrait on the frontispiece is from

a calotype taken of Dr. Knox in his fiftieth year; and
the portrait at page 140 is from the pencil of his
famed pupil, Professor Edward Forbes; and both have
been ably reproduced by the autographic process, by
Messrs. Maclure, Macdonald, and Macgregor, 37, Wal-
brook; the emblem on the title-page, from a drawing
of my own, showing *inter alia* the head of Aristotle,
has been faithfully copied by Mr. James D. Cooper,
188, Strand, London.

H. L.

CONTENTS.

CHAPTER I.

CHAPTER XVII.

CHAPTER XVIII.

CHAPTER XIX.

CHAPTER XX.

LIFE OF ROBERT KNOX.

CHAPTER I.

The Knox Family.—Robert.—*Dux* of the High School of Edinburgh.
—His Graduation.—Army Surgeon.—Waterloo.—Cape of Good Hope.
—Paris and Cuvier.—Contributions to Medical Literature.—Ethnologist
and Naturalist.

JOHN KNOX, the Reformer, was a conspicuous figure in
an epoch unusually prolific of intellectual thought and
revolutionary change. As preacher, polemic, and icono-
clast, he stands pre-eminent among the Scottish worthies
of the 16th century. His abjuration of Papal authority,
his pulpit denunciations, and "first blast of the trumpet
against the monstrous regiment of women"—so directly
aimed at the Court of Holyrood—exercised a marked
influence in achieving the Scottish Reformation. Knox,
like his co-religionist Calvin, was a fiery, contentious
spirit, rude in speech and ruthless in action. His harsh
words often brought tears to the cheeks of "bonnie
Queen Mary;" and he would have been nothing loth to
burn any Romish priest caught lingering by the ruined
altars of his church, after the sway of the "Congrega-
tionists" had become paramount in Scotland.

North of the Tweed, those who bear the cognomen of Knox are disposed to trace their origin to the historic man of that ilk, or the more ancient Knoxes of Ranfurly, in Renfrewshire, to which the Reformer may also have belonged. This is natural enough, as ancestry and clanship are wholesome provender to the Scottish mind proud of its nationality; and a "lang pedigree" aye helps to sweeten the bread, if it does not largely fatten the brose, of life. Among others who held for the blood of the Ranfurly or Haddington Knoxes were a family of farmers located by St. Mary's Isle, Kirkcudbright, early in the 18th century.

Mr. Knox, who concerns this narrative, was a tenant farmer of the Earl of Selkirk. Of himself and wife scarcely anything is known beyond their having a son Robert, a lad of promise, who was sent to Edinburgh to obtain the best education of the country. There the youth showed excellent parts, and proved himself no mean mathematician and scholar. About the year 1775, this Robert Knox married Mary Sherer or Schrerer, a farmer's daughter whose family were of German extraction, and some of whom had become enrolled as citizens of the "gude auld toun" of Ayr. For a time the young couple appear to have resided in the Stewartry of Kirkcudbright, and were favourably received at the Hall of the Earl of Selkirk.[1] Possessing loftier aims than the

---

[1] In 1778, whilst the Earl was from home, "My Lady Selkirk" would entertain her neighbours at dinner. Mr. and Mrs. Knox were present on this eventful, and more or less historic, occasion. The cock-a-leekie soup and the choice salmon of the Dee had been served, when a naval Captain and party abruptly entered the dining-room, and begged permission to join her ladyship's circle. The Blue Jackets proved their relish of the viands

bucolic life of his family, Robert Knox left "Mill-knowe," or the " Little Mote," his father's residence; and bidding adieu to St. Mary's Isle, the banks of Dee, and Solway's silvery sands, sought his fortunes in Edinburgh. There he taught some branches of natural philosophy : he was also the mathematical master at George Heriot's Hospital. As a leading Freemason, he is said to have taken part with Dr. Cullen and other notabilities in laying the foundation-stone of the University of Edinburgh (November 16th, 1789)—on a day ever memorable to the cause of education in Scotland. On the first outbreak of the great French Revolution, he became an ardent admirer of the new order of things, and joined the "Friends of the People;" in whose ranks the free-spoken British spirits of the day were enrolled. His patriotism was not so exuberant as to permit his incurring the martyrdom that fell to many of the Edinburgh worthies for their advocacy of the politics of Marat and Saint Just; so he had the discretion to retire in good time within the safe fold of the autocratic Dundas and the lines of constitutional government. Of the character of

and Bordeaux. When the ladies retired to the drawing-room, the Captain and his men swept the sideboard of its silver plate, and, laying hold of all that was valuable and portable, decamped from the hall, laden with spoil and good cheer ! They offered no apology for this bold procedure, they made no promise to pay, much less to return ; but, as a mark of condescension, the Chief of the piratical crew left his card inscribed—" Paul Jones, of the *Ranger.*"

" Paul Jones," or, more correctly, John Paul, was the son of a gardener, once in the employ of the Earl of Selkirk. A silver ladle or spoon used to be shown by Dr. Knox as the gift of Paul Jones to his mother, as a *placebo* to her outraged feelings on discovering in the Scoto-American pirate the son of a neighbour of decent worth.

this Robert Knox, mathematician, Mirabeauan, or mo-
ralist, little more need be written, nor is there much
definitively known of his life beyond his ability, acumen, and citizenship. He had six sons and three
daughters by his wife Mary: the eldest child and son,
born in September 1776, was named John, after the
great divine; 2, William; 3, Archibald; 4, Mary; 5, Isa-
bella; 6, Paxton; 7, Janet; 8, Robert; and 9, Frederick
John, whose name betrays the family regard for the
ancestral John of national repute. All are dead but
the youngest, Frederick John, who emigrated to New
Zealand about thirty years ago. The eighth child, and
fifth son of Robert and Mary Knox, was born on the
4th September, 1791,[1] and named Robert, after his father:
his history is the one to be discussed in this volume.

Robert Knox, "the darling boy of the family," is said
to have been good-looking, of fair complexion, with soft
flaxen hair and large blue eyes. At an early age he
had smallpox in a virulent form, which cost him the
vision of his left eye, and involved him in delicacy of
health for years. After a good educational training at
home, he was sent to the High School of Edinburgh,
where he had to contend with the best youths of the
city and surrounding district. Few juvenile institutions
could boast of more distinguished names than Francis
Horner, Henry Brougham, and Henry Cockburn; and
on the long roll of illustrious alumni of the High
School scarcely one showed more brilliant parts than

[1] Dr. Knox's birth is taken from the Family Bible, and the same date is
to be found in the records of the Royal College of Surgeons, Edinburgh.
In some documents and brief biographical notices of the Doctor, the year
1793 has been assigned to his birth.

Robert Knox. Apparently without effort, he rose to the head of every class, and came out as Gold Medallist in 1810—leaving other competitors far behind him in the race for the "blue ribbon" of the year. *Robertus Knox* figures on the wall of the Academy among the "*Duces Classis Græcæ et Latinæ*," vi. Aug., 1810. The gold medal was inscribed "*Roberto Knox puero optimo merito condiscipulorum* DUCI ;" and on its obverse "*Præmium Murræanum in Schola Edinburgensi.*" On the day of distributing the prizes to the scholars of the High School, the Lord Provost and Town Council presented Knox with a large folio volume of the Works of Virgil, "*ex editione Petri Burmanni*," to mark their approval of his superior abilities and conduct.

Robert Knox joined the medical classes of Edinburgh in November 1810. His literary and historical studies, his partiality for the collateral as well as the direct medical sciences, and not less his rhetorical powers, led him to take a prominent part in the hebdomadal discussions of the learned Societies assembled under the shadow of his *Alma Mater*. He had evidently won his spurs early in the Royal Physical Society, as prior to his graduation he had twice occupied its presidential chair,—an honour so rare as to be almost, if not altogether, unprecedented in the history of the Society. Owing to the loss of "the Minute Book," no clue can be had to the Essays which he contributed to the Royal Physical Society, or to the mode in which he had distinguished himself so far beyond his compeers.

It is said that, on his first examination for the M.D., Knox was plucked for his anatomy. Such a *contre-*

temps at the threshold of a promising career brought
out his Saxon mettle and roused him to a thorough
sense of duty, that not only saved him from the opprobrium of a second rejection, but the more damaging
position of medical mediocrity. As the anatomical
teaching of Monro *tertius* had been of poor service,
Knox went to Barclay to make amends for lost time.
Under a fresh teacher arose a fresh zest for a study
the cultivation of which revealed a large field of inquiry,
of absorbing and increasing interest to a man of comprehensive mind like Knox. Allured to the ranks of
anatomy, his course became clearly established; he
abandoned the dialectics and rhetorical encounters
of the Societies for practical anatomy — the basis of
surgical art and the best of all introductions to the
study of natural science. His second appearance before his Examiners is said to have been more startling
than his previous rejection; he had anatomy at his
finger's end, and could set forth his knowledge in the
choicest Latin—the language in which the examinations were at that time conducted. He graduated in
1814. His thesis—"*De Viribus Stimulantium et Nar-
coticorum in corpore sano*"—though brief in extent, and
professedly written in haste, showed originality of
thought : it contained observations on the effects of
walking upon the pulse ; and the influences exercised
upon the frame by alcohol and other stimulants, as
well as the narcotics in common use. His experiments
made to ascertain the effects of equestrian and pedestrian exercise on the state of the pulse, came to be
more fully investigated before the close of the year.

In October 1812, Mr. Knox, the father of Dr. Knox, died ; his mother, Mrs. Knox, lived till 1838. After his father's death the Doctor was looked upon as the head of the family.

In January 1815, his essay " On the Relations subsisting between the Time of the Day and various Functions of the Human Body, and on the Manner in which the Pulsations of the Heart and Arteries are affected by Muscular Exertion," appeared in the *Edinburgh Medical and Surgical Journal,* vol. xi. pp. 52–65 and 164–167. To settle the interminable disputes concerning the *stimulant* and *sedative* powers of foxglove, Knox was induced to think of the preparatory steps in the inquiry—the various conditions of the healthy pulse. Dr. Cullen had been of opinion that an acceleration of the pulse happened twice a day, at noon and in the evening, and somewhat resembling a febrile paroxysm. On the contrary, Knox always found his pulse and that of the subject[1] of his 100 observations diminish in velocity as the day advanced ; thus it was 72 at 11 A.M., 64 at 5 P.M., and 58 at 8 P.M. ; and, in the intervals, the pulse lost one pulsation and a fraction hourly. The morning pulse was counted before breakfast, and the evening pulse after exercise of mind and body, and after food and drink ; yet its frequency was less than in the morning, when everything favourable to a rapid state of the circulation was carefully guarded against. He held the pulse to be more excitable in the morning ; after breakfast and before 10 A.M., its average

---

[1] The subject of his experiments was about 22 years of age, of moderate height, and somewhat muscular. He was easily excited by stimulants of almost every kind.

was 72; after dinner, before 5 P.M., 74·22; and after supper (with more or less alcohol), between 10 and 12 P.M.,
64·388. These observations were so opposed to those
Fodéré had recorded in his *Essai de Physiologie Positive,*
as well as Cullen's, that Knox could only explain the
great diversity of opinion by saying that Fodéré, Cullen,
and others had framed their hypothesis on the diurnal
revolutions of the pulse from unhealthy persons, or the
febrile, or phthisical. It required but few experiments
to convince Knox that animal food raised the pulse much
more than vegetable. The excitation of the pulse by wine
is still greater, and that from spirituous liquors greatest
of all. Along with the "daily diminution of velocity in
the functions of the sanguiferous system," there appeared
to Knox a similar revolution in several other functions
of the human frame. Thus, beyond all doubt, our per-
ceptions in the early part of the day are clearer, our
minds more acute, and our intelligence more active. The
same may be said of our stomachic functions. "Were it
lawful for me to speculate," wrote Knox, "in this experimental age, I would venture to support an opinion—at
present, I allow, somewhat antiquated, and very *unfashionable*—that early rising may be conducive to long life, as it
most certainly is to the perfect enjoyment of all our faculties." He believed that "the most powerful stimulant
which can be applied to increase the action of the heart
is exercise," the increase in the number of arterial pulsations being greatly influenced by the debility of the individual. He did not fail to point out the pathological
relations of this fact, and how the slightest muscular
exertion tries the frame weakened by disease, the loss

of blood, fever, &c. He dwelt upon the increase of the
pulsations occasioned by change of posture, and the import of this knowledge in studying the different phases
of disease. Whilst Knox felt anxious for the solution
of the physiological problems, his eye was constantly
directed to the application of his views to pathological
medicine.

In 1815, Dr. Knox obtained his commission as assistant-surgeon in the army : at that period, the junior members of the medical staff were styled " hospital assistants."
Professor Duncan and others, in giving Knox introductions to Sir Walter Farquhar and Sir Gilbert Blane, then
at the head of the Public Medical Departments, called
special attention to the merits of his graduation thesis.
Knox was sent to Brussels to render aid to the wounded
of Waterloo, and in after-years was wont to speak of the
valuable experience he gathered there. He was attached
to the Gens d'armerie Hospital, where "hospital gangrene" prevailed and proved so fatal, owing, as Knox
supposed, to the small confined rooms of the building,
which had formerly been a Nunnery. Secondary ampu-
tations were extremely unsuccessful : only one of Sir C.
Bell's lived ! The people of Brussels, according to Knox,
spoke in disparaging terms of the English medical department ; and he himself admitted that skill and attention were not very rife in the surgical wards ; nor did
the English doctors prove a knowledge of the French
language equal to the necessities of the hour. He looked
upon the hospital gangrene sores as differing but little
from those met with in the wards of St. Bartholomew's,
London. He returned to England in charge of ninety

wounded, and was for a time attached to the Melsea Hospital, in Hampshire.

Being gazetted to the 72nd Highlanders, Dr. Knox, early in April 1817, sailed to the Cape of Good Hope, where he remained till the autumn of 1820. In sailing out to the Cape he made "Observations on the Temperature of the North Atlantic Ocean and the Superincumbent Atmosphere between the Latitudes of 50° 2′ and 20° 24′ N." (*Edin. Philos. Journal,* vol. v. p. 279). It was during the month of April. He used a mercurial thermometer (Fahrenheit's scale), and his observations were made at 6 A.M., at noon, and at 6 P.M. His tables show the remarkable equality of temperature enjoyed as well by the great ocean as by the superincumbent atmosphere. The air and the sea seldom differed more than three or four degrees, and often only one degree of Fahrenheit. He ascribed to the mildness and equability of marine air its extreme salubrity in phthisis; and therefore objected to phthisical patients sailing along a coast or an inland sea where the temperature of the marine air differs but little from that of the neighbouring continent or island. He cited the fact of the Baltic being often frozen when the great ocean, ten degrees further north, is open and the weather mild. Also that seamen were made aware of the vicinity of land by the sudden cooling of the air and of the sea. He considered that the atmosphere resting on the great ocean, by the equability of its temperature, and the uniformity of its qualities as to moisture, will under very few circumstances affect the human frame as the inconstant air of a continent or large island, subject to endless variations from the change of seasons, and even by the alternations of day and night. He called in question the doctrines of *Marsh Miasmata*, and looked upon fevers as resting more on the change in the constitution of the atmosphere regarding its temperature and moisture; and, in corroboration, pointed out the district of Lammermuir, about twenty miles south of Edinburgh, where agues disappeared as soon as the forests were cut down.

Whilst on duty at the Cape, or in "the wilde" of Southern Africa, he seems to have entered with great zest into the arts and practice of soldierly life. To equip himself for real service he became a thorough horseman, swordsman, and "shot." How many old friends and pupils of an after period would have had their eyes gladdened could they have seen Knox in his regimentals, with cocked hat and feathers and high decoration! Practising the soldierly attributes in the plumes and plush of military conceit, Knox must have surpassed himself in grand externals and lofty walk.

As a man of thought and observation, Knox looked beyond the confines of his hospital engagements, and aimed for the light which fresh countries and travel afford. He examined the charts of the Cape territory, and was able to correct and extend them. He studied the physical geography and meteorology of each district, and not less the Fauna, if not the entire natural history under his survey. His observations in these varied walks, as well as medicine proper, will presently be noticed. It was not enough for Knox to look upon the prairies, and the wild untamed denizens of the forest, when so visibly under his cognizance antagonistic races of men were playing their game of humanity—the Saxon encroaching, and the Caffre as daring and impetuous in repelling the foe. There were the Hottentots and their hybrids, and the lethargic Dutch in the field; whilst commercial "John Bull" would take part in the fray only for the interests of civilization, and, of course, "missionary glory," that grand myth of the would-help Providence, and at any cost or sacrifice, of the credulous Britisher. Early in his African experiences the ethnological faculty seemed strongly manifested in Knox, so that he came to look upon the Caffre on the defensive, the Dutch Boer growing cabbages, and English fighting men, lovers of order and organization, as so many forces gathered on an African plateau, and there manifesting to those who could observe, the characteristics, the tendencies, and the antagonisms of race.

Natural history pursuits engaged his spare time; he marked the habits of wild animals, then shot or entrapped them ; he employed men to skin the beasts, and to aid him in the preparation of artificial or natural skeletons. He collected specimens from every division of the animal kingdom. Man, however, was his chief study, and, as war brought its usual contingencies, he took every opportunity thus afforded of dissecting the Caffre and Bosjeman, not without regard to those differences of organization supposed to exist between these savage tribes and the European settler. Had his notes and observations on the anatomical characters, the mode of living, and other physiological traits of the Aborigines around the Cape been arranged, along with the zoological and other scientific data he had gathered, they would have constituted a valuable monograph. Though this was not done, a great deal of what he saw in Africa came to be worked up in magazine articles, whilst the anthropological *memorabilia* formed interesting details for his anatomical classes, and were afterwards woven in graphic colours with his " Fragment " on the Races of Men.

No African traveller could surpass Knox in story-telling. Mounted on his famous Arabian mare, that could travel ninety miles "apparently without the slightest fatigue," and armed with a rifle of marvellous aim, Knox single-handed achieved wonderful things. The palm of the " dead-shot," however, he did not claim for himself, but nobly awarded it to a Dutch farmer and his son ; the examples he recounted of the "dead-shot," and the value assigned to such unerring aim in encounters with the *carnivora*, were grandly piquant to every circle of listeners, as was every narrative of his African experiences—charmingly told and beautifully coloured throughout.

The following extracts from a letter written by Dr. Knox to his brother Frederick are worth quoting for their characteristic touches. The Doctor was then by the banks of the Great Fish River, Cape of Good Hope. The letter bears date 10th September, 1818 :—

" MY DEAREST BROTHER,—By your letters, I perceive that neither time nor absence has in the smallest degree diminished the affections of my relations, or attachment of my friends. How happy am I, and yet how wretched ! Delighted to hear of your health and prosperity, yet miserable at the thoughts of the wide-extended ocean which rolls between us. . . . I am in tolerable health, and as far as regards all the comforts of life every way content. You know, and to you I may say it with-

out vanity, I generally acquire friends wherever I go, and the Cape forms
no exception to the remark; indeed I know nothing but the first society. . . . My banishment cannot last for ever, and I have already
taken such steps as will probably allow of my returning before June 1819.
I begin, my dear brother, to 'lack promotion :' life is short, and excessive
studies have not a little impaired my constitution. It is true, that in this
country I could settle advantageously for life, nay, perhaps acquire a
fortune in ten or fifteen years; but will this recompense me for so long a
deprivation of European society?—the separation from all those whom I
hold most dear, from friends, from relations, from my beloved parent? All
the wealth of India could never reconcile me to this. Home I must
and shall, life permitting, once more behold. . . . Had I, my dear
Frederick, that command of language I once possessed, that readiness of
diction, acquired by a long familiarity with literary subjects, I would, and
perhaps ought to have written, to her ladyship,[1] but I have been neces-
sitated to resign the pen for the gun; to acquire the art of managing the
reins of my horse whilst travelling on the parched roads of Africa, or pur-
suing at full speed the swift antelope over pathless flats, whose termination
the weariest eye searches for in vain. The amusements of the chase,
though interesting at first, soon grow irksome to one whom education and
habits of life have led to different pursuits. Finally, continue to love and
respect as your best friends on earth, our only surviving parent and sisters;
you shall see me before June. Farewell!"

In the same enclosure :—

"MY DEAREST MOTHER,—I have not addressed this letter to you, but
you may believe me when I say that it is written chiefly on *your account.*
Nature herself seems to point out that I do not speak falsely when I say
that I am your affectionate son; for behold an involuntary tear has dropt
on the paper.   " ROBERT KNOX."

He added a few words to his sisters Mary and Jessie
—breathing of kindness. In a subsequent letter, not
now forthcoming, addressed to his mother, he gave her
a long history of the topography of the district in
which he was located, the people and their habits, and

---

[1] This was Lady Wemyss, who had shown great interest in Dr. Knox's
success.

all that pertained to the general features—political, social, and agricultural—of the colony.

Busy in every direction that could engage his mental powers, Knox sought by meteorological registers and other data to arrive at some opinions regarding the sanitary condition of the Cape and its inland settlements. Graaf Reynet was selected by him as illustrative of the average climate. At the distance of about 135 miles from the Southern Ocean, in latitude 32° 11 S., and longitude 26° E., stands the village of Graaf Reynet, about 1,100 feet above the level of the sea, in one of the north-eastern districts of the colony of the Cape. Here were kept the thermometrical tables ; and, with the exception of the Cape Peninsula and the southern mountainous tract, Knox believed the said tables would be found very generally applicable to every part of the colony. From May 1818 to May 1819, the general annual temperature was 62·19 Fahr. ; the lowest monthly mean temperature was 53·79 ; and the highest 71·30 Fahr. The observations were made by J. Ernst, and commented upon and made applicable by Knox. There were 76 rainy days in the year, and of these eleven were stormy ones. Knox maintained that, whatever might be drawn from the tables just noticed, the climate of South Africa was one of the healthiest in the world. Epidemics and fevers of marshy countries were unknown. He admitted the existence of bilious fevers in the young, and during the hot part of summer, and did not recommend the Cape Colony for phthisical patients ; and further observed that the disease (consumption) was not infrequent with the colonists and the Hottentots.

Knox was by no means undistinguished as a surgeon;
his removal of half of the lower jaw of a sergeant, an
operation that several surgeons refused to undertake,
and other creditable efforts, gained him considerable
éclat, both in civil and military service.   He stood in
special favour with the Dutch settlers, who solicited him
to become chief surgeon to the Dutch Free States.
Having aided in planning one of the principal roads towards the interior, caused him to be looked upon as an
authority in such matters, and, marvellous to say, he was
offered the post of surveyor to a part of the colony.

His skill as a surgeon, his zeal in biology and the
varied walks of Natural History, the attention he bestowed upon the climate of the Cape and its sanitary
relations, and the marked interest he had shown in all
that bore upon the material progress of the colony—
traits of character so unusual in a subaltern officer—won
him golden opinions in various ranks of life.   Had he
consented to remain a dozen years at the Cape, there
was no post of honour in the hands of the colonists that
he might not have attained, and, independently of official patronage, would have achieved both position and
fortune there.   Long after his sojourn amongst them, the
Cape colonists spoke in high terms of his transcendent
abilities and exploits in the field.   Influenced either by
home sickness, or health, or a higher ambition than could
find scope in an African colony, Knox left the Cape of
Good Hope on the 22nd October, and, sailing in the brig
Brilliant, arrived in England on Christmas Day, 1820.

He was at home in Edinburgh early in 1821, and joined
the Wernerian Natural History Society, then under the

presidency of Professor Jameson, and became one of its chief supporters. On March 10, 1821, he communicated to it some particulars relative to the Caffre Albino, lately seen by him at the Cape of Good Hope (*Edin. Philos. Journal,* vol. vi. p. 172).

On the 26th September, 1821, Knox obtained permission from military head-quarters to go abroad, and be absent from the United Kingdom for one year. Next month (October) he received the thanks of the Army Medical Department through Sir James McGregor, Director-General, for his chart of the eastern frontier of the colony of the Cape of Good Hope—the execution of which Sir James deemed so creditable to Knox's "industry, zeal, and talents," and for which he (Sir James) always expressed a high appreciation. Knox's object in seeking leave of absence was to enable him to study in the medical schools of the Continent.

In the French capital, to which he now repaired, Knox found every department of natural science, as well as medicine and surgery, ably represented. Cuvier's researches had awakened a fresh love for geology and that grafting of zoology upon it now known as Palæontology ; nor was Geoffroy St. Hilaire's *Philosophie Anatomique* less attractive to the human anatomist seeking for an interpretation of abnormal forms in the general unity of type. Knox was well qualified by his earlier studies, and still more by his love of osteology and natural history, to enter upon the new fields of investigation opened out by the French *savans*. He examined the data upon which Cuvier based his great reputation ; he listened to Geoffroy St. Hilaire expounding his views of the higher anatomy, and became a convert to the new doctrines ; though his great idol, Cuvier, opposed them *in toto.* The French indoctrination had a powerful influence upon Knox, who, for long, if not through life, spoke of Paris as the great school of modern ideas in science. Knox made valuable friendships in Paris with those just named, also De Blainville, Baron Larrey, and others. He joined the Freemasons, in Paris, on the 22nd of April, 1822.

Dr. Knox's " Observations on the *Tænia solium* (tapeworm), and on its Removal from the Human Intestinal Canal by Spirits of Turpentine " (*Edin. Med. and Surgical Journal,* July 1821, vol. xvii. p. 384), showed that in Oct. 1819 the *Tænia solium* had become so general among the British troops stationed at the Cape of Good Hope as to resemble an epidemic. Of a detachment of eighty-six men, thirty-eight were affected ;[1] of these, two had the *Ascarides lumbricoïdes,* and the remainder *Tænia solium.* Young and healthy, old and debauched, were alike sufferers. The presence of this parasite was evidently attributable to the use of unwholesome or diseased meat. Spirits of turpentine proved thoroughly effectual in destroying the parasites. He did not believe in any combination of matter being capable of converting itself into intestinal worms—a theory occasionally prevalent—for, " were we satisfied

---

[1] This was a very large proportion. Knox's observations as to bad meat being the *fons et origo mali* are confirmed by Wauruch, of Vienna (*Lancet,* May 13, 1843), who, in treating of 206 cases, states that 52 of the patients were women cooks ; the rest were butchers, and eaters of large quantities of meat, bad mutton and pork.

with such explanation, the origin of men and all other animals would be readily accounted for from a peculiar arrangement and combination of organic molecules placed under peculiar circumstances, and the story of the Python would be no longer a fable." Had Knox lived till these latter days, he would have seen "protoplasm" endowed with the pythonic force in the hands of both French and English physiologists.

In the same (17th) volume of the *Edinburgh Medical and Surgical Journal*, p. 567, he reported "Cases of Inflammation of the Pericardium; with Remarks on the Adhesion of Serous Membranes." Comparatively little was known of pericarditis at the time, but Knox gave sufficient interest to his cases to call forth an editorial note from Professor Andrew Duncan. Curiously enough he quoted the "instructive case of pericarditis, mistaken for rheumatism," from M. Pelletan's surgical works— the patient was the celebrated Mirabeau — without, however, recognizing the importance of the supposed mistake in the diagnosis.

His "Observations and Cases illustrative of the Pathology and Treatment of Necrosis" (*Edin. Med. and Surg. Journal*, Jan. 1822, vol. xviii. p. 62), were mainly drawn from military practice. His theory of necrosis ran counter to the experiments of Duhamel and Troja, and the observations of most practical surgeons who attached the greatest import to the periosteum; thus he stated: "In no dissection performed by myself or others, has the new bone, in cases of necrosis, been found to depend for its origin on the periosteum, or surrounding of the parts, but, on the contrary, it has

uniformly appeared to be a secretion from that portion
of the old bone which remained alive."

In the same volume (p. 564) he had a few " Observations relative to the Action of the Heart in Fishes,"
evidently made on his voyage out to the Cape. Sharks,
bonitos, and dolphins were the subjects of his experiments; he marked in these animals the contractions of
the *cavæ*, the creeping, vermicular, tremulous action of
the auricle, and the violent convulsive-like action of the
ventricle of the heart, the regular succession of these
motions; and as life gradually became extinct the
auricle sometimes moved without a corresponding action
of the ventricle, but the contrary of this never happened.
The influence of *stimuli* upon the contractions of the
different portions of the heart was also noted.

The *Edinburgh Medical and Surgical Journal* for
April 1823 (vol. xix. p. 210) contained " Observations
on the Regeneration of Bone, in Cases of Necrosis and
Caries," being a supplement to the Memoir published in
January 1822. He had been to London to examine
the Hunterian Museum, and the pathological specimens
in the Military Hospital at Chatham; also to the
School of Medicine at Paris and the collections of
pathological anatomy at Alfort; and from these last-
named he described two specimens of great interest—
the necrosed clavicle presented to the French Academy
by D'Augerville, and a necrosed scapula from Alfort—
to support his views of regeneration of bone from bone
in necrosed conditions.[1] He discussed Haller's and

[1] There is no desire on my part to uphold or contravene Knox's opinions,
as to attempt such would require large space and comment; here and there,

Hunter's opinions, and other authorities, and objected to the torturing experiments made on pigeons and animals so far removed from man in structure.

His history, so far as his military life is concerned, may be conveniently stated here. On the 31st of December, 1822, he wrote to the authorities for his half-pay, due since Christmas 1820, and wished it to be paid in Edinburgh; showing that his mind was made up to settle in his native city, unless the war-cry should again call him to the tented field. He continued to draw his half-pay till Lord Fitzroy Somerset wrote on the 17th Nov., 1831, to Sir J. McGregor on the subject, when it became needful that Knox should resume his duties or retire from the service. On the 2nd Aug., 1832, he did retire, receiving £100 as a commutation, so that Knox may be said to have fared extremely well at the hands of the Government—his five years' active service being rewarded beyond its term with nearly thirteen years of half-pay and a handsome bonus..

however, a note may not be unobjectionable. Few subjects have been more fully discussed than the formation and regeneration of bone; and experiments after experiments have been adduced in support of special doctrines; indeed the highest surgical authorities have been opposed to each other : to-day it is bone; to-morrow it is periosteum; and so the changes have rung from the days of John Hunter to the present time. The matter, it may reasonably be supposed, is within the compass of solution. Each tissue has its own sphere of action deriving its pabulum of growth from the blood elements. Looking at the external covering of bone, its inner membrane, and the Haversian and innumerable other canals connecting both; may it not be that this *intermediate structure*—marked in the embryo, soft, vascular, and permeating the osseous substance and carrying the capillary nourishment everywhere—constitutes the nidus by which bony secretion is effected? Surely it fulfils the physiological growth and aids most materially those operations which Nature is called upon to perform in repairing the pathological necessities of bone.

CHAPTER II.

Contributions to the Wernerian Society.—Comparative Anatomy of the Eye,
    Lacteal Vessels of Cetacea, &c.—Museum of the College of Surgeons
    of Edinburgh; its Conservatorship.—Dr. Barclay resigns his Classes
    to Knox.

FIVE years of practical experience as a military surgeon
would have satisfied less observant men than Knox of
the thorough import of anatomy to professional work.
He had seen enough, and more than enough, of medical
dilettanteism at the bedside of the Waterloo victims, and
on the plains of Caffraria, to guard him against the error
of neglecting the basis of physiology and surgery. His
ethnological and natural history inquiries at the Cape,
to which by the way he had no guide, formed an excellent introduction to his studies in the Jardin des
Plantes and the schools of Paris. Here the exercise of
his best powers, aided by a special culture, was needful
to grasp the philosophic teachings of Cuvier, St. Hilaire,
and De Blainville—men in whose hands the extinct forms
of an antediluvian past, compared with the living organisms on the earth's surface, became as plastic material
upon which to construct a theoretical basis or plan, typi-
cal of the whole world of life. Elated by the presence,

and still more by the personal recognition, of these great masters, whose bold inquiries had penetrated the arcana of science, and revealed to mankind fresh realms of thought, Knox longed to soar above the stereotyped formulas of medicine and to take part in the extension of the new philosophy. Amid the zoological treasures obtained by Napoleon, and the osteological collections of Cuvier, Knox became imbued with a grand emulation for biological study. This spirit was manifested in all its freshness on his settling down in Edinburgh at Christmas 1822, and continued unabated through life.

He had only been at home a few days when he read (on the 28th December) to the Wernerian Natural History Society, a "Notice relative to the Habits of the Hyæna of Southern Africa" (*Trans. Werner. Soc.*, vol. iv. p. 383, or *Edin. Philos. Journal*, vol. xviii. p. 386). He doubted Dr. Buckland's explanation of the bones of various animals being found in the cave of Kirkdale, Yorkshire, being dragged there by hyænas; the lion and panther, he believed, carried off their prey, but not the hyæna or wild dog. Hyænas do not congregate; they are solitary, according to Knox. He had often roused the hyæna from his lurking-place, but assuredly these places bore no resemblance to charnel-houses. He also seemed disposed to call in question the nature of the bones found in the Kirkdale cave, and thought they might be the remains of bears, tigers, as well as hyænas.

His "Observations on the Anatomy of the Beaver (*Castor Fiber*, Linn.) considered as an Aquatic Animal," appeared in the same (4th) volume of the *Wernerian Transactions*, p. 548. He pointed out an extensive "sinus," or receptacle for the blood, situate close to and above the liver, into which entered the *lower cava* and hepatic veins, and from it arose a single trunk conveying the blood to the right side of the heart. The Eustachian valve was very perfect, and another similar valve was found at the entrance of the *superior cava* into the right auricle of the heart. Knox went largely into the history of the venous sinuses, and indicated that the power of suspending respiration possessed by aquatic animals is attributable to the peculiar formation of their venous system. Referring for a moment to the human structure, he stated that he had observed valves at the mouths of the *venæ cavæ* in man.

On the same evening, April 19, 1823, and to the same Society (*Trans. Werner. Society*, vol. v. p. 206), Knox stated the results of his "Inquiry into the original and characteristic Differences of the Native Races inhabiting the extra-tropical part of Southern Africa." He showed a Caffre's cranium, a drawing of which accompanied the paper. According to Knox, there were three distinct races of men in that part of Africa situated to the south of the tropics. Firstly, the Anglo-Dutch colony of the Cape, a mixture of almost all the modern nations of Europe, the Dutch predominating, who had pushed before them and partly exterminated (secondly) the race of Hottentots, or Bosjemans ; and, thirdly, the Caffres. He arranged the Bosjemans with the Mongolian, and the Caffre with the Ethiopian varieties of Blumenbach. The Bosjeman had uncommon powers of vision, which seemed lost by inter-marriage with another race. The cranium, viewed vertically, is nearly equal to the well-formed European head.

Judging from the inspection of a fine collection of skulls

collected by the banks of the Ganges, the property of Professor Jameson, Knox was disposed to question the association of the Hindoo race with the Caucasian variety.

The vast antiquity of the Mongolian hordes of Africa seemed to be proved. It also appeared to Knox that these tribes had penetrated into Europe and Southern Africa, and not improbably modified by their presence some of the races of Central Africa. He further stated that " the peculiar Mongolian face is very strongly marked in many families[1] now inhabiting the Highlands of Scotland, and more particularly the Hebrides."

On April 26, 1823, Knox read a paper "On some Peculiarities of the Structure of the New Holland Cassowary" (*Edin. Philos. Journal*, vol. ix. p. 390).

In the years 1822 and 1823, Knox communicated to the Wernerian Society four memoirs on the anatomy of *Ornithorhynchus paradoxus* of New Holland. In addition to the organs of sense, espcially considered, and the internal viscera of digestion, &c., he described a femoral gland and duct leading to the spur on its heel. This anatomy he held to be original, and the spur to be connected with the organs of generation. (*Trans. Wern. Soc.*, vol. v., or *Edin. Philos. Journal*, vol. ix. p. 390.)

His paper on the Cassowary mentioned above constitutes Article xxi. of the *Edinburgh Philosophical Journal*, vol. x. p. 132; whilst Article xxii. of the same journal, pp. 137–40, is entitled " Additional Observations on the Structure of the Trachea in the Cas-

---

[1] Without being aware of this special observation of Knox's, I have occasionally been surprised to see what are deemed Mongolian features in the faces of the British in other parts of the United Kingdom.

sowary Emeu of New Holland," with a drawing of the
trachea. He looked upon the gallated cassowary found
in the Indian islands as distinct from the species lately
discovered in Australia, and distinguished by the name
of " Emeu Casuary." He gave the anatomy of both
birds at some length, and described for the first time a
remarkable appendage of the trachea in the cassowary
of New Holland—a large muscular bag, about the size
of a man's head, into which the windpipe opens by a large
orifice, occasioned by a deficiency of a part of the circumference, in about thirteen tracheal rings. He knew no similar structure or appendage being attached to the trachea
of any of the feathered tribe, nor of anything analogous
to it in any other animal excepting the chameleon, to the
upper portion of whose trachea there is appended a comparatively large membranous bag. Knox thought it
enabled the bird to swim and preserve life among the
extensive marshes composing Central New Holland.

The interesting paper Knox furnished to the Wernerian
Society on the Foramen of Sœmmering bears date June
20, 1823, but was not read till the 15th November, 1823.
(*Trans. Werner. Soc.*, vol. v. p. 1.) In his " Account of
the *Foramen centrale* of the Retina, generally called the
Foramen of Sœmmering, as seen in the Eyes of certain
Reptiles," Knox stated that Cuvier and De Blainville
had described it in man and the monkeys, but he had
found it in a class of animals differing widely from man,
namely, the lizard tribe of reptiles. The first time he
noticed it was in the *Lacerta superciliosa* of naturalists ;
then the *Lacerta calotes* and *Lacerta striata*. In the
Gecko, the *foramen centrale* was wanting, and also in the

lizard called by naturalists "Lanius" (the *Lacerta ma-buya*) ; so that the *foramen centrale* was present in some and wanting in others. He did not find it in the crocodile. On the following week, Nov. 22 (p. 104 of the same volume of the Society's Transactions), Knox announced the existence of the *foramen centrale* in a large chameleon sent to the Edinburgh University by the Marchioness of Hastings, and in a much more developed form than in the human species. His communication was illustrated by beautiful preparations. (*Edin. Philos. Journal*, vol. x. p. 171.)

It will readily be seen from the above list of contributions that Knox was among the most active supporters of the Wernerian Society during the year 1823. The Society showed their regard for his work by placing him on the Council.

Knox, seated in the family attics in Nicholson Square, and secure from all interruption, made excellent use of his opportunities in Edinburgh. He was a thorough enthusiast, and spared neither time nor money to gain anatomical knowledge. Though comparative osteology was his chief attraction, he surveyed the whole field of anatomy, and laboured in every direction, from the minute textures of the human eye upwards in the scale of magnitude to the elephantine crania. He sought the acquaintance of gamekeepers and river conservators for the game and fish he wanted for special investigation ; and held the Newhaven fishwives in favour for the opportunities he might gain of the marine fauna of the Forth. To him nearly all the oddities found in the fishing-nets of the neighbouring Firth were brought.

He paid well, and knew how to divert the fishwives.
If a difficulty arose with Knox as to an anatomical
structure, he never rested till it was solved.   His giving
fourteen shillings for a brace of grouse, and in Scotland,
too, the great habitat of the bird, showed how regardless
he was of the outlay of money when science demanded it.

The anatomy of the eye must have claimed his attention in Africa, or he could hardly have produced the
valuable essay he read to the Royal Society at Edinburgh, on the 17th of June, 1823—"Observations on the
Comparative Anatomy of the Eye" (*Trans. Roy. Soc.*
vol. x. pp. 43–70).   It was to elucidate the nature and
distribution of the nervous system that led him to inquire into the structure of the eye, and there is good
ground for believing that his first observations were
made at the Cape ; for there only could he have seen
the organs he examined in a fresh state.   In this paper,
drawn from a wide field of comparative anatomy, based
on numerous dissections admirably made by a master
hand, Knox endeavoured to demonstrate that the adaptation of the eye to different distances is effected by
means of the ciliary muscle, or that body which anatomists had hitherto called the " ciliary ligament "—
Annulus albus, &c.   Though furnished only with a
simple lens, he maintained that the *Annulus albus*
showed no ligamentous fibres, but " comparatively large
branches of nerves ; that it did not resemble any of the
textures of the eyeball except the iris, but that here the
resemblance was so close that they could with difficulty
be distinguished."

" Having discovered that in birds, and in the deer, the

so-named (ciliary) ligament received numerous nerves, that its texture bore no resemblance whatever to ligament, that it became rudimentary in those animals whose sight was feeble, which would not necessarily happen were it simply a ligament for the suspension of the tunics and humours of the eye, the conclusion was irresistible that the *Annulus albus* is a muscle, that it is the muscle by which the eye adapts itself to the perception of distant objects; and that by it, in conjunction with the iris, all the changes which take place in the interior of the eyeball are effected."

He remarked that "the development of the ciliary muscle followed the ratio of the strength of vision, or rather of the accommodating powers of the eye in the various classes of animals; *id est*, it is strong in birds,[1] in men, in the *Quadrumana*, and in the deer; weaker in some others of the *Ruminantia*, as the ox; still more so in the horse. Lastly, in most fishes it is completely rudimentary, and is reduced to a mere ligament." He considered that an examination of the eyes of birds and of fallow deer would satisfy any anatomist that the ciliary muscle could not possibly be a ligament.

At a meeting of the Anatomical and Physiological Society of Edinburgh, in 1836, Knox referred to the *Archives Générales* of that year, containing an analysis of various German monographs on the structure and physiology of the eyeball, and the confirmation of his views on the *Annulus albus* by Arnold. Professor Alison, of Edinburgh, the most cautious and philoso-

---

[1] Knox believed that it was by sight only that the vulture was led to discover his prey, and not by the sense of smelling.

phic physiologist of his day, believed in Knox's observations and deductions, but English writers, so far as I
know, make no allusion to them.

Professor Donders,[1] of Utrecht, evidently unaware of
Dr. Knox's observations in 1823, attributed the discovery of the muscular character of the so-called ciliary
ligament to Professors Bowman of London and Bruecke
of Vienna.   This opinion is no longer tenable, as to
Knox is really due the honour ; and the honour is all
the more, that the achromatic microscope had not come
into use, and the nature of muscular fibre was then
unknown.   His extended anatomical observations and
correct reasoning upon the facts so obtained led Knox
to the true nature of the ciliary muscle. He endeavoured
to unravel the anatomical connection of the sclerotica
and transparent cornea, and, looking to the distribution
of the inner membrane of the cornea in connection with
the anterior layer of the iris, he believed that during the
strong contraction of the pupil in viewing objects placed
close to the eye, the form of the aqueous humour must be
considerably affected.   He looked upon the marsupium
in birds and fishes as simply a reflected membrane of
the choroid ; he had traced its functions and the cause
of its disappearance in the *Mammalia.*   He viewed the
ciliary fibres placed immediately over the Capsule of
Petit as membranous folds quite analogous to the folds
of the inner membrane of the choroid coat, and ultimately terminating in processes also analogous to those

---

[1] " On the Anomalies of Accommodation and Refraction of the
Eye," p. 23, by F. C. Donders, M.D.   The New Sydenham Society,
London, 1864.

termed ciliary. In describing the mode in which the optic nerve enters the eye, Knox considered the eye of the deer as approaching in many respects that of the bird. The eyes of birds, of *Quadrumana*, and of man himself, showed him that the ciliary muscle was not a nervous ganglion or plexus.

A supplement to the above paper was read to the Royal Society on the 15th of March, 1824 (*Trans. Roy. Soc.* vol. x. pp. 231–252), entitled " An Inquiry into the Structure and probable Functions of the Capsules forming the Canal of Petit, and of the Marsupium Nigrum, or the peculiar Vascular Tissue traversing the Vitreous Humour in the Eyes of Birds, Reptiles, and Fishes." He had examined the eyes of an executed criminal eight hours after death, and found the *foramen* of Sœmmering " remarkably distinct, and of a deep yellow tinge ; *there was no fold*, a fact which proves the appearance to be a *post-mortem* one, and that Sœmmering had on this point misled all anatomists since his discovery. The retina was transparent." He further stated that the pulpy layer of the retina terminates by a well-defined margin, near to the place where the internal ciliary processes (*Zonula ciliaris* of Zinn) commence, but the inner layer of the retina may be considered as advancing forwards towards the lens, and uniting with the other transparent tissues to form the internal ciliary processes, and the internal parietes of the Canal of Petit. He admitted that this opinion rested on analogy. By the employment of delicate vermilion injections he showed the ciliary process of the vitreous humour (the *Corona ciliaris* of Zinn) to abound with blood-vessels. Of the 47 injected preparations exhibited to the Royal Society, 34 were deposited in the Anatomical Museum of the Royal College of Surgeons, Edinburgh ; the remainder were consigned to a distinguished Edinburgh oculist.

The " Royal " and " Wernerian " Societies of Edinburgh were by no means favourable channels for conveying anatomical and physiological discoveries to the medical profession of the kingdom, and it is doubtful if they were of greater significance to the more philosophic inquirer, either at home or abroad : hence a great deal of Knox's work contributed to the Edinburgh Societies was never heard of south of the Tweed. Even now when physiological compilations are the order of the day, the science that Knox developed and the many valuable papers contributed by him on various subjects are seldom recognized by writers. It is pleasant to find a notable exception to the preceding statement, and that the discovery of the *foramen* of Sœmmering by Knox will no longer be questioned. Mr. J. W. Hulke, F.R.S., of the Middlesex Hospital, one of the latest and best writers on this subject, says (*Journal of Anatomy and Physiology*, vol. i. p. 103): " The first notice of the existence of the *Foramen centrale* in reptiles, which I can find, is by Knox, in the Memoirs of the Wernerian Society, 1823, where he describes very accurately the *macula* and *Foramen centrale* in the chameleon, and says that he has also seen it in *Lacerta superciliosa, L. scutata, L. calotes,* and *L. striata.* There was recently in the Anatomical Museum at Frankfort, a preparation of the chameleon's eye with an inscription in Sœmmering's handwriting, describing the *foramen*, which proves it to have been known to this great anatomist; and there are also in the Museum of the Royal College of Surgeons, London, two old preparations of the chameleon's eye (undated, Hunterian?) which time has spoiled, but which, the catalogue says, are intended to display the *foramen*. These preparations and Knox's memoir were overlooked by later investigators, and till very recently it was commonly taught that the *macula* and central *fovea* were peculiarities of the human retina, and of that of some apes. In 1862, the error was for ever set aside by H. Müller's remarkable memoir on the chameleon's eye, in which he described with great exactness the *macula* and *fovea*, and two sets of vertically and obliquely radial fibres here so conspicuously distinct."

On the 24th of January, 1824, Knox addressed the Wernerian Society " On the Mode of Growth, Reproduction, and Structure of the Poison Fangs in Serpents " (*Trans. Soc.* vol. v. p. 411).

On April 3, 1824, he communicated a paper to the same society on the supposed discovery of Professor Tiedemann and Dr. Fohmann relative to the non-existence of the *Vasa efferentia* in the *Phoca vitulina*. His views are given at greater length in three letters addressed to Dr. Duncan, junior, inserted in the *Edinburgh Medical and Surgical Journal* for July 1824, vol. xxii. p. 23. The vessels conveying the chylous fluid from the intestines to the mesenteric glands, anatomists had agreed to call *Vasa afferentia*, those conveying the same fluid from the glands into the thoracic duct, *Vasa efferentia* : the existence of these latter vessels had been denied by Tiedemann, who stated that the chyle poured into the glands by the *Vasa afferentia* is absorbed by veins only, arising from these glands, and thus conveyed directly into the blood without passing along the thoracic duct. Knox got a specimen of the common seal (*Phoca vitulina* —Linn., *Sheeund* of the Germans), from which Tiedemann had borrowed his description, and found the *Vasa efferentia* quite distinct.   He repeated his dissections upon the seal and porpoise, and discussed Mr. Abernethy's views on the anatomy of the whale and the lactiferous vessels, and concluded by affirming that the anatomy of the seal and the porpoise do not furnish any argument against the long-established doctrine of the transmission of the chyle by *Vasa afferentia* to the mesenteric glands, and *Vasa efferentia* from the glands to the thoracic duct.[1]

On the 17th of the same month he offered a few observations " On the Black Colour of the Periosteum in the *Colymbus septentrionalis*, or Red-throated Diver."

In June 1824 he communicated to *Brewster's Journal of Science*, vol. i. p. 96, " Observations on the General Anatomy of the *Gymnotus electricus*, the Electric Eel of America ; and on the Philosophic Anatomy of the Electric Organs."

His paper on the theory of the existence of a sixth sense in fishes, supposed to reside in certain peculiar tubular organs found immediately under the integuments of the head in sharks and rays, is to be found in

---

[1] Professor Turner (*Journal of Anatomy and Physiology*, vol. ii. p. 77), in his paper on the Anatomy of the Pilot Whale, confirmed, from actual observation of the lacteal vessels filled with chyle, the opinions entertained by Knox, and showed that in the Cetacea, as in other Mammals, the chyle is conveyed by a system of lacteal vessels.

Brewster's Journal of Science, vol. ii. p. 12. Knox examined the opinions of Jacobson (of Berlin), Treviranus, and others, and looked upon the tubular organs as organs of touch, modified, however, so as to hold an intermediate place between the sensations of touch and hearing, but approaching nearest to hearing. The undulation of the water by a tolerably-sized ship might affect these organs at a distance, and thus apprize the shark of the presence of a moving body.

He communicated to *Brewster's Journal of Science,* vol. iii. p. 193, a paper " On the Limits of the Retina in the Eye of the *Sepia loligo,* one of the Cephalopoda Mollusca."

Mr. J. W. Reddock, of Falkirk, having found "the bones of a quadruped in a bed of clay, near Camelon, 90 feet above the present level of the Firth of Forth," brought them before the Wernerian Society, and read a paper upon them. Knox, at the following meeting, in January 1825, showed that the bones were those of a seal, of the species still inhabiting the Firth of Forth (*Phoca vitulina*). At the meeting of the Wernerian Society, on the 14th of May, 1825, Knox exhibited specimens of bones of various animals found in the cave at Oreston, near Plymouth ; being chiefly bones of large oxen, and very large deer, and which, being almost completely deprived of their animal matter, appeared as if calcined.

The preceding pages of this chapter—embracing but a general record of Knox's work from Christmas 1822 to 1824—afford abundant proofs of his zeal and aptitude for original research. During these two years, he took part in the discussions of the "Plinian," the "Royal Physical," and "Medico-Chirurgical" Societies ; and was among the most prominent leaders of the "Wernerian" and "Royal" Societies, to both of which a higher status or excellence was attached. Everything betokened well for Knox's social and scientific position in his native city, when all at once he threw away an important chance or element of success. A world of promise was before him, and he inconsiderately put shackles to his social progress by marrying a person of inferior rank, some time in the year 1824. This marriage was kept a secret. In Scotland this could easily be done, as no ceremony civil or religious, no notice before or after publication, no writing, and no witnesses, are essential to the constitution of marriage.

Dr. Knox became a fellow of the Royal Society of Edinburgh on the 1st December, 1823. He also joined the Medico-Chirurgical Society, and continued to manifest as much interest in surgery and medicine as the keenest follower of both. Occasionally he did a little practice, and might have done more had not his private dissections absorbed so much time. His studies in the Museum of Natural History made him known to Professor Jameson, who was glad to receive the aid of a promising naturalist for his *Quarterly Philosophical Journal*, then in its infancy.

The Museum of the Royal College of Surgeons, in the "Old Hall" of the "Incorporation of Chirurgeons," was a very poor affair in 1823. Along with its relics of the "Art of Chirurgerie," the fleams and cutting instruments of the barber surgeons, and other crude apparatus, surgical and obstetrical, stood dwarfed forms and other deformities, gathered as curiosities from a superstitious past. Its modern collection, or specimens of health and disease, and a few natural history examples, belonged almost entirely to the nineteenth century, and these scarcely numbered 300 in all. This condition of affairs might well shock Knox, fresh from the Parisian School, and he longed above all things to redress it.

On the 2nd April, 1824, Dr. Knox submitted to the College of Surgeons a plan for the formation of a Museum of Comparative Anatomy, having felt, as he said, more than most anatomists the great want of a proper Museum and of an Osteological collection. The letter proceeded : " Towards the formation of a Museum of Comparative Anatomy I am willing to bestow my whole labour and time, with that energy which the cultivation of a very favourite pursuit naturally gives ; the attending expenses of presses, glass, spirits, &c., to be borne by the Royal College of Surgeons. I am, moreover, willing that the Museum so erected be considered as the property of the College, and intended for the use of its Fellows (as is at present the Pathological collection), reserving to myself during my lifetime the use of the Museum for the furtherance of my favourite pursuits and studies." [1] This handsome offer on the part of Dr. Knox was accepted by the College at their meeting on the 15th May, and the " scientific arrangement and active management " of the additional collection of Comparative Anatomy necessarily devolved upon him.

[1] Extracts from the Minutes of the Royal College of Surgeons, Edinburgh.

At this period in its history the College Museum was
under the charge of a Committee of Fellows—called
"Curators," whilst two other Fellows held the special
office of "Keepers," or what might be termed unpaid
Conservators. Both Curators and Keepers were annually elected to their respective offices. On the 11th of
September, the College, on the notice of the President,
voted their thanks to Dr. Knox "for the labour and
attention he had bestowed in regard to the Museum."
His work pleased the Fellows so well that, on the 13th
of January, 1825 (within eight months of his accepting
office), a proposal was made to him "to take charge
of the Pathological Museum, in co-operation with the
'Keepers,' and under the direction of the Curators, at
a salary of £100 a year," he to defray the expense of
assistant. Knox accepted the offer, and was now considered "Conservator of the Museum, or, to speak more
correctly, of its pathological portion."

No better choice could have been made, for, restless
in his ambition to see his College progress with the
times, and in possession of a Museum worthy of the
great school it sought to lead in surgery, Knox was con-
tinually urging upon the chief men of the Institution the
need of amplifying the collection of both the physiological and pathological series. It was probably his
example and promptings that led the College to consider
the proposal offered it in November 1824, by Mr. (afterwards Sir C.) Bell, of disposing of a large part of his
Museum in Windmill-street, London, for £3,000. Dr.
Knox and Mr. Watson being deputed to go to London,
reported most favourably of the Bell collection. On the

15th February, 1825, the day on which the Bell negotiation was recommended, the College agreed to give Dr. Knox and his colleague £21 each for their trouble in going to London. Knox courteously declined the money, on the ground of its being a remuneration for services which he conceived to be a duty he owed to the College as its Conservator. The purchase of the Bell collection being completed on the 22nd July, Dr. Knox was authorized on the 5th August to proceed to London, and arrange for its safe removal to Edinburgh, for which service the sum of fifty guineas was voted to him.

So valuable a collection as Bell's gave a fresh, or rather entirely new, character to the Surgeons' Museum, and led to important changes in the management—the end of which was the appointment, on the 15th May, 1826, of Dr. Knox as Conservator of the entire Museum, at a salary of £150 a year.

Anatomy was not an ordinary occupation or mere intellectual pastime with Knox, but viewed by him as an object of high philosophic research. He was early to recognize the two divisions—anatomical science and anatomical art: the former embracing the elucidation of the nature or structure and organization of animal bodies; the latter comprehending all those means and contrivances, manual or potential, by which organisms can be unfolded and demonstrated. Whether or not he had studied Constant Dumeril's *Essai sur les Moyens de perfectionner et d'étendre l'Art de l'Anatomiste*, 11 Fructidor, an. xi. (1803); and Gilbert Breschet's *De la Dessication et des autres Moyens de Conservation des Pièces anatomiques*, 1819; Knox looked first to Expo-

sition ; second, to Preparation ; and, thirdly, to Conservation, as the grand objects to be attained in anatomical
art. There might be no novelty in the mode of
museum construction pursued by Knox, but its application to the Edinburgh College of Surgeons[1] was
unquestionably new. The labours of Eustachius, De
Graaf, Ruysch,[2] Riolenus, Glisson, Willis, Swammerdam,
Bellini, Lieberkühn, and others had not been overlooked
by Knox in his initiative efforts to secure a good
groundwork to his anatomical art.[3]

Knox's work in the College of Surgeons' Museum
was well done. Deriving but little aid from others,
he classified and catalogued the whole collection, and
strove to make it available to the medical student and
practitioner. He gave a new direction to the Com-

[1] Under the quaint but expressive title of the "Anatomist's Knife,"
Michael Lyserus, the student of Simon Pauli and Thomas Bertholinus, at
Copenhagen—the latter of whom was helped by Lyserus in the discovery
of the chyliferous absorbents—had done much to aid the construction of
Museums as far back as 1653.

[2] Ruysch's Museum was described as a perfect necropolis, all the inhabitants of which were asleep and ready to speak as soon as they were
awakened. "The mummies of Ruysch," said M. Fontenelle, in his *Éloge*
of the anatomist, "prolonged in some degree the visible duration of life,
while those of ancient Egypt prolonged only the appearance of death."
Peter the Great bought Ruysch's Museum for 30,000 florins, and was so
struck with the life-like countenance of a child that had been preserved by
Ruysch for many years after it had ceased to breathe, that he actually laid
aside both Imperial dignity and Muscovite severity, and kissed the apparently animated features.

[3] The whole subject of Conservation is most curious, and Egyptian art, in
this particular, far excels the civilized nations of the Christian era. How
cautious Englishmen should be in boasting when the arts of colouring,
the process of embalming, the raising of Monoliths and Pyramids 5,000
years ago and upwards, far surpass the greatest of modern efforts.

parative Anatomy series, and added to its variety by
several preparations of his own.   One of the novelties
introduced by Knox was a collection of specimens to
illustrate Human and Comparative Pathology—the
more desirable that a School of Veterinary Surgery had
just been opened in Edinburgh.   He obtained every
zoological example within reach, as he maintained that
the field could not be too large and varied to be
inviting to the student.   Of his familiarity with the
surgical part of the museum, his anatomical classes had
frequent opportunities of judging, and benefiting thereby.
Knox's seven years' service (1824-31), like a diligent
apprenticeship, in the College Museum, fairly entitled
him to the honours of Master.   He placed it in
methodical order, and worthily left his own impress
upon every department.   Unfortunately a great part of
Knox's catalogue that cost him much labour has been
lost, and no one knows how, but there are portions left
to show his painstaking character and his thorough
knowledge of the work.   When Knox entered upon
office, in 1824, there was but a shell of a collection, but
by Bell's purchase and Barclay's noble bequest, with
presentations from the Fellows of the College—Knox's
own probably the largest contribution—the Museum, in
1831, had become worthy of a Royal College that had
its Bells, Listons, and Symes, as exponents of modern
surgery.   This excellence was largely owing to its distinguished curator.

For some years the fame of the Anatomical School
of Edinburgh had rested with Dr. John Barclay—of
whose character and position it is needful to say a few

words. John Barclay, the son of a Perthshire farmer, was educated for the Scottish Church, and duly licensed to preach ; but his leaning to anatomy[1] and natural history led him to study medicine and to become an Edinburgh graduate in 1796. In the following year he gave his first course of Lectures on Anatomy, in the High School-yard, adjoining Surgeon's-square, Edinburgh. His mode of teaching was a great improvement upon that of the Monros, and his pleasant manners and thorough zeal in anatomical research added to his popularity and success. When Monro (*secundus*) retired in 1808, and his son, Monro (*tertius*), began his long and tedious reign, Barclay got a large class which was not much affected by the appearance in the field of an able lecturer, Dr. John Gordon—a man of great promise, but unfortunately of short career.

Dr. Barclay was an enthusiast in anatomy, and devoted his whole time to its pursuit. He was vigilant and painstaking as a teacher, faithful in collecting data, and sagacious in their interpretation; he framed a new anatomical nomenclature, wrote admirably on biological questions, and established an excellent museum. He made Human Anatomy attractive, and seems to have

---

[1] Barclay, as a preacher, was for some weeks the *locum tenens* of the Rev. G. Baird, of Bo'ness. Mr. Baird, wishing to ascertain how his parishioners liked Barclay, asked the opinion of a shrewd villager. "Gey weel, minister, gey weel," quoth Sandie ; "but everybody thought him daft." "Why, Sandie?" "Oh, for gude reasons, minister; Mr. Barclay was aye skinning puddocks" (frogs). It used to be said that dogs avoided Barclay's path from an instinctive dread of his dissecting them. If it be true that he was disliked by animalities, he was much loved by his contemporaries and friends.—GOODSIR's *Memoirs*, vol. i. p. 25.

been the first teacher in Britain to give a direction to the study of Comparative Anatomy. His lectures were greatly in advance of his time, and helped to sustain the character of the Edinburgh School.

After sixty or more summers, thirty of which had been devoted to science, the dim shadows of life began to steal over Barclay, and with these tokens came anxiety for the continuity of his school—its fame and its honours. Should his anatomical and physiological teachings, the growth of so much labour,[1] be left to chance and time's effacing fingers, or should search be made for an eminent disciple to whom the Barclayan standard might be consigned ? Barclay had excellent assistants in his time—Robert Nasmyth,[2] Sir George Ballingall, Robert Liston, A. Dickson, and others, who had obtained honourable positions at home and abroad ; but none were exactly at their master's call in the year 1825.

In his visits to the Museum of the College of Surgeons, Dr. Barclay came in immediate contact with the new

[1] Henry Brougham, on the staff of the *Edinburgh Review*, asked Barclay to give him half an hour's talk on anatomy, to enable him to write a critique on one of his (Barclay's) works ! The anatomist might well express surprise, as well as refusal, at the audacity of a Scotch barrister, who had never handled a part of the anatomy, offering to review a work that had cost him years of thought. Such sheer impertinence was very characteristic of Henry (afterwards Lord) Brougham, who always wished to be considered a man of science, yet never had a drop of scientific blood in his veins but what he got by transfusion. Brougham's ambition for omniscience gave him the effrontery of Serjeant Buzfuz.

[2] From my kind friend Mr. Nasmyth, the father of Scottish Dentistry, I have heard much of Barclay ; and in days gone by, also from my friend Sir G. Ballingall, who wrote a brief biography of Dr. Barclay, prefixed to his "Introductory Lectures," published in 1827. [With unfeigned sorrow I have to add that the good Mr. Nasmyth died May 12, 1870.]

conservator, Robert Knox, in whom he saw a person of precision, method, and expertness, a growing naturalist, and an excellent human and comparative anatomist. Moreover, Knox was one of his own pupils, rising in fame and large in promise. Many thoughtful men had gone into the great field of medical competition armed with the Barclayan method, but no one offered more sterling qualifications as an anatomist than Robert Knox. Accordingly, Barclay offered a co-partnery to Knox, the terms of which were agreed upon and signed on the 2nd March, 1825. Knox agreed to relieve Barclay " of the whole labour in every branch of the Institution whatsoever during the continuance of the co-partnery," Barclay having the option of taking any part agreeable to himself. Provision was made in case Knox should get a professorship in any University—a fact in the record that implied the probability of such an advancement. Knox was to retain the position and emoluments of his College of Surgeons' Conservatorship. As the contract was to terminate on the death of either of the parties, and Dr. Barclay died (aged 66 years) in the autumn of the following year—24th August, 1826—Knox came into possession of the class and profits after eighteen months' service. Barclay gave the introductory lecture to the session 1825-26, and took no further part, but in all respects showed the highest regard for Knox's well-doing, and stipulated by will that his Museum, wherever deposited, should be accessible, or rather available, for Knox's use in lecturing.[1]

[1] The Barclayan collection of comparative and physiological anatomy occupies a prominent position in the Royal College of Surgeons' Museum

It now became incumbent upon Knox to join one of the Royal Colleges to secure the proper recognition of his lectures, and he naturally preferred the Surgeons, whom he joined on the 19th April, 1825. His probationary essay for admission to the Fellowship of the Royal College of Surgeons, Edinburgh, was "On the Causes and Treatment of Lateral Curvature of the Human Spine." It bears date April 1825, and consists of 52 pages 8vo, and was dedicated to John Henry Wishart, F.R.S. Edin. His notion was that lateral curvatures of the spine were "the direct results of civilization —arising from an abuse of sedentary employments, an excessive manufacturing population, and a total neglect of the physical education of youth." He believed that in the crowded population of large European cities only one out of twenty could show a perfectly erect spine, formed on the model which "nature originally bestowed on man, and which Grecian art transmitted to admiring posterity." He traced the history of the subject from Hippocrates downwards. He dwelt upon the erroneous system of education demanding of children efforts beyond their strength, by which the muscles supporting the spine daily lose their energy for want of relaxation and a correct system of exercise. He did not object to corsets during school hours, nor did he declare against mechanical aids in the treatment of lateral curvature ; but his great preventive and panacea was exercise and living according to nature's dicta.

in Edinburgh. There is also a bust of the worthy donor, who loved and practised science as few men ever did, and whose many good qualities of head and heart had won him golden opinions in society.

Dr. Knox's first course of lectures on anatomy and physiology, delivered in 1825-26, was a great success, and fairly sufficed to establish his character. With Knox, as Thomas Carlyle would say, the clock—making its advance to the meridian—did not strike one, two, three *gradatim*, but sounded twelve at once. He eschewed the puerile, formal methods of lecturing, and sought the free, expressive, and higher academical; and partly followed the course of his predecessor, which had drawn excellent classes of excellent men. He kept to the lines of his master, but in the adoption and use of a decorative art gave to the Barclayan conception an æsthetic colouring no less warm than effective ; thus, whilst Barclay completed the walls and cornice with just proportion and skill, Knox furnished the panels and frescoes that gave lightness, tone, and consonance to the whole apartment.

Knox's public appearance might well excite attention. Here was a first year's lecturer, of marked individuality in style, treating anatomy as a pastime of the hour, yet giving to its demonstration a practical aim and philosophic character. To attempt to follow Barclay in any direction implied courage and experience, and to claim the privilege of succeeding so able a man augured the possession of talents of no small magnitude. Knox was more than a successor to his distinguished master; he was himself, and soon came to be designated by his class as " Knox *primus et incomparabilis.*"

CHAPTER III.

ANTIPATHY to dissection after death is a natural and primary feeling that has been manifested by all nations, creeds, and peoples; the Egyptian and the Greek, the Roman and the Jew, the Christian and the Mahometan. This instinctive aversion rose to a superstitious dread, under the fostering care of a wily priestcraft ever operating on human minds, from the rise of the Nilotic dynasties to the fall of the Roman Empire; nay, down to modern times, and the Victorian era. The primitive Christians, as is evinced by the epitaphs on their tombs, left anything but blessings to the disturbers of their remains in the Roman Catacombs.[1] As the Koran forbade dissections, whatever the Mahometan instructors taught of anatomy was borrowed from the Greeks. Pope Boni-

---

[1] My own notes on this subject, made in 1858, are not forthcoming; but Dr. McCaul's able work on the "Christian Epitaphs of the First Six Centuries" (Bell and Daldy, 1869) affords examples of the text above, thus: "*Male pereat, insepultus jaceat, non resurgit cum Judâ partem habeat, si quis sepulchrum hunc violaverit.*" A heathen epitaph shows a twin feeling of benediction: "*Si quis violaverit ad inferos non recipiatur.*"

face VIII. issued a Bull prohibiting even the preparation of the skeleton. The pious wish of King Robert the Bruce to have his heart deposited in Jerusalem, did not shelter the act of "cutting out and embalming" from sacrilegious condemnation at the hands of Pope Benedict XII. Luther, ascribing the majority of diseases to the influence of the devil, dealt out hard blows against the physicians; and so the world went on—theological dogmatists ever standing hostile to the advancement of science. Popes and anti-Popes sanctioned the lowest empiricism, whilst they acted towards medicine as if it were a "black art" of no better repute than sorcery or alchemy, the emanations of Satan.

Now and then a bold man appeared in history like Democritus of Abdera, the friend of Hippocrates, and Galen, attracted to Alexandria by its possessing two human skeletons; but how rare are such examples in ancient history! The dark clouds of the Middle Ages were passing away when Italy, true to her repute as the leader of science, came forth with Mundinus, Achellini, and Berenger (Carpi), to rescue anatomy from its degraded position. These were followed by Leonardo da Vinci (*l'uomo universale*), who, apart from its medical relations, pursued anatomy as a branch of science worthily associated with the revival of modern letters. France had her Jacques Dubois and Charles Etienne; but these and many others were eclipsed by Andrew Vesalius— the great anatomical light of the new era,—a Fleming by birth, in reputation an Italian, who adorned the great schools of Pisa, Padua, and Bologna, and left an imperishable name in history.

At the dawn of the sixteenth century, Edinburgh, though consisting of little more than a long street connecting its ancient Castle with Holyrood Palace, evinced a laudable desire for anatomical knowledge. The rudiments of medicine had got some acknowledgment in the previous century, or the "Guilde" or *craft* of "Surregeanis" and "Barbouris" [Surgeons and Barbers] could hardly have obtained a charter of incorporation from the Town Council on July 1, 1505, that received the sanction of King James IV.[1] the following year. To know the "anatomea nature and complexioun of every member In manis bodie" was imperative on all applicants for admission into the "Incorporation," and it was also set forth that "We [the Surgeons] may have anis in the year, ane condampnit man efter he be deid [2] to make

---

[1] James IV. was partial to the practice of physic ; he is described as "weill larned in the airt of medicine and a guid Chirurgiane." In the lists of the expenditure of the Lord High Treasurer (February 9, 1511-12) there is an entry of a payment in the following terms :—"Item to ane fallow, because the King pullitfurth his twtht [tooth], xiiii. *s.*" The King was paying for his education, and fourteenpence for pulling a tooth was handsome remuneration to any "fallow." The doings of King James are touched upon in an interesting historical work of Sir J. Y. Simpson's, "Antiquarian Notices of Syphilis in Scotland in the Fifteenth and Sixteenth Centuries."

[2] The words "efter he be deid" will sound strangely to the modern reader. They indicate that cases had occurred prior to the reign of James IV., where the dissector had anticipated death. Vesalius incurred the odium of the Inquisition for examining the body of a Spanish nobleman before muscular life had disappeared. In the Minute Book of the London Barber-Surgeons, dated July 13, 1587, there is a distinct order relative to the disposal of "any bodie which shall revyve or come to lyve agayne, as of late hathe been seene." As the bodies of criminals were the only ones available to the anatomist, the hanging had been but an incomplete strangulation, so that the application of restoratives now and then succeeded. History records several such revivals—Ann Greene in Oxfordshire, Margaret

E

anatomea of quhairthrow we may haif experience Ilk ane
to instruct uthers And we sall do suffrage for the soule.[1]"

It is curious to note how anatomy got a footing in
Scotland, and that it was made to hinge upon the work
effected by the gallows, or rather to complete that work
in the eyes of the law—a circumstance that tended more
than anything else to bring dissection into bad repute
with all classes of society for three succeeding centuries.[2]

Dickson in Edinburgh, in 1728, and Patrick Redmond in Cork, in 1766.
Sir William Petty restored Ann Greene to life, and, oddly enough, she was
proved to be an innocent woman. Margaret Dickson got married, and lived
thirty years after her hanging! Redmond was recovered by Glover, a play-
actor who had some knowledge of surgery. The same evening Patrick
Redmond, inspired by gratitude as well as by whisky, went to the play-
house, and on Glover's appearance jumped upon the stage, and returned
thanks to his preserver, to the no small terror and astonishment of the audience.—*Researches in the South of Ireland,* by T. CROFTON CROKER, p. 191.

[1] This charter had a religious bearing, as by it the Surgeons were bound
to "uphold ane altar in the College Kirk of Sanct Geill [St. Giles] in the
honour of God and Sanct Mongow our Patron." See Dr. John Gairdner's
able "Historical Sketch of the Royal College of Surgeons, Edinburgh,"
published in 1860; also his "Sketch of the Early History of the Medical
Profession in Edinburgh," 1864, from which the quotations in the text have
been taken.

[2] The fact of hanged criminals being "left for dissection" increased the
natural horrors against it. A strong instance may be adduced. Upwards
of forty years ago a man was hanged in Carlisle ; and the friends of
the culprit determined to revenge themselves on the doctors who engaged
in the post-mortem examination. All the medical men sustained personal
injuries, and of a severe kind. Mr. Anderson, whom I knew so well in
after years, was shot in the face, and carried the marks of this diabolical out-
rage to the grave. Another surgeon was found dead by the side of a lofty
bridge, over the parapet of which, it was believed, he had been thrown. As
a child I remember the great excitement that prevailed, for poor Anderson
was shot within a hundred yards of my father's door. Hanging in chains on
the public roads, to be dissected by vultures, seemed less frightful to the
condemned criminal than knowing he would be " cut up" by the doctors !

Edinburgh, to her great credit be it said, made her first advance to a knowledge of surgery nine years before the birth of Andrew Vesalius, the father of modern anatomy; four years before that of Ambrose Paré, the great French surgeon; and one hundred and twenty years prior to Harvey's setting forth the discovery of the "Circulation of the Blood." The early start was more propitious than the progress of the cause; for, consistently with the feeling of the times, the avenues to learning were beset with suspicion; science and magic were almost synonymous, and both stood in a black-balled position to theology. As anatomy wore a questionable aspect, it had to be pursued with a caution and reserve by no means favourable to its development and success. Fifty years of "Incorporate" life had given no great character to Scottish Physic, or Jerome Cardan would not have been brought from beyond the Alps to cure the Archbishop of St. Andrew's in 1552. Nay, a century and a half after obtaining their chartered footing, the Surgeons had only small acquaintance with the basis of their art, as is shown by the following quaint record, semi-pious and semi-anatomical, copied *verbatim* from the Archives of the University of Edinburgh :—
"*Res Rariores sive Naturales sive Artificiales Donatæ vel Acquisitæ.* A skeleton of a Frenchman brought from Paris by Doctor Michael Young, who, physician-like, frighted us at first sight, and then to dissipate Fear and make this sad spectacle very familiar and Monitory of what we must all be at last, presented the Colledge therewith 1671. It is neatly and cleanly done, and covered with a white sheet, and wants three teeth above

E 2

and four below, and the forefinger or joynt of the right hand is dropt off. He hangs in a very convenient oblong box of timber which, opening with three doors, exposes all parts of him to view."

The cranium — so it is affirmed — of the Scottish historian George Buchanan and this French skeleton constituted the entire "*res rariores anatomiæ*" of the University; yet, previous to this, William Wormius had published (1665) the *Museum Wormianum*—a catalogue of the rare and curious objects of Natural History established by his renowned father Olaus Wormius; and Nehemiah Grew was busy with his *Museum Regalis Societatis;* and Frederick Ruysch had made Amsterdam famous by his great anatomical collection.

Edinburgh had but a small population, and a trade nearly limited to the making of "quhanzears" (swords), so that, in setting up a claim for anatomy some years prior to the establishment of Walter Chapman's printing-press within the walls, the citizens showed their participation in the fresh intellectual force ushering in the dawn of the sixteenth century. Art[1] had come boldly forth, and Science was trying to divest herself of the shackles

---

[1] Almost synchronous with Edinburgh's first advance towards anatomy, Da Vinci was engaged in some of his grand works, evincing an intimate knowledge of external form and human physiognomy; and in the very year of the Surgeons' Charter of Incorporation (1505), Michael Angelo had finished his cartoon of the "Bathing Soldiers" for the great hall of the Palazza Vecchio, in Florence—a work that fully exhibited the result of his twelve years' study of myography. Nor was Raphael a whit behind his predecessors and compeers in his adornment of the *Camera della Signatura*, and in his creation of Madonnas of imperishable glory in art; indeed, the greatest efforts of his genius rest on a just appreciation of the human form divine.

that had so long bound her to alchemy, astrology, and priestly dogmas. In this general assertion and awakening of the European mind, the close alliance existing between the French and Scottish Courts in the sixteenth century would essentially aid in the creation of a medical faculty of observation in Edinburgh. Scotland, however, for many long years, was too much engrossed with her political status, her theological feuds, and the burning of witches, to give much heed to scientific culture.[1] The Reformation, though based on moral and spiritual aims, was more a political than an intellectual movement; its theology was dogmatic, if not mystical; and it too often came visibly forth that "New Presbyter was but Old Priest writ large." The Kirk, the ruling power in Scotland, was busy with its "godly discipline," and hurling excommunications right and left upon its refractory members. Everything that exalted the intellect, or betrayed a love for physical and æsthetic enjoyment, was viewed as critical or dangerous to the soul's welfare, and liable to be treated as heresy. Even minstrels and pipers had to cease their vocation, lest they harped ungodly tunes, or brought the sons and daughters of Eve in too close harmony of person; and as late as 1569 two poets in

---

[1] See Buckle's "History of Civilization," Lecky's "History of Rationalism in Europe," Sir W. Scott's "Demonology," and Mrs. E. Lynn Linton's "Witch Stories." Paganism had as much credit as medical science in the outlying districts of Scotland. Thus the register of the Presbytery of Dingwall, in the year of grace 1678, shows that several members of the Mackenzie family were cited for "sacrificing a bull in a heathenish manner on the Island of Rufus, commonly called Ellam Mowry in Lochen, for the recovery of the health of Constance Mackenzie, who was formerly sick and valetudinaire."

the Scottish "land of song" were hanged, possibly "*pour encourager les autres.*"

It was not till 1694 that an effort was made to establish a School of Anatomy in the Scottish metropolis, by asking the Town Council to grant the dead bodies of foundlings, and such as die of violent deaths and have none to own them, for dissection. Three years previously (1691) Paul Martin, a distressed French Protestant, had commenced the manufacture of surgical instruments in Edinburgh. In 1705, a Professor of Anatomy was appointed, with a salary of £15 a year, to teach the chirurgeon-apothecaries! In 1720 Alexander Monro succeeded to the professorship and its emoluments. He (*primus*) had studied in Paris and Leyden;[1] and of his fame it is unnecessary to speak, as everybody is aware that he and his son Alexander (*secundus*) laid the foundation of the Anatomical School of Edinburgh.[2]

Before the days of the Monros, the supply of "subjects" was so inadequate, that the surgeons' apprentices

[1] The anatomists had to seek the Continental Schools, yet all the while there was plenty of *matériel*, could it have been but utilized, in Edinburgh. The number of persons condemned for witchcraft alone would have afforded a superabundant supply. In 1664 no less than nine women witches were burned together at Leith! (Dalzell, "Darker Superstitions of Scotland," pp. 669, 670.) The Presbyteries held that the element of fire was necessary to the purification of the "Satanic progeny." It might have been supposed that the "puir Deil" would have been allowed to deal with his own progeny and in his own way. Oh, Religion! what crimes are committed in thy name!

[2] There are no pretensions in these pages to an historical account, but only to note a few salient points bearing upon the Knox narrative. Professor Struthers has carefully collated most of the facts pertaining to the medical school in his "Historical Sketch of the Edinburgh Anatomical School." (Maclachlan and Stewart, 1864.)

and young barbers determined upon the adventurous step of procuring them from the graveyards. The Old Greyfriars, containing the sacred dust of the Martyrs and Covenanters, was still the chief sepulchral ground of the city, and to this place of interment the said apprentices resorted. How long they had practised the system of body-snatching is not known ; but the secret oozed out in 1711, as on the 20th May of that year the College of Surgeons recorded a minute, that " of late there has been a violation of sepulchres in the Greyfriars churchyard, by some who most unchristianly have been stealing, or at least attempting to carry away, the bodies of the dead out of their graves." For a few years subsequently nothing more was heard of grave-desecration ; but with the success of Monro's teaching arose suspicions of a return to the " unchristian practices," to guard against which the College of Surgeons, on the 24th January, 1721, ordered that a clause should be put into all the indentures of apprentices against violation of the church-yards. Notwithstanding this, in April 1725, a further disturbance of graves became known, and, in the fearful tumult that arose, the populace nearly demolished Monro's anatomical establishment.

The framers of the English language had not provided against the contingency of such a special artisanship as that of robbing graves. So deeply grafted was the sacred-ness of " God's Acre," that the removal of a body from its walled precinct was viewed as nothing less than an interference with the " plans of Providence" and the " great Resurrection." Hence, probably, arose the name of " Resurrectionists," to designate the body-snatchers.

For a time the apprentices and gravediggers were the only resurrectionists; but at the beginning of this century a distinct class of men engaged in the work, and earned great wages in Edinburgh, owing to the popularity of its medical school attracting a majority of English and Irish students. The demand was so much greater than the supply afforded by the northern resurrectionists, that Dr. Barclay, in 1806, and subsequently,[1] sent to London for "subjects:" this was a precarious, and necessarily costly, speculation. The trading smacks plying between London and Leith were oft detained by adverse winds, and the boxes of mortalities, marked "perishable goods," seldom reached their destination in a satisfactory condition.

Though the dissection of brute forms, particularly those of the higher mammals, have furnished much anatomical information, and served greatly to elicit the general principles of physiology, human bodies are essential to the true anatomy of man and the practice of pathology and surgery. Anatomical teaching, to be successful, or at all applicable to the pursuit of the healing art, required the use of "mortal remains," and these were sought for and obtained at all hazards. The non-profes-

---

[1] In the Diary of a London Resurrectionist, for 1812 and 1813, which I had the opportunity of examining in the Royal College of Surgeons' Library (London), I found ample confirmation of what is recorded above. Occasionally twelve bodies were despatched to Edinburgh by one sloop. Of all diaries extant, this of an English Resurrectionist seems the most remarkable. The notes are written in a good hand, and each chapter in the book is introduced with fine caligraphic flourishes; these stand in striking contrast with the fearful data contained in the record. Thus : "Drunk, Ben and Tom and Jack with me." "Did nothing last night; came to the Moulders' Arms, and got drunk." "Got six—packed three to Edinburgh."

sional reader will ask if it had not been the custom to provide the anatomist with the unclaimed dead of prisons, hospitals, and poor-houses, as well as the executed criminals ; why, therefore, should he resort to the cemeteries ? To which the anatomists of forty years ago could only have replied : " Our legitimate source hardly amounts to units in the scale of wants, and is therefore totally inadequate ; our professional status does not receive any recognition at the hands of the Legislature ; and, in self-defence of interests, affecting the general weal more than ourselves, we are forced to associate with the most abandoned of characters—the Resurrectionists."

To revert for a moment to an antecedent period, it may be stated, that among the social and political reforms engaging England after the peace of 1815, Medicine, whether viewed *per se* or in its hygienic and State relations, could not wisely be overlooked. The Navy and Army Medical Departments, and not less the general public, were solicitous for a more skilful class of doctors than the old apothecary and phlebotomist of an un educated age. Looking to the labours of John Hunter and Matthew Baillie in the field of anatomy as suggestive of a more philosophic surgery and pathology than England had yet obtained, the Royal Colleges of the United Kingdom, as trustees of the profession, advocated an extension of the anatomical courses and instruction in their medical curriculum. With this salutary move in the way of medical reform, sanctioned too by the ruling powers, it was hoped that anatomy would obtain a legalized footing in Britain, and so be able to hold its

own against the more complete organization prevalent
in the medical schools of Europe. The hope was futile :
the English Executive endorsed the wishes of the profession for a higher standard of anatomical proficiency,
nay, made it imperative upon all students of medicine ;
but took no steps whatever to facilitate the acquisition of
the knowledge they demanded. Thus it played fast and
loose with the profession. The law of Britain against
the practice of exhumation was kept in full force all the
while ; there were no less than fourteen convictions in
one year in England : fines, imprisonment, and in one
case transportation for seven years was awarded by the
Essex quarter sessions, where the guilt was far from being
established. Whilst the Eldons and Castlereaghs had
their minds fixed upon party and personal interests, the
State Church and our "glorious Constitution ;" Medicine,
the most valued of all sciences, was left out in the cold,
or resolutely thwarted in its progress by the rule of Tory
fogyism !

Under circumstances so humiliating to the national
fervour, what was the anatomist to do ? He had long
"prayed and petitioned" the Jupiters of his constitutional Pantheon for help ; he had offered incense at the
shrine of municipal and parochial boards, and humbled
himself to the nod of corporates great and small, even as
low as the plush of Beadledom ; but realized only the
"*non possumus*" and the "circumlocutions" of office. No
wonder the question, from time to time, arose—Was the
profession of medicine to be sustained in this country as
a noble calling based on anatomy ; or was it to revert to
that of the barber-surgeon, intertwined with the herbalist

and bone-setter? Every intelligent person knew that, as
the rule and the square were to the architect and builder,
and the compass to the sailor, so was anatomy to the
surgeon ; yet the means for its practice had to be obtained furtively, with that rare exception, the carrying
out what might be designated the final *in terrorem* of the
law against malefactors. If medicine merited a place in
English civilization, had it to march *pari passu* with the
progressive science of the day, and enjoy the privileges
due to well-directed efforts in the cause of truth, or to be
" cabin'd and confined" by legislative enactments till it
sank back to the level of scholastic mediævalism? Was
man, in his infirmity and suffering, to fare no better in
nineteenth-century England than the wounded and half-
dead victim of the Jericho thieves did at the hands of
the priest who passed by on the other side? Happily
for the English name, the love of science and the greater
love of humanity made suitable response. The followers
of the healing art stepped forward as good Samaritans,
nerving themselves to a work both imminent and painful,
hoping that the day was not far distant when the State
would imitate the continental Governments, and make
anatomy available to the cultivator of science.

The schools of Paris and Vienna, being well supplied
with " subjects," attracted the more enterprising English
student; and if means of travel had been as available
forty and fifty years ago as now, the anatomical institutions of this country would have been reduced to the
lowest possible ebb. Whilst Protestant England, boasting
of her advanced civilization and constitutional liberties,
was rabid in her opposition to the pursuit of human

anatomy, the great Catholic countries of France and Austria, lent every aid to promote the cause of medical science in their respective capitals.

No greater hardship could have overtaken men of feeling and education than being brought in personal contact with the Resurrectionists—a crew of unequivocal Ishmaelites. Whilst reprobates and thieves formed the van, others credited with better demeanour joined the ranks, and shared in the lucrative pay attending grave-robbing, or, as it might be, coffin violation. The guardians of the peace, the servants of the Church, the exacting undertakers, as well as the Pharisaical " mutes " and other parties engaged in the last rites paid to mortality, not only connived at the doings of the Resurrectionists, but readily took their bribes. How the " well-greased " palm could change the doleful whine of the sexton's " Amen," and open the gates of the sacred precincts to the thief of the night! Numbers were implicated in this traffic, and possibly viewed it in the same light as Jerry Cruncher, "honest tradesmanship of an agricultooral character." Paid members of the funeral *cortége* would occasionally respond in words to the " hopes of a glorious resurrection for our dear brother here departed," who knew that the coffin lowered in the dust contained no "brother" at all, but an equivalent weight of soil and rubbish. Amidst the crime and sacrilege of their operations, these monsters never scrupled to exact heavy deodands from the anatomist, whereby to drink and dissipate and drown the cares of life.

All sorts of schemes were resorted to for the carriage of bodies by sea and land from distant districts to the metropolitan schools. The Resurrectionists personified drysalters, pork-curers, purveyors of animals for museums, even apple-dealers and blacking-makers. Nothing was too base for them to do. Their countenances betrayed a sinister expression, and their dress, always shabby, neither resembled the artisan nor the lowest of tradesmen ; they were nondescripts in person, as they were in character. They did their best to avoid recognition, and always seemed in a hurry to place their box in the coach "boot," or to get their casks on board ship. They lacked the art of packing and the use of antiseptics : hence the frequent disclosures of their traffic on the quays of Dublin and Glasgow, and in coach transit[1] from the provincial towns of England. Had prudence or common decency guided these men, the world might have gone on for a time without being much wiser of the relations between the doctors and their purveyors ; but the increased demand and higher pay for *matériel* generated sad reckless- ness and brutality. Quarrels arose over the spoils: the jealousy of success, the rivalry of the factions of the different schools, and the frequent attempts of the Resur- rectionists to outwit each other, led to personal denun- ciations and a fearful publicity.

Nothing could well be more incongruous in the history of legislation than enforcing "practical anatomy" upon every medical probationer, whilst his seeking the means

[1] The danger of discovery was greatest in the towns where the stage coach stayed for the night. Several inquests were held at Carlisle on bodies thus detected, and meant for the Edinburgh school. The deci- sions of the juries on these occasions—"Found dead in a box "—used to amuse the Scottish jurists and anatomists, and naturally threw discredit on the proceedings of all "Crowners' quests."

of its pursuit involved the risk of fetters to his heels and
a lasting opprobrium to his name. The law of England
resembled the Venetian as laid down by Shakespeare's
" Portia ;" it exacted on the bond the pound of flesh, yet
denied the operation of removing it. The law, as it bore
upon anatomy, typified the goddess of Justice with one
eye professedly open to the wants of the public service,
the other eye in a state of occlusion to the evils of a great
social abuse that disturbed the domestic quiet of the
realm, and shocked the tenderest feelings of humanity.
The law virtually proclaimed that the surgeon should
possess aptitude and powers as well as a formal licence
to practise ; nay, it went further, and subjected him who
failed to display " proper skill " to pecuniary forfeiture
in the civil courts at the instigation of any dissatisfied
patient ; yet the only mode of- acquiring that skill,
namely, from dissections of the dead clandestinely obtained, was in the criminal court held to be a misde-
meanour, punishable by fine and imprisonment !   There
was no steering between the Scylla and Charybdis of the
law. Think of the youthful cultivator of medicine seeking
anatomical expertness by opportunities, the detection of
which would send him to a felon's cell ; or, if he grew up
a dunce rather than risk such a contingency, finding himself in after years charged in a civil court with want of
proper knowledge, and cast in heavy damages ! Instances
of both these forms of forfeiture could be adduced from
the history of the English and Scottish courts.

    Whilst legal enactments and the indignation of the
lower orders were allied against dissections, the student
daily listened to the academical expression of anatomy

being a *sine quâ non* to his advancement, the map or globe of the medical geographer *ab initio*. The indoctrination of his teachers came with all the more force when the historical examples of professional superiority, derived from the renowned men of the past as well as living surgeons, were shown to rest on the higher achievements in anatomy. It could be truly said that without anatomy England would have had no Cheselden, no John Hunter, and no William Lawrence in surgery, and might have ranked no higher in the biological sciences than some petty States beyond the Alps ruled by ecclesiastics, Austrian satraps, and other oppressors of human thought.

With such recognized data on the chart of his studies, no wonder the novitiate in medicine evinced so strong a feeling for the means of anatomical research. Prompted, as all true students were, by a high sense of duty to their calling, no difficulty seemed too great to enable them to obtain the special desideratum in their education. With such fervour in the class-rooms, the enthusiasm of the hospital surgeon seeking the highest honours in his own walk may be readily inferred. To be *au courant* with the improvements in his art, and to make the service of his patients the solicitous care of his life, were constant objects of consideration with all good and humane surgeons. The hazardous surgical operations of fifty years ago[1] were seldom attempted by the most skilful of hands

---

[1] Between 1820 and the passing of the Anatomy Act of 1832 some of the boldest operations in surgery were performed in Edinburgh. British Surgery had no more promising representatives than Robert Liston and James Syme at the time. Soon afterwards Mr. (now Sir W.) Fergusson, Bart., won his laurels in the Edinburgh Hospital as the reward of a constant and noted vigilance in the pursuit of anatomy.

without a previous preparation on the dead body; and if such opportunity was not to be had, the operators bent upon success had no alternative but to repair to the burial-grounds. There was some justification for the step, provided the feelings of living relatives were in no wise trespassed upon : *here*, in hospitals and in the homes of a large city were the maimed and diseased crying for relief ; *there*, in graveyards, fast mouldering into dust, were resources which, rightly used, might prove highly beneficent to living mortals. The restoration of one life of real value was worth the sacrifice of many cadavera. The professional ardour that prevailed[1] has been much overlooked in discussing the history of these times of peril to British Surgery ; it stood forth as a ruling passion affecting men of the highest moral and intellectual endowments—the Bells, Barclays, and Coopers —and what they sanctioned as aids to a cause they served so nobly might well be excused in their successors, pending the introduction of legislative measures to correct a large and still growing evil.

For some years prior to the catastrophe that brought the anatomical affairs of Britain to a crisis, considerable

---

[1] This enthusiasm was well proved during the cholera visitation of 1831-32. Whilst the strongest of minds were filled with alarm as to the contagious pestilence in the city, and coffins and bearers could hardly be had wherewith to bury the dead, the Edinburgh anatomists laid hold of every unclaimed cholera subject. For a time Knox's Rooms contained no other than those holding the virus of the disease. Courting the "bubble reputation at the cannon's mouth" was not more fraught with danger than the dissection of cholera bodies fresh from the wards of an hospital. The bodies of fever patients contained the seeds of contagion. Dr. Murchison, the author of the best work on fever now extant, caught the disease in this way in Edinburgh. He had not been near any fever patient.

apprehension existed as to the safety of the dead both in town and rural districts; even the secret sources by which the anatomist pursued his art were no longer to be connived at by the public authorities. Rumour, with its thousand tongues, magnified the horrors of the situation, whilst the imagination of the sorrowful as to the fate of their lost ones helped to pile up the agony far beyond the real facts of the case. In Edinburgh, the civic authorities were called upon to act with greater vigilance; "detectives" were placed near the anatomical rooms, and all visitors of questionable purpose were traced to their residences. The "minions of the moon" felt the surveillance most keenly; they were marked men to whom no quarter or mercy could be shown, if caught *flagrante delicto*. Being ferreted out of their old haunts by the terriers of the law, and finding no shelter or safety in the worst slums of the Old Town, these outlawed caterers for science were forced to make raids across the Borders, or take ship to Ireland. Almost everywhere within the realm the cry of "Death to the Resurrectionists!" resounded, and to such purpose as materially to affect the existence of the anatomical classes of Barclay and Monro.[1] The cry, so exultant and menacing out of doors, caused reaction as defiant within the anatomical rooms; and this was but a prelude to heroic action, well developed and well sustained. The students, organized in bands and under good leadership, set out on Vesalian crusades, and succeeded beyond

[1] Mr. James Syme, the well-known Professor of Clinical Surgery in Edinburgh, taught Anatomy for a time, but, finding it impossible to obtain bodies, retired from the field at the beginning of the Session 1828-29.

F

expectation ; the greatest triumphs fell, however, to more experienced hands, and one Lecturer especially signalized himself in these times.   He was a Napier in action, bold, dexterous, aye ready, and in the van of danger, and single-handed equal to any three of the regular staff of workmen.   Thus one night, when a party of medicals headed by this surgeon saw they were discovered in a city churchyard, the chief actor laid hold of two large " adults " that moment disinterred, and, carrying one under each arm, escaped by a door which led into the garden of a private Institution.   Perhaps no man in Edinburgh could have done such a feat of strength, or made so good a retreat, whilst under "the cover" of blunderbusses.   Strategy and foresight were quite as much in request as brute force, and men of intelligence succeeded where the Resurrectionists failed, as in the following instance.

A country lad whose disease had excited large interest, and upon whose case numerous medical men had been consulted, at length succumbed to hydrocephalus, and his body was buried in the exposed cemetery of a fishing burgh on the shores of the Firth of Forth.   Having strong suspicions of the doctors, the friends of the deceased engaged trustworthy watchers of his grave—men who for night after night, and week after week, resisted every overture of bribes and whisky offered them by the Resurrectionists. The agents of Monro and Barclay and others were all intent upon what in the language of the schools was termed a " rare osteological specimen ;" money was abundantly lavished, and every artifice and intrigue put in force to obtain the subject ; but all to no purpose.

Weeks had gone over, and the excitement of the contest between the "watchers" and the besieging force of Resurrectionists had passed away, when one evening at dusk two well-dressed gentlemen, smoking their cigars, drove up in a dog-cart to the chief hostelry of the little burgh : they alighted, and requested that their horse might be taken care of for an hour. The "whip-hand" gentleman told the ostler that he expected a livery servant to bring a parcel for him, which could be put in the box part of the conveyance, to which the key was attached. In a short time a man in smart livery came to the stable-yard, deposited a bag under the seat of the dog-cart, pocketed the key, and walked off—" a canny silent man, or dull o' hearing." Presently afterwards the two gentlemen returned to the inn, ordered out their " trap," and trotted off at a brisk pace. The sharp-eyed stable-boy could not help remarking that the " liveryman" who brought the bag was deuced like the off-side gentleman, and fancied he saw a bit of the scarlet lining under the said gentleman's brown overcoat. " Haud yer tongue, Sandie," said the lad's superior; "ye're aye seeing farlies." Whilst the unknown gentlemen were trotting homewards at full speed, the watchers of the night, or rather the guardians of the hydrocephalic body, were approaching their post of duty. As usual on entering the cemetery, they looked at the grave to see that all was right ; but to their astonishment found that it had been disturbed; nay, more, that the coffin was broken, and that the body was gone ! What! abstracted in daylight—impossible, yet too true ! The reader will have surmised that the " dog-cart gentlemen" were the depredators, and most expert ones too ; for they had done a piece of work that had baffled the ingenuity of the most experienced Resurrectionists of Scotland. Availing themselves of the twilight just before the watchers appeared on the ground, they succeeded in disinterring the body and carrying it off in thirty minutes. Two such accomplished artists in their own line, as Liston, the Edinburgh surgeon, and Crouch, the London Resurrectionist, the world never saw before, and, now that " Othello's occupation's gone," cannot possibly see again. A terrible hue and cry was raised in the burgh, that soon extended to Edinburgh ; detectives, search-warrants, and all the agencies of the law were put in force, but no clue could be had to the den of Cacus, and of course *non habeas corpus.* Years rolled on ; the contents of the big sack, having in the meantime become manipulated beyond " all mortal ken," found a resting-place in the noblest anatomical collection of Britain—the donor's name being worthily attached to the *chef d'œuvre* of his body-snatching exploits. The many thousands who during the last thirty years have looked upon this remarkable skeleton, No. 3,489, little fancy that its history from first to last would afford materials for a tale of thrilling interest—the truth in the record being stranger than any fiction that could possibly be woven around it.

A case of almost equal import could be instanced from the Fife coast, where watchings and counter-watchings, sentinel-ism and subterfuge, contended for long ; but victory eventually rewarded the anatomists. Horses fleet of foot, and mounted with panniers simulating the old " pack-saddle" of other days, were stationed near the field of action; as soon as the saddle-bags got filled, men of bold enterprise hastened to the coast, where a boat was ready to receive the Charon-freight, and to set sail for the southern banks of the Forth, and nearest to Edinburgh. All attempts to overtake or discover the delinquents invariably failed.

Independently of the doings of the Resurrectionists, this volume might be filled with stories of dangers by flood and field incurred by educated. men for the sake of professional excellence, and the safer practice of a humanitarian art. One instance more may be cited, as it brings out both the "plot and counterplot" of the Resurrectionists, their scandalous conduct at the grave-side, and their discomfiture with a vengeance by more knowing masters in the same field. Messrs. L. and M., anatomical teachers, walking about midnight in the direction of a churchyard, discovered flitting lights among the tombstones, and soon heard human voices in angry tone and violent dispute—Resurrectionists, of course! One party had nearly raised a body when another set of men appeared on the scene and claimed *it* as their special privilege ; a row followed, and blows were very freely exchanged by the combatants. Now was the time for honest interference, and who could seize the vantage-ground with more skill than Mr. L., who, stealthily approaching behind the tombstones, suddenly struck the fiercest leader of the fight, and felled him to the ground. The presence of the "deil himself" could not have produced greater consternation ; the cowardly ruffians took to their heels *sauve qui peut,* leaving their tools and *cadaver* to the "gentleman in black," whom they avowed, in defence of their awful fright, to have been possessed of something more than a cloven foot.

With the external signs of daring effrontery and of devils incarnate, the Resurrectionists showed a vast amount of cowardice; even a lunar shadow scared them at times. Their schemes for getting money from the anatomists which they never meant to pay, their knavish artifices, their betrayal of each other, their wholesale brutality, marked them as little less than caco-demons. Two "noted hands" called one night at Knox's rooms, and asked the assistant on duty if he would take "an adult" which they had "close by." Agreed, and in ten minutes the body was brought in and paid for. Next morning Mr. Lizars' anatomical class was in great excitement on learning that a "fresh subject" had been carried off during the night from the tables of their dissecting-room. Lizars himself was in a terrible rage, and interrogated Peter, the janitor, very closely. "You say you bolted and barred all the doors, and found them the same this morning?" "Yes, sir." "Then how the devil could the body be got away?" "Well," quoth Peter, "I dinna ken, unless it was the deil's ain work, for there's neither a chink in the door nor a flaw in the window for an imp to creep in by." As no clue could be had to the body, the superstitious Highland student saw a deeper meaning than the mere abstraction, nothing less indeed than a *bonâ fide* resurrection of a new prophet for his Scottish Israel. The burglary was in every way outrageous. A body stolen from the grave is sold to Lizars; it is re-stolen from his dissecting-room, and sold again within the hour. The villains netted £25 by their work, and had no fear of indictment.

As showing an utter disregard not only of all moral and sacred standards, but of the shadow of decency, among these fellows, the following may be narrated :— During the prevalence of cholera in Edinburgh, 1831-32, one of the last of the Resurrectionists ever seen about his old haunts was found on the street in a comatose state. The police, supposing him to be dying of cholera, carried him off to the Cholera Hospital, where he was treated by Dr. McIntosh as a patient in the last stage ; viz. by venesection, the Doctor's favourite remedy. Next morning the despaired-of choleraic was wonderfully recovered, and Dr. McIntosh pointed with delight to the last happy illustration of the good effects of his system ! The patient, whose only remembrance of the previous night was being " awfu' fou" at Sandy McTavish's dram-shop, was as much surprised to find himself in the presence of nurses and doctors, as the latter could possibly be at his " marvellous recovery" from cholera ! He was too knowing a rascal to mis-understand the interest taken in his case, and played his cards accordingly, by pleading weakness and soliciting brandy and nutriment. On his entire restoration from a " drunken bouse," he showed his gratitude by debauching every comely nurse in the wards of the Institution !

Such were the practices in vogue to secure provision for the anatomical schools when Dr. Knox succeeded to Dr. Barclay's Lectureship in 1826 ; nay, had been in existence for a century ; yet Knox was spoken of as originating the system ! To clear away some clouds of

prejudice, this semi-historical chapter became imperative. It is needful for the lay reader to bear in mind
that in these painful transactions, the Anatomists, ranking
amongst them so many excellent and honourable persons
as Sir C. Bell and Sir George Ballingall, had to deal with
matters affecting medical and scientific interests as they
best could and not assuredly as they wished, and not
as they were in the habit of dealing with the ordinary
affairs of life. Everything indeed was exceptional. If
Barclay, the preacher, good citizen, and philanthropist,
could be a party to these practices, Knox, a younger
man, might well pass unscathed ; for if Barclay had difficulties in the way of supply to his rooms, Knox, with
a larger class, had unquestionably more to contend with.
Edinburgh and its environs were almost in a stage of
siege *quà* anatomy, so the area of operations had to be
greatly enlarged. Ireland was found to offer greater facilities than either England or Scotland, and Knox had
large dealings with the Dublin resurrectionists. As
a teacher, he placed himself *en rapport* with his class,
sharing in its enthusiasm and scientific ardour, and, to
gratify these aims, thought nothing of the trouble or
expense he might incur in furnishing his anatomical
rooms ; hence No. 10, Surgeons' Square, had a supply
which no other establishment possessed.

CHAPTER IV.

Hare and Burke.—The Murder's out.—Excitement and Alarm everywhere in the Land.—Knox defamed and in danger of Martyrdom.—A Committee of Inquiry: their Report, and Knox's Letters of Exculpation.

" Specus et Caci detecta apparuit ingens
Regia, et umbrosæ penitus patuere cavernæ."
ÆNEID, lib. viii.

ON the 29th November 1827 an old pensioner of the name of Donald died in Tanner's Close, West Port, Edinburgh. He died in debt to the extent of £4, and William Hare, his creditor, in whose lodging-house he had lived, saw but one way of reimbursing himself, and that was by disposing of the old man's body to the doctors. Hare found a ready accomplice in William Burke, another of his lodgers. The body was removed from the coffin, and a bag of tanners' bark took its place; the coffin lid was screwed down, and all made decent for the bearers. Several neighbours, who had listened to the old man's stories of the war, respectfully joined the funeral procession, little conceiving that their tears at the grave-side were shed over deal boards and tanners' bark. The same evening Hare and Burke stealthily repaired to the college, and, meeting a student in the quadrangle, asked for Dr. Monro's rooms. On discovering their errand, he, being a pupil of Knox's, advised them to try Dr. Knox's, 10, Surgeons' Square. There they sold the pensioner's body for £7 10s. So big a sum and so easily got proved sadly ominous : the two Irishmen loved their labour less and their whisky vastly more from that hour of " selling their friend's carcase." They had not courage to attempt the mode of the Resurrectionists, and, as waiting for another casualty at home was "awfu' tedious," Hare, the vilest of the two monsters, suggested a fresh stroke of business, namely, to inveigle the old and infirm into his den and " do for them."

Prowling about the streets in search of a victim, Hare met an old woman from the neighbouring village of Gilmerton " fresh with drink ;" he asked her to his house, and gave her lots of whisky ; she got merry and garrulous, sang her favourite ditties, drank more deeply, and then became comatose. Now was the fit opportunity. Hare placed his hands firmly over her nose and mouth to stop respiration, while Burke laid himself across her body to ensure stillness. The operation succeeded—the woman of Gilmerton was dead. The body brought £10!—a gold sovereign for every minute of time spent in the work. Verily this realized De Quincey's notion of " murder being one of the fine arts." The expertness and surety of the mode enhanced the blood-money ; the vampirian thirst now took possession of Burke and Hare and their paramours who shared in their devilish gains. Widows, orphans, streetwalkers, and imbeciles were allured on various pretexts to the houses of Burke and Hare, and there dosed with whisky and suffocated. Dante's *Lasciate ogni speranza, voi ch' entrate*, should have been inscribed over the door leading to this den of infamy in the West Port. Thuggism and other horrid forms of Eastern fetichism found their counterpart in atrocity during the year 1828 in the " Heart of Mid-Lothian," the capital of " moral and Christian Scotland." Emboldened by their repeated successes, Burke and Co. murdered their victims in daylight, and drank and danced in the midst of death. The " deil's luck " befriended them fifteen times ; the sixteenth turn of the wheel proved fatal to the horrid fiends. A woman of the name of Docherty was invited from the street to spend the " Halloween "[1] in Burke's house, hoping no doubt to meet there with

> " Hearts leal, and warm, and kin'."

She danced and sang, and joined in the revels of the night, that were wound up by her roaring " a horrid murder shout,"

> " In dreadfu' desperation !"

Next morning her dead body is seen under some straw by two lodgers, who gave information to the police. Burke and Helen McDougal and Hare and his wife were then apprehended on the charge of " Wilful murder."[2]

---

[1] The character of " Halloween," as kept in Scotland, will be best obtained from Burns's famous poem. " All Hallow Eve, or the eve of All Saints' Day, is thought to be a night when witches, devils, and other mischief-making beings are all abroad on their baneful midnight errands." Burns little fancied that his poetical definition would be realized to the full by devils in human shape, living in the year of grace 1828 under the shadow of Edinburgh Castle.

[2] At the trial of the prisoners (December 24, 1828) Hare, the most hideous of scoundrels, and his wife turned approvers, and so escaped the

The reader may conceive the astonishment that prevailed in the city of Edinburgh when it became known on the 2nd November that a woman had been murdered for the sake of her body, and that it was found in Knox's rooms. The deed itself was sufficiently horrifying; it was but a nucleus, however, to a hundred suppositions equally dreadful and alarming. The air was filled with suspicions of the direst kind, and dismay like an epidemic spread over the land. Edinburgh got the credit of being the head-quarters of the new Thuggism. History was ransacked for parallel instances of human immolation; and religious history was specially appealed to for an interpretation of the events that had made " the Halloween" of 1828 the saddest on record. Who could have designed this latest and "fatalest sort of devildom ?" Burke and Hare were Irishmen; they were also Roman Catholics; might they not be agents of the Jesuits? Were the days of Philip the Second of Spain to have a secret revival in Protestant Scotland, with an anatomical Inquisition to complete the horrors? The smothered embers of the old Covenanters' hate of both Papacy and Prelacy were again lighted up by "auld grannies," ensconced by Scottish ingle-nuiks, reciting from their infantile recollections stories of persecutions long gone past, to willing and excited listeners. Super-

gallows, only to be hunted, however, from town to town like wild beasts. They returned to their native country (Ireland), and were no more heard of except in the pages of fiction till a few months ago, when Hare was reported as being seen in London. Burke was hanged and dissected; his skeleton is to be found in the Anatomical Museum of the University. His cranium resembles that of a woman, and could hardly have been taken for that of a murderer. Helen McDougal's guilt was "not proven." She is said to have died in Australia in 1868.

stition and love of vaticination—known attributes in the
Scottish character—lent no small aid to the disquieted
state of the public mind. Some had lately seen in the
display of the aurora borealis, generally so beautiful in
October nights in the North, portentous streaks of red
and blue. The West Port discovery was dreadful, but
were not worse things in store for poor Scotland? In
the perfect unanimity of opinion that there was something
" rotten in the State of Denmark," everybody in authority
came in for a share of blame, from the wicked George
IV. down to the hateful exciseman. The "General
Assembly of the Kirk," the religious Parliament of
Scotland, was accused of having lost its sterner attributes. The pulpit was not so warm and edifying in its
exhortations to the elect, and not sufficiently vehement
in its denunciations of the sinner. The common folk were
crying for reform and reading newspaper trash, instead
of reforming themselves and studying "The Book."
Burke and Hare were but the carnal weapons of Satan ;
their concubines the alluring servitors of Romish priests,
keenly alive to the selection of fitting instruments for
plotting and effecting mischief.

This terrible tragedy afforded such provender to
garrulous men and gossiping women, and the prejudiced
of every rank and age and sex, that each reputed
version of the facts showed more sombre and sinuous
lines of villany. Newspapers, forty years ago, were
limited very much to towns and the higher and middle
ranks of life; the lower orders had to trust to the piquant
" broadsides " and the ribald ballad for a large part of
the current news. The "Burking affair" was clothed in

brackish prose and rhyme,[1] and meant for the *profanum
vulgus;* the old Gaberlunzie filled his wallet, and the
pedlar his basket, with these "full, true, and particular
accounts," and after inundating the villages and hamlets
with them, sought the byeways, across hill and muir,
even the solitary bield, and everywhere they met
with a welcome that had never been awarded them
before, and entirely due to the special horrors contained in their fresh budget of news. A reign of
social terror prevailed. Every household gathered
its members within doors before dusk ; working men
walked home from their night's toil in groups ; the
streets were scarcely frequented even by the "unfortu-
nates," lest they should share the fate of " Bonny Mary
Paterson." If Buonaparte, early in the century, had
been the bugbear of naughty children, and "Bonny's
coming" was a dread, the winters of and succeeding
1828-29, in which were heard "Burke and pitch-plasters
to your mouth," assured a more effective call to order
and obedience in every domicile.

In the midst of all the excitement, unfortunately
the name of Knox mingled with that of Burke, and
the British vocabulary was ransacked for epithets of
defamation to his character. At the corners of streets, at
the mouths of narrow wynds, and issuing from lairs of
iniquity, women half nude, half drunk, and more than

---

[1] Here is a specimen :—

> " Down the Close and up the Stair,
> But and ben wi' Burke and Hare.
> Burke's the butcher, Hare's the thief,
> Knox the man that buys the beef."

half savage, stood in groups, clamorously egging on both men and lads to act a desperate part towards Knox. The lowest rabble of the Old Town, full of menacing oaths and ferocity, rushed out to Newington and attacked Knox's house in the expectation of securing his person and hanging him along with his effigy, by the lamp-post in front. Here was a surging *plebs* in all its wrath like a hostile mob with a " No Popery " cry, and rising with the occasion of having a philosopher instead of a Captain Porteous to burn and destroy.

Knox was daily exposed to Jeddart-law justice, which means hang your victim first and try him afterwards; yet all the while there was not a single circumstance in his behaviour to which blame could be attached, much less any act of criminality. The Procurator-Fiscal of Edinburgh had made his searching inquiry ; the Lord-Advocate of Scotland had fathomed all the facts of the case; but nothing could be adduced to show Knox in any way accessory to the West Port atrocities.

Next to the physical force enemies of Knox was the Press, which, with few exceptions, blamed him. Then his rivals in the Anatomical School, who pretended they saw in the Burke supply his vantage-ground and success, and who tried to damage his reputation to the utmost. Lastly, and pretty strongly, came the religious probing of his character by a people who are nothing if not religiously critical of their neighbours. If Knox sanctioned such and such practices, what was to become of his soul ? Then, who had his soul in keeping? or under whom did he sit (*Scotticè* for saying whose religious ministry did he attend) ? or of what congregation was he a communicant? The name of Knox was Scottish, Presbyterian, and historical ; but Robert the anatomist was not to be found among "the Elect" of his great ancestor's "Reformed Church." What a relief to the Fathers and Elders of the Kirk of Scotland! Was he Episcopalian or Dissenter ? No! Robert Knox ranked with no sect or congregation of religionists ; so all the Churches breathed freely. Whilst none had the privilege of excommunicating him, every class of the "unco guid" was ready to condemn the "miserable sinner." Some in charity asked if his penitence and public avowal of past errors could not be brought about. Let those who knew Robert Knox in the glory of his strength and intellectual independence—with an eye that penetrated every artifice of statecraft and priestcraft— fancy the Anatomist subjected to an inquisition of conscience by a Padre, and paying cash and credence to a successor of Pope Joan ; or, in sackcloth and ashes, receiving the Athanasian admonitions of a thirty-nine articled canonical! Think for a moment of Knox standing upon the "cuttie stuil" of repentance in St. Giles', Edinburgh, and repeating aloud a Westminster formulary. Such a sight would have startled both gods and men, and shaken high Olympus to its base !

Relying upon his entire innocence in the "Burking business," Knox allowed the winter of a nation's discontent to pass over without making any public declaration that might have appeased the raging clamour. He expected the excitement to subside, and that the better classes would never believe in so dire a motive as his connivance with criminal acts of fearful enormity, much less his associating with monsters of the deepest dye of infamy. He calculated wrongly for himself. Silence cannot be comprehended by a clamorous mob. The people were infuriated that he had not been indicted along with the West Port murderers, and not less maddened with disappointment at Hare's escape ; so Knox had to bear the whole weight of the city's wrath, increased by covert enemies in every quarter. Two months after Burke's condemnation, and his confession exonerating Knox from all blame whatsoever had been given to the world, *Blackwood's Magazine*, in its "*Noctes Ambrosianæ*" (March 1829), written by John Wilson, Professor of Moral Philosophy, *alias* "Christopher North," made every effort to blast the character of the anatomist. Literary ruffianism is too mild a term to apply to the foul words used by Wilson, who, not content with holding up Knox to public execration, rushed with the savagery of the warwhoop and tomahawk upon an unoffending anatomical class for showing an affectionate regard for their great teacher.

Knox's silence over January and February 1829 might not be good policy, but his refusal to bring his enemies to account when he could have obtained heavy damages for their foul libels, was peculiarly creditable to his feelings and forbearance. His regard for science amounting almost to a passion, his hope that the late atrocities would induce the Government to take immediate steps *quoad* the supply of the Anatomical Schools, and his belief that justice would be done to his character sooner or later by the thinking minds of England, served to restrain his pen for months. The appointment

G

of a committee of distinguished citizens to inquire into
the whole affair caused Knox to break his long silence
by the following letter :—

"To the Editor of the 'Caledonian Mercury.

"Sir,—I regret troubling either you or the public with
anything personal, but I cannot be insensible of the
feelings of my friends, or of the character of the profession to which I have the honour of belonging. Had
I alone been concerned, I should never have thought of
obtruding on the public by this communication.

"I have a class of above 400 pupils. No person can be
at the head of such an establishment without necessarily
running the risk of being imposed upon by those who
furnish the material of their science to anatomical
teachers ; and, accordingly, there is hardly any such
person who has not occasionally incurred odium or suspicion from his supposed accession to those violations of
the law, without which anatomy can scarcely now be
practised. That I should have become an object of
popular prejudice, therefore, since mine happened to be
the establishment with which Burke and Hare chiefly
dealt, was nothing more than what I had to expect.
But if means had not been purposely taken, and most
keenly persevered in, to misrepresent facts and to inflame
the public mind, that prejudice would at least have stood
on right ground, and would ultimately have passed away,
by its being seen that I had been exposed to a mere misfortune which would almost certainly have occurred to
anybody else who had been in my situation.

" But every effort has been employed to convert my misfortune into positive and intended personal guilt of the most dreadful character. Scarcely any individual has ever been the object of more systematic or atrocious attacks than I have been. Nobody acquainted with this place requires to be told from what quarter these have proceeded.

" I allowed them to go on for months without taking the slightest notice of them ; and I was inclined to adhere to this system, especially as the public authorities, by never charging me with any offence, gave the only attestation they could that they had nothing to charge me with. But my friends interfered for me. *Without consulting me,* they directed an agent to institute the most rigid and unsparing examination into the facts. I was totally unacquainted with this gentleman ; but I understood that in naming Mr. Ellis they named a person whose character is a sufficient pledge for the propriety of his proceedings.

"The result of his inquiries was laid before the Dean of Faculty and another Counsel, who were asked what ought to be done. These gentlemen gave it as their opinion that the evidence was completely satisfactory, and that there was no want of actionable matter, but that there was one ground on which it was my duty to resist the temptation of going into a court of law. This was, that the disclosures of the most innocent proceedings even of the best-conducted dissecting-room must always shock the public and be hurtful to science. But they recommended that a few persons of undoubted weight and character should be asked to investigate the matter, in order that, if I deserved it, an attestation might be given to me which would be more satisfactory to my friends than any mere statements of mine could be expected to be. This led to the formation of a Committee, which was never meant by me to be anything but private. But the fact of its sitting soon got into the newspapers, and hence the necessity under which I am placed of explaining how that proceeding, in which the public has been made to take an interest, has terminated.

" I have been on habits of friendship with some of the Committee; with others of them I have been acquainted; and some of them I don't even yet know by sight. I took no charge whatever of their proceedings. In order that there might be no pretence for saying that truth was obstructed from fear, I gave a written protection to every person to say what he chose about or against me. The extent to which this was in some instances taken advantage of will probably not be soon forgotten by those who witnessed it.

"After a severe and laborious investigation of about six weeks, the result is contained in the following report, which was put into my hands last night. It is signed by every member of the Committee except one, who ceased to act long before the evidence was completed.

"I cannot be supposed to be a candid judge of my own case, and therefore it is extremely probable that any opinion of mine on the last view adopted by the Committee is incorrect, and theirs right. If it be so, I most willingly submit to the censure they have inflicted, and shall hold it my duty to profit from it by due care hereafter. My consolation is, that I have at least not been obstinate in my errors, and that no sanction has ever been given in any fair quarter to the more serious imputations by which it has been the interest of certain persons to assail me. Candid men will judge of me according to the situation in which I was placed at the time, and not according to the wisdom which has unexpectedly been acquired since.

" This is the very first time that I have ever made any statement to the public in my own vindication, and it shall be the last. It would be unjust to the authors of the former calumnies to suppose that they would not renew them now. I can only assure them that, in so far as I am concerned, they will renew them in vain.

" I have the honour to be, &c. &c.

(Signed) " R. KNOX.

" EDINBURGH, 10, SURGEONS' SQUARE,
    17*th March*, 1829."

REPORT OF THE COMMITTEE.

" The Committee who, at the request of Dr. Knox, undertook to investigate the truth or falsehood of the rumours in circulation regarding him, have gone into an extensive examination of evidence, in the course of which they have courted information from every quarter. They have been readily furnished with all which they required from Dr. Knox himself; and though they have failed in some attempts to procure evidence, they have in most quarters succeeded in obtaining it, and especially from those persons who have been represented to them as having spoken the most confidently in support of these rumours ; and they have unanimously agreed on the following report :—

" 1. The Committee have seen no evidence that Dr. Knox or his assistants knew that murder was committed in procuring any of the subjects brought to his rooms, and the Committee firmly believe that they did not.

" 2. On the question whether any suspicion of murder at any time existed in Dr. Knox's mind, the Committee would observe that there were certainly several circumstances (already known to the public), regarding some

of the subjects brought by Burke and Hare, which, now that the truth has
come out, appear calculated to excite that suspicion, particularly the very
early period after death at which they were brought to the rooms, and the
absence of external marks of disease, together with the opinion previously
expressed by Dr. Knox, in common with most other anatomists, of the
generally abandoned character of persons engaged in this traffic.   But, on
the other hand, the Committee, after much anxious inquiry, have found no
evidence of their actually having excited it in the mind of Dr. Knox, or
of any other of the individuals who saw the bodies of these unfortunate
persons prior to the apprehension of Burke.

" The bodies do not appear in any instance to have borne *any external
marks* by which it could have been known whether they had died by
violence or *suddenly from natural causes*, or from *diseases of short duration ;*
and the mode of *protracted anatomical dissection practised in this and other
similar establishments,* is such as would have made it *very difficult* to ascertain *the causes of death, even if special inquiry had been instituted with that
intention.*

" No evidence whatever has come before the Committee that any suspicion of murder was expressed to Dr. Knox by any one, either of his
assistants or of his very numerous class (amounting to upwards of 400
students), or other persons who were in the practice of frequently
visiting his rooms ; and there are several circumstances in his conduct, particularly the complete publicity with which his establishment was managed,
and his anxiety to lay each subject before the students as soon as possible after its reception, which seem to the Committee strongly to indicate
that he had *no suspicion* of the atrocious means by which they had been
procured.

" It has also been proved to the satisfaction of the Committee, that
no *mutilation or disfigurement* of any kind was ever practised with a view
to *conceal the features,* or abstract unseasonably any part of the body, the
presence of which might have facilitated detection ; and it appears clearly
that the subjects brought by Burke and Hare were dissected in the same
protracted manner as those procured from any other quarter.

" 3.   The Committee have thought it proper to inquire further, whether
there was anything faulty or negligent in the regulations under which
subjects were received into Dr. Knox's rooms, which gave or might give a
peculiar facility to the disposal of the bodies obtained by these crimes ; and
on this point they think it their duty to state their opinion fully.

" It appears in evidence, that Dr. Knox had formed and expressed the
opinion, long prior to any dealings with Burke and Hare, that a considerable supply of subjects for anatomical purposes might be procured by

purchase, and without any crime, from the relations or connections of deceased persons in the lowest ranks of society.

"In forming this opinion, whether mistaken or not, the Committee cannot consider Dr. Knox to have been culpable. They believe there is nothing contrary to the law of the land in procuring subjects for dissection in that way; and they know that the opinion which Dr. Knox had formed on this point, though never acted on to any extent in this country, has been avowed by others of the highest character in the profession. But they think that Dr. Knox acted on this opinion in a very incautious manner.

"This preconceived opinion seems to have led him to give a ready ear to the plausible stories of Burke, who appears from all the evidence before the Committee to have conducted himself with great address and appearance of honesty, as well in his conversations with Dr. Knox, as in his more frequent intercourse with his assistants; and always to have represented himself as engaged in negotiations of that description, and occasionally to have asked and obtained money in advance to enable him and his associate to conclude bargains.

"Unfortunately also Dr. Knox had been led, apparently in consequence of the extent and variety of his avocations, to entrust the dealings with persons supplying subjects, and the reception of the subjects brought, to his assistants (seven in number) and to his doorkeeper indiscriminately. It appears also that he directed or allowed these dealings to be conducted on the understanding (common to him with some other anatomists) that it would only tend to diminish or divert the supply of subjects to *make any particular inquiry of the persons bringing them as to the place and mode of obtaining them.*

"In these respects the Committee consider the practice which was then adopted in Dr. Knox's rooms (whatever be the usage in this or other establishments in regard to subjects obtained in the ordinary way) to have been very improper in the case of persons bringing bodies which had not been interred. They think that the notoriously bad character of persons who generally engage in any such traffic, in addition to the novelty and particular nature of the system on which these men professed to be acting, undoubtedly demanded greater vigilance.

"The extent, therefore, to which (judging from the evidence which they have been able to procure) the Committee think that Dr. Knox can be blamed on account of transactions with Burke and Hare is, that by this laxity of the regulations under which bodies were received into his rooms, he unintentionally gave a degree of facility to the disposal of the victims of their crimes, which under better regulations would not have existed,

and which is doubtless matter of deep and lasting regret, not only to
himself, but to all who have reflected on the importance and are therefore
interested in the prosecution of the study of anatomy.   But while they
point out this circumstance as the *only ground of censure* which they can
discover in the conduct of Dr. Knox, it is fair to observe, that perhaps the
recent disclosures have made it appear reprehensible to many who *would not
otherwise have adverted to its possible consequences.*[1]

> (Signed)
>
> "JOHN ROBINSON   "W. P. ALISON.
>   (*Chairman*).   "GEO. BALLINGALL.
> "M. P. BROWN.   "GEORGE SINCLAIR.
> "JAMES RUSSELL.   "W. HAMILTON.
> "J. SHAW STEWART.   "THOMAS ALLAN.

"13*th March*, 1829."

The gentlemen who formed the Committee were Mr.
Robinson (afterwards Sir John), Secretary to the Royal
Society; Mr. Brown, Advocate; Mr. Russell, Professor
of Clinical Surgery; Mr. Stewart, Advocate; Dr. Alison,
Professor of the Theory of Physic; Sir Geo. Ballingall,
Professor of Military Surgery; Mr. Sinclair the younger
(or Sir George), of Ulbster; Sir W. Hamilton, Bart.,
Professor of Universal History; Mr. Allan, banker, in
Edinburgh.

[1] With a view of facilitating reference to this important document, I have
placed some passages in italics.

CHAPTER V.

WHILST Knox was assailed by the public press, and
threatened with "Lynch law," but small sympathy was
extended him by the professional ranks in his native
city. Such ungraciousness was the more reprehensible,
that no fault could be attached to his mode of conducting
his establishment. Compared with some medical teachers,
he really stood on vantage-ground. He never went out
on body-snatching expeditions ; he abhorred the Resurrectionists; moreover, he had suggested to the Edinburgh
School to form a joint action with London and Dublin
in seeking the aid of the Legislature on anatomical affairs.
It was by the merest accident—the meeting of a student
when the pensioner's body was to be disposed of—that
Knox was brought in relation with Burke at all ; and his
contemporaries should have remembered that *his* misfortune might have been *theirs*, and was within an ace of
being Monro's. Had the West Port subjects gone to the
University Rooms, as Hare intended, the odium that fell
upon Knox would have been cast upon Professor Monro

or Mr. W. Mackenzie, his assistant and factotum. Had such come to pass, Monro *tertius*, then in his decadence, would hardly have been able to stand against the popular wrath, and his professorship would most probably have fallen to Knox. Such a consummation, devoutly wished by those who compared the two rivals from 1825 onwards, would have been of vast import to the anatomical chair and the medical interests of the University at large.

Jealous of the exaltation of Knox, his contemporaries preferred to indulge their private pique rather than make common cause with him for anatomical interests. He had been a luminary to the student, whilst their feeble lights were being gradually put out. He had won the honour of the Barclayan succession, and each year proved his ability to cope with its responsibilities and to extend its fame: moreover, he had two-thirds of the whole medical school in his class rooms; and this fact of itself was enough to engender a covert uncharitableness, if not open hostility, towards him.

Knox had for months borne the burden of vituperation; at length he spoke his mind pretty freely of those who had almost obsequiously attached themselves to his sleeve on his onward course to fame, but on the first recoil, arising from the Burke relations, were disposed to fall away from his side, then to carp at and malign him. He owed nothing to the medical corporations, who might have stood by a man of his promise, if it were only for their own interests and the reputation of the Edinburgh school. Without provocation on his part, slander, and other unobtrusive machinations, were put in force by jealous rivals to crush Knox—the idol of the student, the leading mind and lecturer in the School. In future pages of this memoir, the cynical attitude of Knox himself will be seen in bold relief; up to 1828, however, the period now under discussion, there were no indications, as far as I can ascertain, of his indulging in the satirical methods that afterwards characterised him so strongly. His course from 1825 had been prosperous; the cares of a large class occupied him nine months, and the remaining three months of the year were bestowed upon museum work. His devotion to science had helped to keep him aloof from the snares of medical coteries. Most of the attacks sustained by Knox in the professional walk originated with disappointed rivals. He was at bay for a time, but when he took up the glove that his enemies had thrown down while the Burke excitement overshadowed his position, he challenged each by turn, and seemed to say, in the words of Macbeth:

> "Lay on, Macduff,
> And damn'd be he that first cries ' Hold, enough ! ' "

One of the charitable constructions put on Knox's conversation was, " Ah ! Knox used to say he could always command subjects ; now we have the explanation : he had the West Port villains in pay." The " commanding of subjects," to which he had incautiously referred, simply meant that bodies, like other things purchasable, could be had at a price.[1] Before Burke and

[1] Sir A. Cooper, in his examination before the Select Committee on Anatomy in Parliament (1831), said : " The law only enhances the price, and does not prevent exhumation ; nobody is secured by the law ; it only adds to the price of the subject." Sir Astley knew that everything in this world had

Hare's operations, Knox had a vastly better supply of bodies than his neighbours, owing to his more liberal offers. The skilful Resurrectionist sought his rooms because he got better pay and prompter payment; and, moreover, could rely upon the doctor's faithfulness at all times. A Dublin agent, in 1828, writing to Mr. S., of Edinburgh, who had retired from anatomy and wished to retire too soon from his money responsibilities in Ireland, hesitated not to draw the marked contrast, by saying : " Knox's word once passed I have never known him to violate." Again : " Knox is honourable in all his transactions." If the ordinary price was 10*l.*, Knox in need would give 15*l.*, and on one occasion actually paid 25 guineas rather than see his class disappointed. Nobody but himself would make such pecuniary sacrifices, for when he was paying 15*l.* or 20*l.* he was charging his pupils according to a scale of prices that was regulated by a much lower standard. He was so lavish and regardless of his own pocket, that in one session he lost the almost incredible sum of 700*l.* or 800*l.* by " subjects " alone,—a loss vastly surpassing some anatomical lecturers' entire gains. Without wishing to outbid rivals richer than himself in money means, he could not, with 400 pupils around him, bear to see empty tables, much less to hear the importunate solicitations of his class seeking for professional opportunities that were denied them away from a medical school. Inspired by the genius of their teacher, Knox's

its price, and that, during the days of the Resurrectionists, the body of a spiritual peer could be obtained as readily as the pauper, if the anatomist was disposed to pay the cost.

students were largely devoted to anatomy, and of course all the more difficult to restrain.

The circumstances recorded in the preceding paragraph afford sufficient proof of Knox's immunity from the charges of "commanding subjects" so unscrupulously laid at his door. It may well be asked, Would Knox have sent 200*l.* to Ireland for supplies (a sum, by the way, entirely lost), if he had so profitable a yield in the West Port? Would he have despatched the ablest of his assistants to Dublin in October 1828, to arrange for the approaching session, if he had had any reliance upon, or wished to offer any encouragement to, those who could procure victims *ad libitum* in the slums of Edinburgh? The visits of Burke and Hare to the anatomical rooms were not so frequent as to claim special notice from the assistants, much less from Knox, who saw them there but twice in all; moreover—and the fact should be duly noted—Burke's contributions did not exceed *one-sixth* of the whole number obtained during the session. In dealing with a large establishment, the monsters knew that they ran less risk of detection.

It has been frequently averred, and as generally credited by some, even to this day, that the bodies were received by Knox; that they were so fresh as to be warm to the touch, and not seldom marked about the head and neck; and that there was no internal disease to account for death: statements obviously meant to indicate a wilful oversight on Knox's part to the *modus operandi* of Burke and Hare. The Doctor did not receive the bodies; this was done by his assistants and the janitor of the establishment. If the bodies had been bruised—no such

indications, however, existed about the face and neck—
it by no means followed that these signs betrayed the
infliction of injuries during life. Contusions and marks
were by no means uncommon upon bodies furnished from
hospitals as well as cemeteries. The "Burke" mode
was by suffocation of the victim already dead drunk, and
grasping of the neck or throttling was not resorted to.
The nose and mouth were kept tightly closed, and the
smothering was soon effected. Burke's own declaration
after his conviction was very clear on this point, and
his also maintaining that marks were not to be seen on
the neck from his and Hare's operations.

In the woman Docherty, Professor Christison, the
medical witness for the Crown, found the ligaments
connecting the posterior parts of the vertebræ torn,
and some blood effused among the spinal muscles.
This fact was much dwelt upon at the trial of Burke,[1]
and afterwards advanced to show the blindness or
extreme incautiousness of those who dissected the
murdered bodies. Exception might have been taken
to the Docherty instance, particularly as she struggled
hard with her murderers, and her body was forcibly
pressed into a tea-chest,[2] but this was unnecessary, as

[1] Dr. Christison admitted that the injury of the spine, along with the
effusion of blood among the spinal muscles, "might have been caused
quite as well after death as before it;" and that the forcible pressure of the
body into the tea-chest might produce the conditions just described. In
cross-examination he further admitted that the appearances in the body
taken *per se* were "merely suspicious" of death being caused by violence.
(Trial of Burke and McDougal, taken in shorthand by Mr. John Macnee,
Writer, pp. 121—123. Edinburgh : Robert Buchanan.)

[2] Now Docherty's body was brought to Surgeons' Square on a Saturday,
and next morning the police had to cut the ropes binding the tea-chest

similar conditions were found in bodies obtained from the cemeteries. This statement is made on the authority of those who pursued anatomy in the Resurrectionists' times, and who had charge of practical rooms and very large experience upon which to found their opinions.

The cause was not far to seek. In the disinterment of bodies considerable force was required, and this was mainly exerted round the neck by means of a cord and other appliances. Now, withdrawing the contents of a coffin by a narrow aperture was by no means an easy process, particularly at dead of night and whilst the actors were in a state of trepidation : a jerking movement is said to have been more effective than violent dragging, and this would necessarily subject the cervical vertebræ, in which the body had been so strongly squeezed : in other words, the body had not been touched by the anatomist. If the spine of other "subjects" had been similarly affected, it is doubtful if such would have been detected, owing to the usual delay in examining the deeper parts of the anatomy. Four weeks would elapse before the ligaments of the neck got dissected. The same remark will apply to the non-recognition of some internal pathological changes—the viscera being seldom seen before decomposition had affected the structures. Daft Jamie struggled most of all with his murderers, yet there were no signs of violence or injury done to his body. A distinguished Professor speaks of having dissected "Jamie" without recognizing his features.

Speaking from some experience, I may be allowed to say that post-mortem examinations reveal conditions that are by no means easily solved. Whilst associating with my lamented friend Professor John Reid—then acting as pathologist to the Edinburgh Infirmary—we occasionally saw bruised surfaces and torn muscular fibres beneath, in bodies which had been merely transferred from the wards below to the pathological room above. Comparisons were made between these abnormal conditions and what had been observed in the bodies provided by the Resurrectionists, as well as that of the woman Docherty; the general result of which was to show that the greatest caution should be exercised in forming opinions as to the proximate cause of some post-mortem appearances.

or rather their connecting fibres, to a severe test. Burke and Hare suffocated their victims, and as a rule the bodies would show less external marking than cemetery subjects : not that any such comparison was ever instituted, as no suspicion of foul play rested on the *cadavera* offered by them any more than on others. It may be safely affirmed that there was nothing but freshness of appearance upon which to found the slightest suspicion of Burke's victims being sooner in possession than the bodies of the Resurrectionists, and in this particular some excuse might be assigned.[1]

All bodies were known to be got surreptitiously. They were generally brought to the anatomist at night, and immediately consigned, in Knox's establishment at least, to a cold damp cellar. Burke brought three of his bodies in the daytime : this, instead of exciting, was calculated to disarm suspicion, as it corroborated the statement he had made once or twice, that he got bodies from lodging-houses and took the earliest opportunity to transfer them to the rooms. The assistant in waiting, tired and worn with his many hours of labour in a tainted atmosphere, could hardly be expected to make a close scrutiny of a corpse when all that was required to be known was the probable age, the sex, and its general applicability to the wants of the class.

[1] Every experienced medical practitioner will be able to recall examples of bodies retaining their freshness for several days after death. Two such cases cross my mind at once. On the seventh and eighth days respectively I was asked to allay the fears of those who could trace no perceptible change in the freshness of the complexion or character of the features of their deceased relative. One was a lady of sixty-three years; the other a gentleman upwards of seventy years.

On the following or sometimes second morning, the body was placed on the table of the dissecting rooms. Everything was done openly and above board at Knox's establishment; no corpse was hidden from the public class, and no steps were ever taken to mar its features, or in any way to destroy its characteristics. As thieves and lawless villains were concerned in the work, it would have been sheer folly to interrogate them on the smallest matter that bore upon their practices. No circumstance had arisen by which suspicion might fall on the character of Burke and Hare's transactions, any more than upon the Resurrectionists in general with whom they were naturally associated. Without tangible reasons—and none whatever existed—it would have been highly impolitic on the part of the anatomist to pry too closely into the acts of those who served his class. Moreover, no good could have arisen, as these rascals dealt only in lying and deceit. The persons who subsequently to the catastrophe used to talk of " grounds of suspicion," " natural mistrust," and the like, knew nothing whatever of the management of anatomical rooms. The most guarded behaviour cannot meet the circumventions of rogues in whom rascality was the genuine type or predominant feature. It does not require any great mental effort to be wise after the event ; with the prosy and prophetic, however, it is the only opportunity they have of proving their vast abilities to the world. Knox had as chief assistants T. W. Jones, William Fergusson, Alexander Miller, and four juniors : the three just named came in for a share of the abuse heaped upon their master. If there had been incaution or any blame in the transactions with Burke, it obviously rested with them, and not with Knox; but nothing ever transpired to show that they had the remotest idea of the "Burking system."

Knox's assistants were just out of their teens, and could not be expected to act with the sagacity of age, or to show that mistrust which the world too often engenders; they were alternately on evening duty, and too often absorbed with special work upstairs to give much heed to the "last comer." The doorkeeper or porter[1] of the establishment was the person to receive the bodies and to deposit them in the mortuary, and then report the essential particulars to the assistant. Had Knox himself been in such close relations with Burke and Hare as his subordinates, his keen eye, equalling that of a French detective, would most probably have penetrated the veil that hid the doings of these monsters. In his hands

---

[1] David Paterson, Knox's doorkeeper, who admitted seeing Docherty's body in Burke's house, incurred a vast amount of condemnation. To try and mitigate the popular wrath he wrote an exculpatory pamphlet, and also addressed the Lord Advocate on the subject. The tenor of his writings was to cast doubt on Knox's assistants, who peremptorily replied, and by more than a *tu quoque* accused him of associating with Burke and Hare. They first showed that he was "a menial servant hired by the week at 7*s.* and dismissed at pleasure," and not a "keeper of Knox's Museum," as he had represented himself; and then stated that he (Paterson) "was going to enter into an agreement with Burke or Hare, and become his partner, and intended, nay, actually tried, to make a profit on the subjects procured from the West Port." Their letter in the *Caledonian Mercury* concluded: "This (Paterson) is the person who says he suspected Burke and Hare, and determined to watch them! And this is the person who said the body of the woman Docherty presented marks of violence; yet this was the same body to sell which he was in treaty with a lecturer for 15*l.*, saying his master (Knox) would not give more than 12*l.*"

their exposure would have been most complete; and what a sea of troubles would have been saved thereby!

Burke's contributions were observed to be "fresh;" and to obviate any doubts on this score, he made no secret of his dealings with the relatives of the deceased, or the owners of lodging-houses. When his attention was drawn to two apparently newly dead, his glib tongue and feasible statement served his purpose so well as to lull all doubts. One of these was warm, on touching which the assistant expressed himself much horrified. Burke, being challenged in the strongest terms, admitted the warmth, "for the person died only a few hours previously, and for secrecy the body had been in close contact with the fireplace." His open manner and ready excuse when so boldly taken to task, told immeasurably in favour of the accuracy of his statement.

It is needful to revert to the mode of procuring "subjects" from lodging-houses, to show the grounds for believing, as all Knox's men did, that Burke and Hare trafficked in the dead of unclaimed strangers. If the artisan or tramp, the sma' pedlar, the gaberlunzie, and other waifs and strays, decrepid and aged, classed as unknown vagabonds, died in a lodging-house where ten or more persons slept, the removal of the corpse became an urgent necessity. The Resurrectionist, aided by his scouts, chiefly abandoned women, often stepped in and proffered his services, and by means of a few pints of whisky discreetly given, "to hold the wake," succeeded in getting the body. Those who knew the Old Town of Edinburgh, its wretched "wynds," its hovels, or rather styes, its whisky shops and dens of iniquity, could have

no difficulty in comprehending the frequency of casualties amid such a frightfully debased population. Life was
everywhere surrounded by the contingencies of death.
The filth and horrors of Paris, as described by Eugène
Sue, had their counterpart in the Cowgate, Canongate,
and Grassmarket. Housed in the sunless and fetid alleys,
or the worse tainted *cul de sacs* or "closes," sheltering by
dilapidated gables and sheds for cattle, or half smothered
amid burrowed ruins and cellarage tenanted with rats
and vermin, men, women, and children huddled together
in brutal fashion. Of what consideration was life to
mortals in the veriest rags and tatters, in the midst of
stench, and feeding on the garbage of the gutters, or
the poison of the dram-shops? Was death not rather a
consummation devoutly to be wished? Human beings
so lost to shame and natural feeling would have sold the
corpse of their neighbours, and as readily that of their
nearest relative, for a few bottles of whisky; nay, their
souls too, if anything like profitable barter could have
been done in that way. The Edinburgh proletarian,
maddened with drink and still longing for more, in whom
all traces of affection for both kith and kin were gone,
would have disposed of "any mortal thing" that could
yield cash and liquor.[1] Now, all bodies obtained in this
way were, of course, but recently dead; the same

---

[1] Examples of persons offering their own bodies to the anatomist on condition of having food and quiet during their last days on earth, could be
adduced from both sides of the Tweed. Mr. Joshua Brookes, a London
surgeon of this century, had an application of this kind; and a Salisbury
surgeon was also written to by a James Brown wishing to dispose of his
"healthy and sound body" for a moderate sum of money. "I shall be
delivered to you on demand, being persuaded," writes Brown, "that on the

remark was applicable, but not so forcibly, to some exhumed bodies removed immediately after the regular interment.

Two of Burke's victims were often cited as instances condemnatory of Knox. One was " Daft Jamie," a poor imbecile in the habit of rambling through the streets of the " Old Town ;" the other was a pretty girl of the name of Mary Paterson. Now, if the anatomist had had the slightest suspicion of murder, would he have exposed " Daft Jamie" in the rooms to which hundreds of students had access ? The brazen audacity of Burke in offering " a town's character" to the rooms showed too truly his devil-may-care conduct, and how strongly ingrained was the thought, as he expressed it after his conviction, that he might as well be hung for a sheep as a lamb. The body of the girl Paterson could not fail to attract attention by its voluptuous form and beauty ; students crowded around the table on which she lay, and artists came to study a model worthy of Phidias and the best Greek art. Here was publicity[1] beyond the professional walk; nay, more, a pupil of Knox's, who had been in her company only a few nights previously, stood aghast on observing the beautiful Laïs stretched in death, and ready for the scalpel of the anatomist. This student eagerly

day of general resurrection I shall as readily find it in your laboratory as if it were deposited in a tomb."

[1] Knox, wishing for the best illustration of female form and muscular development for his lectures, had Paterson's body put in spirit for a time, so that when he came to treat of the myological division of his course, a further and daily publicity was given to Paterson's remains. Mary Paterson formed the basis of many imaginative stories, and one novel, and that highly sensational, appeared in one of the London penny miscellanies.

and sympathizingly sought for an explanation of her sudden death : Burke on his next visit was confronted with his questioner in the presence of two gentlemen, and declared that he bought the corpse from an old hag in the Canongate, and that Paterson had killed herself with drink.[1] He offered to go and show the house if they doubted him. His explanation was feasible ; it rested on the whisky tendency of all such women—and Paterson's body smelt of liquor when brought in—their reckless life and exposure, and their frequent abandonment when at death's door.

It should be stated that a *noli me tangere* feeling guided the anatomist in all his relations to the Resurrectionists : like outlaws, these men were seldom known by their real names, and then only after years of service. Burke and Hare were "fresh hands," and neither their names nor their residence were at all known in Knox's establishment till Paterson, the doorkeeper, came in closer intimacy with them towards the last days of their career. In the book recording the number of "subjects," their date of reception, &c., the names of "John and William" were used to designate Burke and Hare ; whilst Lees frequently appears to be spoken of in his real name, and also others of the "old set." The West Port murderers, especially Burke, were too cunning to allow either their character or abode to transpire till they wished to league with Paterson. They furnished thirteen victims in all to

[1] There are no coroners' inquests in Scotland. The sudden death of either stranger or citizen does not concern the public authorities unless suspicion is entertained and evidence can be offered to warrant the attention of the Procurator-Fiscal, who then makes a most thorough investigation in private, untrammelled by stupid juries and the comments of the press.

Knox's rooms during their eleven months' operations, and never but once brought two bodies at a time.

Newly-dead bodies were not so uncommon in the practical rooms. The Resurrectionists were always on the *qui vive* for dying persons without friends, and to know all about their history, and, if possible, to personify the individual of whom the deceased had spoken in his or her last moments. Marvellous were the expedients resorted to by these false claimants of the unprotected dead, and equally marvellous was their success, considering that all the various personifications of character rested with so small a group as three or four men, one of whom had to profess direct kinsmanship with the deceased. A rascal of the name of Andrew Lees[1] was the leading spirit in the funereal line. He was a tall, gaunt fellow, with a long pale face, the muscles of which were exceedingly pliable to any emotional need—tragedy, comedy, or farce. Grotesque in look and gesture, and wearing a cast-off suit of black that had not been made for his " shrunk shanks," the students named him " Merry-Andrew ; " and over his cups he could maintain the fool's part well. When assuming the character of mourner, his appearance

---

[1] " Merry-lees " was at one time a carrier between D—— and Edinburgh. His dwelling so abutted the country churchyard, that he could enter by his windows and do his resurrectionist work with safety. One night he succeeded in getting three *cadavera*. As a carrier delivering boxes to the medical schools, no one dreamt of his more profitable pursuit. His drunken habits and loose tongue involved him in suspicion, and D—— became too hot for him ; he then headed a party of Resurrectionists. When "subjects" brought double the prices of his first experience, he used to revert to his former facilities when he could obtain them, as he said, " as cheaply as penny pies." This hardened sinner drank sixteen glasses of raw whisky daily ; on great occasions he was equal to as many pints !

was dismal enough ; his pale face, with dropped jaw, set
off by the habiliments of grief, and odd manner, far surpassed any theatrical " get up." His approach to the
house of death was that of a stranger from the country
timidly inquiring for a certain house, on entering which
his bleared eyes, that would have made the fortune of
a London " mute," became suffused with tears. After
dwelling on the virtues of his " dear relative," he would
at length intimate that he wished to convey "the remains"
to the family burial-place in the country; that he and
some friends would return with a cart and coffin towards
evening. His "friends," all in the same line, were,
first, " Spune," as he was called, a little man who shaved
very cleanly, and looked as demure and resigned as a
Methodist preacher—so saintly, and, barring his greasy-
black clothes, of truly " sweet savour;" *secondly,* Mowatt,
who got the name of Moudiewarp (moldewarp) from his
successful imitation of the mole in burrowing the earth,—

> " Well said, old mole ! canst work i' the earth so fast ?
> A worthy pioneer ! "

thirdly, the mock minister or clergyman, who was personified by a deep-dyed vagabond who called himself
Howard, in the hope of hiding his iniquity under a noble
English name. Dressed in a black suit, too seedy for
even a curate by the fell-sides of Cumberland, and with
white choker, the "praying Howard "[1] officiated *à la*

---

[1] With the exception of Episcopalians and Roman Catholics, there is no
" burial service " either at the church or grave-side in Scotland. In lieu of
this, a minister attends the funeral, who offers up a prayer or suitable address
by the side of the bier at the house of the deceased. This solemn and impressive procedure was imitated by the vile hypocrite named in the text.

mode, improving the occasion by calling upon those around the bier to reflect on the uncertainty of life and the need of a spiritual regeneration, for man was but a vain shadow : in using these scriptural words, he looked with becoming gravity upon the thin form of Merry-lees, as if to draw the moral or to warn his friend ! The group of mourners having played their part, the funeral *cortége* moved towards the suburbs. As soon as night and circumstances favoured the change of scene, the black curtain was raised ; the *dramatis personæ* mounted the cart and returned to Edinburgh, and lost no time in transferring the body to the anatomical rooms. With cash in hand, the quaternion had a night of it; and Merry-lees, now seen in his character of the laughing Mercutio, made the welkin ring, till he had put each of his " friends " below the table dead drunk. The same parties played the same game at the Infirmary, and got several unclaimed bodies ; they often dragged in their women coadjutors to aid in the deception practised on the officials of public institutions.

It is but right to state that the West Port murders and the supposed complicity of the doctors formed the basis of several tales of fiction ; some passable enough, others vilely overcharged with malice against Knox and his assistants. Among the romances issued of late years was the " Court of Cacus, or the Story of Burke and Hare," by Alexander Leighton (Nimmo, Edinburgh). Unfortunately for the cause of historical truth, the author had dressed up his story so well, and introduced moral and pious reflections to suit the Scottish mind (surely not his own freer thought), that many mistook his work

for a *bonâ fide* narrative of events! Mr. Leighton's prejudices prevail on every page of his romance. Previous
to the publication of this biography, the only authentic
documents bearing upon the relations of the anatomists
to Burke and Hare were to be found in the report of
the trial of the West Port murderers, alluded to in p. 94,
and the verdict of the committee of inquiry into Knox's
conduct, given at length in pp. 85—88 of this volume.

This painful history of the surroundings of the anatomist belongs entirely to the past, and that past can
never be revived. The Anatomical Act, 2nd and 3rd
William IV., cap. 75, passed in August 1832, annihilated
all secret sources of supply to the anatomical rooms of
Great Britain and Ireland. It cannot be too strongly
set forth in this volume, possibly to be read by others
than the medical fraternity, that the governmental regulations afford the most perfect safeguard against all body-
snatching : nay, more, it not only protects the grave
of all classes, but infallibly respects the wishes of the
humblest of her Majesty's lieges as to the burial of
their bodies after death. The pauper and the peer are
alike safe.

CHAPTER VI.

Knox in danger.—His Courage and Daring—Narrow Escape.—Love of his Class.—Scientific Work.—Cloquet's Anatomy.—Mitchell's Plates.—Beclard's General Anatomy.—Peruvian Lama.

LORD COCKBURN noticed the events sketched in the foregoing chapter thus : "All our anatomists incurred a most unjust and very alarming, though not an unnatural odium ; Dr. Knox in particular, against whom not only the anger of the populace, but the condemnation of more intelligent persons, was specially directed. But tried in reference to the invariable and the necessary practice of the profession, our anatomists were spotlessly correct, and Knox the most correct of them all."[1]   Considering the anger of the populace,[2] it is remarkable that

[1] " Memorials of his Time," p. 257—a charming book on Scottish manners.   As the popular citizen and one of the ablest representatives of the Scottish Bar, and who could sift evidence and see through human motives with the readiness of instinct, Lord Cockburn's words, based on personal knowledge of all the facts, are of great weight in establishing Knox's freedom from blame.   Had this page been appropriate to an *In Memoriam*, I should have said much in grateful remembrance of Lord Cockburn's kindness, and of his eldest son Archie's hearty companionship of other days, at Bonaly.

[2] Possibly the savage feeling that prevailed against all the anatomists might have been assuaged had the public known the many dangers sur-

Knox escaped violence. His private residence and public class-rooms were no secret; his physiognomy, however, was known only to a few of the upper and middle ranks of life, and rather as a man of science in the learned societies of Edinburgh. There were fewer opportunities for publicity forty-five years ago than now. The philanthropic schemes for making men virtuous and women angelic, and regenerating society at large, were not then in vogue ; neither were the peripatetic Congresses, those

rounding the art of dissection.   An infinitesimal part of a drop of poisoned human virus entering the skin by the merest abrasion, or through the instrumentality of the finest needle, is enough to affect the whole system, and cause death in less than fifty hours!   Every winter session used to afford instances of this kind, and often young men of great promise were the victims.   It may be added, that the morbid secretions of living men affect in a similar way.   At this moment an eminent provincial surgeon cannot use his hand, owing to his having opened an abscess, upwards of sixteen months ago, without being aware of a part of the integument under the nail being somewhat thin.   In the same city, the house-surgeon of a large hospital lately died from poisoning of his system after a post-mortem examination.   The dread influences and casualties surrounding the art of medicine would fill a chapter of horrors that might possibly interest "Ladies' Associations" arrayed against the Contagious Diseases Acts.

In the year 1847 alone it was calculated that no fewer than 500 medical men in Ireland, or one-fifth of the whole number, suffered from typhus, of whom 127 died !

Professor Christison and two of his colleagues in Edinburgh, during a period of thirty-two years, attended upwards of 280 medical students for fever caught in the Infirmary or Fever Hospital. The number did not include more than a part of those who suffered.   In one month, November 1837, I remember four promising graduates who died in the Fever Hospital.

As the *cadavera* from idiopathic fever used to form a large proportion of the dissecting-room supply, numbers, like Dr. Murchison, mentioned in page 64, caught the disease ; yet all this while there was a clamour against the anatomists, emanating, it is true, from a frothy, democratic class, blind to their own interests, and ungrateful for the many benefits they had received from the medical profession.

free and easy unions of the loquacious and *bas-bleu*, diverted by the presence of "the third sex," as the clergy were designated by the witty Sydney Smith. In short, there was less "platform drumming," but possibly quite as much solid sense in the world. If Knox owed something to his retirement and sequestration from open haunts and popularity, he owed vastly more to his intrepidity and boldness in securing personal immunity. Every means were taken to make him known to the rabid masses by speech-criers of the last horrid doings of Burke and the doctors, headed by caricatured portraits[1]—the penny-a-line narrative and the lamp-black art being alike worthy of the gutters of the Old Town.

Knox was a man of thorough pluck, and this was well exhibited on the night that the rabble assailed his residence and burned his effigy. Seeing that his life was aimed at, he walked out by a back entrance, and on his way to town passed through the midst of the enraged

---

[1] A series of lithographic prints, illustrative of the chief *dramatis personæ* who figured in the West Port tragedy, were published by Nimmo, under the title, "Wretch's Illustrations of Shakespeare," or, as some called them, "Nimmo's Illustrations of Wretches." These prints were mainly directed against Knox. In one of these caricatures the devil is seen in a garden with a pair of big shears in his hand, ready to crop "a Nox-i-ous plant; or an old virtuoso appropriating a new curiosity." The anatomist is portrayed in his lecture-room ; also in effigy, with burning fagots and an uproarious mob ; as Richard III. looking out for a Tyrrel, whom he finds in Burke ; and as Macbeth, in the cavern scene—"Another yet ? A seventh? I'll see no more."

Such drawings were meant to make Knox known to the mob, and to damage his character, nay, to damn him beyond all hopes, either as a citizen or as a lecturer. In justice to the publisher it may be said, the illustrations conveyed but the public sentiment ; that sentiment, every reader of this biography should see, was decidedly wrong.

populace. Unobserved (for who could possibly fancy him in the open street?) he reached the house of his friend Dr. Adams, in St. Patrick's Square, where his presence caused almost frantic surprise. "What in heaven's name, Dr. Knox, has tempted you out to-night, when thousands of ruffians are seeking your life, and ready to burn you with your effigy?" Knox said he knew it all, nay, he had seen the wretches and touched their sleeves on his way thither; but rather than stay at home and become the modern Servetus of a Calvinistic mob, he had braved the danger of being discovered in the open street. Moreover he was prepared for the worst; then, throwing aside his military cloak, and pointing to a sword, pistols, and High-land dirk, he added: "You see my arms, and had I been called upon to defend myself, I would have measured a score of the brutes." Knox seemed less concerned than the kind family who sheltered him, and, after taking supper, talked in his usual easy manner, becoming more emphatic when discussing the historical meanings of the night that had threatened him with destruction; thus he referred, in apt words, to the ostracism and death of the nobler Greeks, the modern instance of Priestley, and unsparingly condemned the uncurbed democracy of every age. He never spoke more eloquently or more calmly.

For some weeks after the Burke disclosures, persons were on the watch for Knox returning home from his evening lecture, and made the High School yards, the only entrance to Surgeons' Square, their place of rendezvous. One night when Knox had attracted a large class to hear him on a favourite subject, the crowd in the ap-proaching street or "yards" mustered in unusual force.

During the pauses in the lecture, the yells and howling outside were distinctly heard in the class-room. The students got alarmed, and kept looking to the doors of egress. Knox perceiving the growing restlessness of his audience, suddenly paused, and then made use of words to this effect :—"Gentlemen, you are disquieted by these noises, to which, no doubt, you attach a proper meaning. Do not be alarmed ! It is my life, not yours, they seek. The assailants of our peace may be big in menace, but they are too cowardly in act to confront such a phalanxed body of gentlemen as I see before me. How little I regard these ruffians you may well judge, for, in spite of daily warnings and the destruction of my property, I have met you at every hour of lecture during the session; and I am not aware that my efforts to convey instruction have been less clear or less acceptable to you." This statement was received with such cheers as never rung through a class-room in Edinburgh, and, as they re-sounded beyond its walls, actually cowed for a time the uproarious mob. Knox resumed his lecture, and, as pleased as ever in manner, rose far above the immediate subject; and now and then electrified his audience by referring to Vesalius[1] and others who had suffered martyrdom in

---

[1] Vesalius died the victim of the Spanish Inquisition. His inspection, with the full consent of the relatives, of the body of a Spanish Grandee, whose heart gave some feeble contraction when divided by a knife, brought him before the tribunal of the Inquisition, and, had not the King interfered, would have led him to the burning stake. Vesalius, compelled to make a pilgrimage to the Holy Land, was shipwrecked on the island of Zante, and died in extreme penury, and most probably of starvation. A liberal gold-smith defrayed the funeral charges, or the remains of the greatest anatomist the world had seen would have been devoured by birds of prey. In the same year of Christian grace, 1564, the French anatomist, Charles Etienne,

their zeal in the cause of anatomy. As he proceeded with the historical exposition, it was easy for the class to draw the parallel instance. The serenity of his manner and the lofty purport of his words, that breathed of a manly, if not an inspired eloquence, touched all hearts ; he surpassed himself that night, and impressed every one with his commanding genius. His cool demeanour on an occasion so frightfully trying—many of those present believed, and with good reason, that his hour was come —recalls Lavoisier's attitude and words when seized in his laboratory, and begging the gendarmes to wait the completion of a chemical experiment, the solution of which concerned him more than the guillotine to which he knew he was about to be hurried.

It was sometimes necessary for Knox to stay in his rooms till the last of the *sans-culottes* dispersed, especially as he declined any protection beyond that of his senior assistants, whose numbers were too small to constitute a body-guard ; they lacked nothing, however, in devotion and promptitude. Thus, one night, some lads issuing from the Cowgate observed Knox turning up Infirmary Street, and of course raised a hue and cry. Instead of seeking protection in the Infirmary, Knox walked on at his usual pace, crossed the great thoroughfare, and took

sharing in the oppressive persecution to which his family were subjected for their religious opinions, died in a dungeon. Only eleven years previously (1553), Servetus, also an anatomist, had been burned at the stake by Calvin's orders, because he denied the Trinity. What a gathering of fagots there would be to-day if all non-Trinitarians were to be so treated ! It makes the heart shudder to record that Andrew Vesalius, Charles Etienne, and Michael Servetus, as martyred souls, suffered the death of persecution at the hands of men professing to be the followers of Christ.

up North College Street; his assistants kept within a short distance, and on the opposite side of the street. The crowd was gathering force, and a strong-boned fellow led the party some yards in advance. The moments were critical, and unless some diversion could be accomplished the rabble would succeed in their foul purpose; it was then that one of Knox's athletic and warmest supporters instinctively seized the only chance of safety left his master, by rushing upon the vociferating leader, and dealing a powerful blow that felled him to the ground. The sudden collapse of the voice and form of the big bravado served as a most effective check to the advancing crew, who were puzzled to account for the fall of their leader; in the meantime Knox and his friends took rapid strides homewards.

Assailed by the press, attacked by mobs, and slandered by Philistines, who but Knox could have stood against such an array of malignities? His only solace, the silver lining to as dark a cloud as ever shadowed a man's position, was to be found in an approving, nay, affectionate class of students. His anatomical establishment, where he toiled from morning to night, however paradoxical it may seem, was his only haven of peace or rest; there he received the morning congratulations of his associates and the smiling greetings of his pupils; and each appearance in his lecture-room elicited heartfelt expressions of sympathy from every side of the crowded benches. No lecturer on science was ever so idolized by a class as Knox during that eventful session of 1828-29; its members hailed his presence with the enthusiasm that would mark the political devotion of a

I

great party to their leader. Moreover, they wished to
give him a lasting proof of their attachment, by presenting him with a handsome testimonial. Knox heard of
this, and, in writing, expressed his objections to the proposal being carried out at such a time, not that he failed
to appreciate the affections of his pupils, for their kindness had contributed powerfully to uphold him in a
situation which required no ordinary support; but he
was afraid of the honour offered him being misunder-
stood. " The absurd imputations against me," wrote
Knox, " by which the public has been industriously
misled, are viewed by you and all reasonable men as
they deserve. But, however extravagant these misrepresentations may be, I have never disguised from myself,
nor shall I attempt to disguise from you, that the connection of my establishment with the late atrocities, however accidental, is a very serious misfortune; insomuch
that, though utterly unconscious at the time of anything
wrong having been done, yet the very recollection of
these shocking occurrences must be ever painful to me."

His pupils, however, could not forego the gratification
of carrying their design into effect; they cited the fact
of Knox having " sacrificed to the accommodation of the
class an extra hour daily (in which the lecture delivered
at eleven o'clock is repeated for the benefit of those who,
from the crowded state of the room, could not be accom-
modated during the previous hour), thereby incurring the
extraordinary exertion of lecturing for three consecutive hours, namely, from 11 A.M. to 2 P.M." On the
11th April, 1829, the presentation of a handsome gold
vase was made to Knox, and a kind letter also accom-

panied the gift, the last clause of which may be quoted :
"We have deeply sympathised with you during the
mental sufferings which you must have experienced in
consequence of circumstances on which we are unwilling
to dwell. That you should now stand acquitted of every
imputation affecting your character, must gratify, but
cannot surprise us. The public voice has at length
exonerated you from charges of which we who know you
from the first moment felt the injustice."

Only once, as far as I can learn, did Knox exhibit
any emotion on account of the connection of his name
with the Burke and Hare atrocities, and his freely alleged
complicity in the transaction. Walking in the meadows
at Edinburgh with his old friend Dr. Adams, their conversation turned upon "outward form" and its relation
to "inward qualities." Knox had a keen appreciation of
the beautiful in form ; and it chanced at the moment
that a pretty little girl about six years of age caught his
notice while at play. She afforded a text for Knox's
comment on physical beauty combined with unusual
intelligence in so young a child, for by this time he had
drawn her into a playful conversation. At length he gave
her a penny, and said, " Now, my dear, you and I will
be friends. Would you come and live with me if you
got a whole penny every day ?" " No," said the child ;
" you would, may be, sell me to Dr. Knox." The anatomist started back with a painfully stunned expression ;
his features began to twitch convulsively, and tears
appeared in his eyes. He walked hastily on, and did
not exchange words with Dr. Adams for some minutes :
at length came a forced laugh, with a questionable em-

phasis on the words "*vox populi,*" which led to a new topic of discourse.

No man could be more thoroughly occupied than Knox was during these years. He retained the Conservatorship of the College of Surgeons' Museum till September 1831, along with the heavy duties of the largest anatomical class ever seen in Britain, or likely to be heard of again within the four seas. He was also preparing manuscript for the press, and building up a museum of his own, collected from every available source. Methodical in the work that was imperative to his position as a great teacher, he never slackened in his devotion to science all the year round. No country medical practitioner—that poor drudge of humanity always at the call of the public, the hardest worked and poorest paid member of the community—had less time for recreation than Knox. He was at his rooms about nine o'clock, and seldom left till seven at night. His simple meals were brought to his museum—coffee and eggs at ten in the morning, soup or Scotch kail containing meat and vegetables at five, but no stimulant. Such laborious exertion and hardly Saxon diet in support proved the fine temper of his constitution, as well as the robustness of his intellect.

Sir Thomas Brisbane, Governor-General of Australia, having sent to Professor Jameson, of Edinburgh, a specimen of an animal much resembling the wombat, the Professor handed it over to Knox for dissection. The animal was new in Edinburgh, and Knox could not ally it with the Phascolome of Peron, brought to France and described by St. Hilaire, with which it had

been confounded by anatomists and naturalists; nor
could it be made to agree with the genus *Koala* of
Cuvier, a marsupial animal, described briefly in the
Règne Animal. Surgeon Bass, the companion of Captain Flinders ("Voyage to *Terra Australis*"), had described a wombat: but Knox believed the specimen in
his hand to differ from it, and, in honour of Flinders,
named it the Wombat of Flinders. According to
Flinders, there were two sorts or species of the wombat;
one inhabiting the islands, which burrows like a badger,
the other living in the tops of trees, and in manners
bearing resemblance to the sloth. Knox, after controverting the opinions of Home and Illiger, went on to
show that as the Phascolome of Peron, Cuvier, and
St. Hilaire had two long incisive teeth in each jaw, ten
molar teeth, and no canine teeth, it could not be the
same as his specimen, which possessed six incisors, two
canine, and ten molar. Other differences he pointed
out: thus the Wombat of Peron had a short and wide
cæcum and an appendix vermiformis; the cæcum of
the Wombat of Flinders was 6ft. 5in. long, tapering
gradually to a point, and without a vestige of appendix
vermiformis. The Wombat of Flinders appeared to
Knox to constitute the link connecting the marsupial
animals with the *Rodentia,* and the form and structure
of its intestinal canal as placing it in close relation with
the beaver and with the class *Rodentia.* Considering
the opinion of the natives of New Holland as to the
generic terms *wombat* and the *koala,* and the species
Koala wombat; and after examining the characters of
the Koala described by Cuvier, Desmarest, and De Blain-

ville, all of whom differed in their descriptions, he proposed the abolition of the term *koala*, and the classification of those extraordinary animals under the genus
Wombat, and of this genus the species *Flinders*, which
he had described, and, secondly, the Phascolome of St.
Hilaire, Wombat of Bass, &c.   His views were read to
the Wernerian Society, January 14th, 1826 (*Edin. New
Philos. Journal*, vol. i. p. 104).

The dental characters and long cæcum of Knox's
Wombat of Flinders agree with those of the Koala
(*Lipurus cinereus* of Goldfuss, *Phascolarctos* of De
Blainville).   Cuvier, it would appear, knew only the skin
and digital characters when Knox wrote on this subject.
In Professor Owen's able paper on the *Marsupialia*, in
Todd's "Cyclopædia of Anatomy and Physiology," vol. iii.,
the reader will find the whole question treated of—the
dentition of the Koala, p. 271, fig. 95; and cæcum of the
same animal, p. 302, fig. 126.

On the 27th of May, 1826, Knox furnished to the
Wernerian Society (*Edin. New Philos. Journal*, vol. i.
p. 130) a notice respecting the presence of a rudimentary spur in the female Echidna of New Holland, in
which he controverted the opinions of Sir E. Home, who
had stated that the spur belonged to the male only.

In July 1827, the Highland Agricultural Society conveyed their thanks to Knox for giving free admission
to the practical students attending Mr. Dick's veterinary
classes, to his valuable lectures on Human and Comparative Anatomy.

In 1829, "A System of Human Anatomy, on the
Basis of the *Traité d'Anatomie Descriptive* of M. H.

Cloquet," by Robert Knox, was issued by Messrs. Maclachlan and Stewart. Knox got 150*l.* for the translation and editing. A second edition followed in 1831. Knox, in his preface to Cloquet, defended himself against the accusation of too forcibly influencing the student's mind, and of dragging it away from other collateral studies, to fix it exclusively on anatomical pursuits. Though somewhat heavy in detail, Cloquet's work in Knox's hands did great service ; it balanced the brevity of the Dublin " Dissector," then so much in use in the rooms, and so far made French descriptive anatomy available to the English student. Knox's name appeared upon the title-page of a new edition of the " Anatomy of the Bones of the Human Body, represented in a Series of Engravings, copied from Sue and Albinus, by Edward Mitchell, Engraver, with explanatory references by the late Dr. Barclay." Mitchell's engravings of the muscles, copied from the folio plates of Jules Cloquet ; of the arteries, after Frederick Tiedemann ; and the cardiac nerves, the eighth and ninth pair of cerebral nerves copied from the *Tabulæ Neurologicæ* of Antonio Scarpa, were all endorsed by Knox's name, and generally went under the designation of " Knox's plates." Some passed through a third edition, owing to his high recommendation of them to his numerous classes. It was Knox's intention to make a more complete work of the engravings of the ligaments that Mitchell had copied from the original works of the Caldanis, beyond the " revised and carefully compared with nature " edition of 1834.

Dr. Knox's views as to the use of figures and plates for

anatomical teaching were almost identical with those of his predecessor, Dr. Barclay. " Figures are exceedingly useful when the originals are not to be had; but to study plates when the originals may be procured, is so far from bespeaking a taste for anatomy, that it scarcely implies an ordinary share of common understanding. Even the best are only aids in studying the originals ; but when they are substituted for the originals their intention is perverted—they serve only to mislead, to diffuse error, and to perpetuate it."[1]   Again says Barclay : " Anatomy is an art, and those who would study it must see it practised : they must see the forms, magnitudes, positions, proportions, and connections of the structures and organs as they are in nature. No figures or verbal descriptions can ever compensate for want of the originals ; they give not the same relish nor interest, nor afford the same correctness of ideas. Even when accurate, they but assist the imagination to conceive the things which they represent; and if they be otherwise, as they frequently are, they tend to mislead it, and become, not unusually, the strongly fortified depôts of error.   In short, at their best they are only shadows in place of the substances ; and if they be faulty, they are worse than shadows, because they are shadows without any substance or prototype in nature."

[1] Barclay's " Introductory Lectures to a Course of Anatomy," pp. 106 and 146-7 (published by Maclachlan and Stewart, Edinburgh, 1827).

Anatomical figures for teaching purposes are supposed to have been in use in the 13th century. At any rate Hermondeville taught anatomy from them at Montpellier in the 14th century. Da Vinci made engravings subservient to the art, and may be held to be the greatest iconographic anatomist up to the 17th century.

Dr. Gordon, of Edinburgh, in 1815, briefly discussed the anatomy of the "common textures" in the first volume of his unfinished "System of Human Anatomy;" and Dr. Barclay strove to familiarize his students with some of the views of Bichat and Beclard; but Knox advanced beyond both his predecessors. The writings of Winslow, Vicq d'Azyr, Prochaska, W. Hunter, Bordeu, the Wenzels, Meckel, and Bichat, were accessible to the higher educated professional ranks, though seldom consulted by them; but no special work on the anatomy of the tissues appeared in an English form before 1829, and that work—"The Elements of General Anatomy, containing an Outline of the Organization of the Human Body," by R. D. Grainger—was Beclard of 1821 repeated and scarcely modified, with Richerand as its physiological authority. About the same time the "French Manual of General Anatomy," by Messieurs A. L. J. Bayle and H. Hollard, was translated by H. Storer. Oddly enough in point of time, Knox the same year issued his translation of Beclard's "General Anatomy:" this work was only a part of the superstructure, the basis of which had been laid by himself in 1826, before a large anatomical class. To Knox, therefore, is mainly due the credit of introducing to the British student the subject of "general anatomy." He made Beclard a household word in Edinburgh, and gave a higher interpretation to the French and German doctrines. In his teaching he discountenanced the physico-mathematical hypotheses of the Boerhaave School, and wished the various speculations that were entertained of the elementary fibres by Haller, Walther, Pfaff, Richerand, and others, to be considered on their own merits as tested by a rigid examination of the tissues themselves. The great disparity prevailing abroad as to the number of the tissues—Haller's mystic three and Bichat's twenty-one—did not seem to give Knox so much consideration, but it might have been supposed that the views expressed by Meyer, of Bonn, as to the cell, the vessel, &c., in his *Histologie*, would have caught his fancy as pointing to a newer version of structure ; as, in all probability, they aided Johannes Müller in his adenological generalizations. The days of Schleiden and Schwann had not dawned.

Knox was partial to the free handling of all anatomical structures, and the examination of them *in situ*, as the best mode of comprehending their nature. It was an essential feature in his teachings ; not that he overlooked the physical and chemical properties of each tissue, their analogous characters and relations, their actions and reactions under the influence of pathological change. The new views on histology have effected a revolution of late years, but as far as the science of the day was known, Knox was an admirable pioneer and exponent of what was then considered " French anatomy," as deduced from the labours of Bichat down to the last authority, Beclard.

At a meeting of the Edinburgh Royal Society (4th January, 1830), Knox read his " Observations on the Structure of the Stomach of the Peruvian Lama ; to which are prefixed Remarks on the Analogical Reasoning of Anatomists in the Determination *à priori* of Unknown Species and Unknown Structures " (*Trans. Roy.*

Soc. xi. 479). The author shows an unusual amount of disquisition and zoological reasoning in this paper, and maintains that, as animal machines were not pieces of human mechanism, the physiological systems built on the design of separate individual organs are so many systems of false philosophy. As the camel had been styled by poets the "ship of the desert," and belonging to the old world, Knox held the lama to be the camel of the new world. He believed the stomach of all animals to be a single organ; but, in conformity with the language used by anatomists, he himself spoke of double, triple, &c. The single human stomach was not infrequently found contracted about the middle, so as to divide the cavity, as it were, into two by means of a narrow constricted portion. He looked upon this deviation from the ordinary human conformation of the simplest kind, and as an irregularity in man, but a regular structure in certain of the lower animals,—that structure being, as it is so often, persistent in them which in him is only fugacious. This reasoning of Knox, as to the "multiple stomachs" being but modifications of the single organ, solves many of the apparent difficulties that have been advanced regarding the formation and variety of the stomach, or its comparative anatomy. This paper, like many others of Knox's, has not been read by the would-be historians of anatomical progress, or we should have been spared the perusal of much that has been written on the double stomach of man

CHAPTER VII.

DR. KNOX was slightly above the middle stature, and his person realized the definition of a muscular, "tight-made man." He showed the nervo-sanguineous temperament of the Saxon, to which race he steadily held for his blood alliance. His wide chest and powerful shoulders, and rather long arms, presented something of the *physique* of the wrestler ; but no such characters for a moment vied with the gentlemanly air and pronounced intellectuality of the man himself. His carriage was upright, his walk firm and soldierly, and both body and limbs showed a free and lithesome action. The rise on the toes, and the apparent restlessness of both his features and framework, bespoke the versatile Frenchman more than the " canny Scot." The atrophied condition of the left eye,[1] the large nose, and full mouth were heightened

---

[1] Though Knox had but one eye, he saw more clearly than most men do, with two eyes. Of him it might be said, as Spenser wrote of one of his heroes, "Faërie Queene," Book iii., canto x. :

> " His halfen eye he wiled wondrous well,
> And Hellenor's both eyes did eke beguyle."

in force by strong lines and a coarseness of features in-
cident to the worst form of confluent small-pox. He
had a strikingly fine head, that shone in all its baldness ;
the prominence of the supra-orbital region and eyebrows
served to place the frontal development in high relief,
and to make the cranial outline appear more dome-like
and massive. His perfect eye was perfection itself, and
an excellent index to his passing thoughts. Like Lord
Brougham, whom he resembled in plainness of visage,
the muscles of Knox's face were seldom at rest when
his brain was occupied. These involuntary twitchings
were far from agreeable, especially those which affected
his under-lip, the crossing of which from side to side
produced a kind of smacking noise. Co-ordinate or
alternating with these facial movements, the neck was
extended, the shoulders raised, and the arm drawn to
the side. Possibly these gestures may have served as
diverticula to his exuberant force ; they cannot be said to
have improved his presence in the eyes of a stranger.

If Nature had been less kind in her gifts to the outer
man, she was lavish in her bestowals upon the social and
intellectual Knox. However harsh if not forbidding in
personality, his courtesy and conversation atoned for all.
He was bland in manner, and full of pleasantry ; he had
a gentle, agreeably-toned voice, and a ready persuasive
tongue that made captive of every listener who could
appreciate colloquial excellence.

Dr. Knox was wonderfully got up in the way of costume, and perhaps the only lecturer who ever appeared
before an anatomical class in full dress. Being a well-
made person, his tailoring was all the more effective for

his display of "the gloss of fashion and the mould of form." A dark puce or black coat; a showy vest, often richly embroidered with purple, across which gold chains hung in festoons; a high cravat, white or in coloured stripes, and the folds of which were passed through a diamond ring; a prominent shirt collar, delicately-plaited cambrics, watch-seals and pendants, set off by dark trousers and shining boots, completed his outer man— significantly gay, if not loud in colouring. Knox, in the highest style of fashion, with spotless linen, frill, and lace, and jewellery redolent of a duchess's boudoir, standing in a class-room amid osseous forms, *cadavera*, and decaying mortalities, was a sight to behold, and one assuredly never to be forgotten.

The door of the lecture-room was seldom more than half open when the bald head and bowing attitude of Knox became visible, as if he were solicitous to bestow a smiling recognition on the occupants of every bench of the amphitheatre. Placing his watch and seals upon the table, he would brace himself up for his work, and again survey the class, as if to be sure that every one was ready to go along with him. His oral communications to his class were among his happiest efforts. Possessing high natural endowments, he strove for perfection in a walk seldom attainable—that of public lecturing—and he achieved an excellence that far surpassed all his contemporaries. Words cannot convey Knox's superiority in this respect. Some lecturers walk unconcernedly to their desk and read off-hand; some are condescending, others are *brusque* in manner; and of the modes of address it may be said—*quot homines, tot sententiæ.* The exits and the entrances of Knox were alike graceful and exceedingly characteristic; nor did he for a moment during the hour of lecture lose his suave demeanour and high respect for his class as a body of gentlemen.

A youth about to take the initiative in medicine, and with reserve approaching the precincts of an anatomical institution, might well express surprise on observing Knox for the first time in his capacity of teacher, a man of smiling courtesies and elegant apparel. The osseous and repellent forms were forgotten in the admiration of the lecturer; the eye, glancing for a moment at the doctor's bald head and gold spectacles, soon centred upon the artist *par excellence* in his showy attire. As Knox passed from side to side in the special area of his lecture-room, demonstrating the anatomy, he showed a rare felicity of movement, now reminding you of the slow and graceful minuet, then the quiet *pose* or soldierly "attention;" and these again were succeeded by the rapid gesture; then his actions were so pertinent and applicable to the matter on hand. After each division of his subject he would readjust his spectacles, draw up the waistband of his trousers—he wore no braces—and then, presenting a steady front to his class, resume his prelection. All this was inimitably done, and thoroughly revealed his powers as a natural dramatist.

If the class appeared a little wearied with the description of a bone, say the sphenoid, the minute portions of which were invisible to all but the front benches, Knox would show his skill in refreshing his audience by a pause ; then saying in a distinct voice, " Gentlemen, the

sphenoid bone is the most important bone in the body."
This assertion, "nowhere writ" in the text-books, startled
the class by its novelty and abruptness ; every eye now
became eager to scan the form and realize the description
of the bone. To support his bold opinion, he would refer
to the relation of the sphenoid to the cranial arch, the
effects of fracture at the base of the skull, or perhaps
touch lightly upon the osteogenesis and morphology of
the bone, to awaken the deeper interest of his advanced
pupils. Nobody could ever say that he gave a dry
lecture, or one that was not specially instructive.

Knox had no real competitor in the medical school
of Edinburgh. His style, his illustrations, and insinuat-
ing speech lent a fascination to the study of human
anatomy ; dissection was not only to be viewed as an
introduction to the practice of surgery and medicine,
but invested with the loftiest aims *quoad* science in
general. He stood before his class the impersona-
tion of lofty intellect and self-possession ; the latter
faculty never for a moment deserted him. The area of
his class-room was to Knox a charmed circle, and there he
exercised a weird influence that traversed from side to side
the thronged benches, and subtly pervaded the mind of
every member of his audience. With many teachers anatomy wore a monotonous, Dryasdust aspect, but in Knox's
hands the descriptive outline was like a pleasant lesson in
geography, with frequent diversions into the history and
manners of the people of the country. If masterly in
action, he was equally specific in his phraseology. "You
perceive, gentlemen," or "you observe," were words
which he happily repeated, and often emphasized by his

raised arm and pointed forefinger, upon which he wore an exquisite diamond ring. In hazarding an original remark based on his own observation and experience, he would with apparent modesty add, " If I may be permitted to say so, gentlemen." He had the art of saying things never said before, and his expressions oft became the talk of the school ; indeed, many of his *dicta memorabilia* would have been worthy of publication, not only as brilliant facetiæ, but as wise saws and modern instances in the Knox philosophy.

There was no circumlocution in his teachings ; he aimed at a clear delineation of the work before him. He was more practical than minute, more suggestive than analytic in his systematic course : rather than linger on points of detail, he indicated the path to be pursued by the student. His mode of teaching was not suited to the "grinding " or " cramming " system ; hence those who sought anatomy for examining boards went elsewhere. His prelections were well adapted to stimulate thought, as he meant them to do. Being a surgeon and pathologist, Knox could significantly apply anatomy to a practical calling ; and as a physiologist of high aim, he looked to zoology as a *sine quâ non* to the study of the higher philosophy of Man himself.

The Knox platform was broad yet specific, and no less philosophical than practical. Those who sought to follow and comprehend the Master—Knox—had to serve a faithful apprenticeship, to be educated, and diligent and aspiring. Schoolboyism would not do, and mnemonics, however artful, could not raise the youth to the Knox standard : on the other hand, lads of keen

K

faculties and comprehension ascended the steep with their chief and rallied under his flag, as soldiers in the fight battling for the colours of their regiment.

As he took warm interest in the progress of his class, and was at all times accessible and ready to offer counsel, he became the guide, philosopher, and friend of every worthy student. His pupils loved him, and lauded him to the skies. He was not slow to befriend the medical candidate in the hall of his college and in the council of other examining boards, and always argued for fewer classes and more practical tuition. His popularity, however, rested mainly on his eminence as a teacher, his enthusiastic pursuit of science, and his vast and crowning abilities. No medical lecturer in the United Kingdom ever enjoyed so much public confidence as Dr. Knox. From 1826 to 1835, over a period of nine years, his students annually averaged 335, and in the session of 1828-9 he had 504 pupils ! No such anatomical class ever assembled in Britain. The old lecture-room of Dr. Barclay would not admit of more than 200 persons, so Knox was obliged to lecture three times daily, and on the same subject each time. Such laborious repetition would seem a terrible task, especially as these lectures were given, for one winter at least, in consecutive hours ; but Knox seemed scarcely affected by a work that thoroughly engaged his heart. He courted popularity, and it had come as a flood ; he was proud of his rhetorical powers, and here in crowded benches was a fulsome adulation to their exercise. When the College of Surgeons vacated their old hall in Surgeons' Square in 1832, he moved there from Barclay's premises and built a very large class-room; even there he repeated his morning lecture the same evening, and men of superior education and character, like Sir George Sinclair, were induced to attend both. No higher proof need be instanced of the general attractiveness of his lectures.

The benches of Knox's class-room were occupied by a scholarly, earnest, and appreciative class; the majority were strictly medical students, but mingling with these were English barristers, Cambridge scholars and mathematicians, Scottish advocates and divines, scions of the nobility, artists, and men of letters. The zoologists and naturalists flocked to Knox for their comparative anatomy and general studies, looking upon him as the great master of his art, and fully endorsing the encomiums bestowed upon him by Audubon and others of still greater eminence, both Continental and Transatlantic. Military and naval surgeons, in active service or on half-pay, oft mingled with the crowd. Some students who had passed through the *literæ humaniores*, logic and philosophy, and with an aim to the Church, carried on a duality of study—medicine and divinity —as if wishing two strings to their bow of lucky adventure in this profane world. These youths, as well as the " probationers," or fully fledged ministers, waiting upon Providence for " a call to the pulpit," occasionally took to physic and became capital practitioners. Of these outsiders—semi-medical, semi-theological, as well as the *dilettanti* of every university—Knox got by far the largest share. The man of travel, the higher class of visitors to Edinburgh, the country parson, the young squire coming up to study agriculture and natural his-

K 2

tory, all sought out the hero of the day. One of the sights or living lions of the Scottish metropolis was Knox in his lecture-room. Men were attracted by his fame, and looked upon his prelections as the greatest intellectual treat afforded them in the " Modern Athens." Even the lecturers of a rival and by no means too friendly school were in the habit of attending Knox's "introductory" to have an hour's thorough enjoyment. Dr. Argyle Robertson, himself one of the most pleasing and popular of lecturers, told me that so great was the pleasure of listening to Knox, he would gladly attend him all the year round.

He gave both character and colouring to his anatomical teachings ; he went further, and indoctrinated his pupils with a love of science for its own sake as well as its professional worth. In his historical disquisitions he brought the great men of the age visibly before his class, and in citing their examples as illustrations of what a powerful incentive could accomplish, did not lose the opportunity of impressing his pupils with a love of medical literature. As Knox the anatomist stood *per se,* so to a certain extent did his pupils stand apart from the rest of the medical community. The greater the intellectual calibre of the student, the more largely did he extol Knox ; and as the anatomical classes in which men were daily thrown together marked the divisions of the school, the "Knoxites" prevailed in point of numbers, and not infrequently in scholarly attributes. The daily plodders or routinists—in other words, the majority of the dull men or slow coaches— went elsewhere, to the brothers Lizars, where they got the A B C of anatomy, as plainly as the largest and most coloured alphabet could be presented to the infant mind in the nursery. The "Knoxites" were everywhere leaders, and for many years may be said to have ruled "Young Physic" in Edinburgh. It was the "Knoxites" who most frequently occupied the presidential chair and took chief part in the discussions of the Royal Medical, the Hunterian Medical, and other societies; it was they who constituted the editorial staff of the *Maga*, a weekly magazine of fun and satire, with Edward Forbes as artist and *rédacteur en chef*. The poesy and art and lively prose of the *Maga* and "Medical and Quizzical Journal" had a decided flavour of Old Surgeons' Hall. It was the Knoxites who originated "the Oineromathic Society," or, more correctly speaking, the "Brotherhood of the Friends of Truth,"[1] and gave fame and celebrity to its character; finally, they may be said to have taken an active part in all matters of polity affecting the medical school and the

[1] The reader is referred to Goodsir's "Anatomical Memoirs," vol. i. p. 60, for a brief account of the famous Brotherhood, among whom Forbes, the Goodsirs, Sam. Brown, J. H. Bennett, John Reid, Geo. E. Day, and others, were enrolled, all of whom contributed largely to the spread of science. Here is a stanza of an Oineromathic song, written by Edward Forbes, the *Arch Magus* :—

> " Some love to stray through lands far away,
>   Some love to roam on the sea ;
> But an antique cell, and a College bell,
>   And a student's life for me.
> For palace or cot, for mead and grot,
>   I never would care or pine ;
> But spend my days in twining lays
>   To learning, love, and wine. "

general interests of the profession. A *corps d'esprit*[1] prevailed among the Knoxites; they were proud of their teacher and jealous of his honours, and lost no opportunity of defending his scientific status in the world of Medicine.

Dr. Knox was a born orator, and by studying the classical examples he became a highly accomplished one. It was supposed that he prepared himself when he had a great work on hand or a higher effort to sustain; and the broad features of the following story used to pass current among a few of his senior students.

At a late hour of a winter's evening, two of Knox's junior assistants had gone down to the dark cellared mortuary for the purpose of injecting the arteries of a new "subject," and, whilst so engaged, were much startled by hearing noises in which vocal sounds faintly mingled with a sort of tramping march. In the full belief that they were the sole occupants of the building, and being quite unable to unravel the unearthly acoustics, and further tried by

> " The horrible conceit of death and night,
> Together with the terror of the place "—

something akin to Juliet's dread stole over them, in a

[1] In all the street rows brought about by the antagonism of the Bakers' lads to the students, the Knoxites shared in the discredit of promoting them, and of abetting other mischief. In the snowball encounters with the populace they were conspicuous, especially in the great riot of 1837, best known as the "Battle of the Quadrangle," described so humorously by Edward Forbes, from the conflict between the students and the police taking place within the University walls. They made a noble stand in the fight, driving the "Peelers" outside the gates, wounding and disabling several : indeed the students only gave way to authority when hard pressed by a body of infantry presenting fixed bayonets to their cardiac regions.

vault amid *cadavera*—one "but green from the earth,
fest'ring in his shroud," others half dissected and showing haggard features and mournfully spectral shapes,
hideous to behold in humanity-form. "Hush !" there
is another heavy beat, a pause, articulate sounds, now
emphatic, now sinking away in a distant cadence, then
followed by stillness. The disconcerted medicals resumed
their operation of tying the aorta as if all cause of
alarm had subsided, when fresh intonations and more
gliding movements returned.

> "What may this mean,
> That thou, dead corse, again "—

deters us from our work ? In breathless haste they
left the charnel-house and rushed upstairs. As they
approached the door of the lecture-room they drew
near to the *locus in quo* of their fears ; they listened,
and detected a human voice, and that voice could be
no other than the weird anatomist's : the "questionable
shape" was discovered to be a "spirit of health," and not
a "goblin damn'd !" Yes ! the syrenic Knox was heard
busily tuning his instruments for to-morrow's "oratorio."
Verily a strange rehearsal, and stranger scene ! Stand
ing in the small enclosure of a big amphitheatre
of empty benches, and in the midst of darkness that
"a farthing dip" rendered visible, Knox was going
through the part of his own Hamlet, practising the
attitudes, now delivering his thoughts in calm and
measured tones, now loudly vehement, as the subject of
his prelection demanded. The skeleton in its tripod
was the only semblance of humanity around him, and
standing by its side and resting his hand upon one

of its acromion processes, he apostrophized the osseous
entirety with as much earnestness as the true Hamlet
did the "canonized bones hearsed in death" of the
Royal Dane. "For one night only" did he attempt a
rehearsal, so it is believed. Had it been at all his practice, it would have been soon heard of, and much dwelt
upon by his rivals. Even if time had permitted of such
preparation, of what import was it compared with the
exercise of his own innate powers, capable of meeting
every emergency? A strong, nay, incontrovertible argument against the habit of rehearsal is to be found in the
fact of his frequently having been called upon to lecture
on a subject foreign to the regular course of things;
besides, all his most notable efforts were quite impromptu, of which many instances could be given from
my own personal knowledge.

In his rhetorical efforts there was nothing pompous,
but rather a Saxon homeliness of speech, combined with
perfect dignity of manner, so that with the familiar inci-
dent or lively epigram readily grasped by every member
of his class, he practised a faultless style and felicitous
expression calculated to please the higher minds. At
times, but rarely, he manifested passion and emotion,
and the force that is generated by these; but there was
nothing of the passion that with uneducated speakers is
apt to be blatant, if not frothy and boiling over. He
was viewed as a consummate actor of his part; but then
his part was always sustained with consummate ability.
His oratory was racy and refreshing to a degree, nor
could it fail to lighten up the path of mediocrity and
dulness that is too apt to be present in every assembly

of the mixed classes of English life. Superior to his contemporaries in possessing an academic temperament, he surpassed them all in creating exaltation of thought and a steady, healthful penchant for educational improvement. If he carried his pupils to the heights of Science, he was not unmindful to note the rough and arduous steep; and, when those fancied heights had been gained, would with significance point to the clouds above and beyond, waiting the light of philosophy to pierce, and thereby to reveal fresh pinnacles and a still higher Olympus. Familiar with the biography of the renowned men of the past, he could throw a beautiful halo of laudation around the labours of the physicists Newton and Laplace, the anatomists Vesalius, Harvey, and Bichat, and the chemists Lavoisier and Dalton. Such men constituted the Knox pantheon, each niche of which seemed to contain a living statue upon whose sculptured form he loved to dwell. Well versed in the literature of his profession, and always fertile in resource, he could interweave his historical readings, or ideas if you will, with the subject of his lectures, in a manner no less exceptional than grandly impressive. Anatomy was his text, and in discussing its general bearings he saw no impropriety, but much advantage, in illuminating his text with every ray of light that could be brought to bear upon the subject under review.

Dr. Knox had a natural and decided aversion to the use of artificial aids for refreshing the memory of the young anatomist. The "private teachers," or "grinders," who prepared candidates for their public examinations, often came under the lash of his satire. The " cramming

system " he held to be little less than an imposture,—
offensive to habits of culture, damaging to the practice
of medicine, and altogether derogatory to man's intellect.
He denounced both the men and the mode, calling the
former " quacks," and the latter a parrot system of
instruction. The small octavos issued by the London
grinders were bad enough; but the *ne plus ultra* of
make-believes was the " Pocket Anatomist." Knox hit
upon a happy method of showing it up. At one of his
introductory lectures (winter session,[1] 1837-38), attended
as usual by crowds of students and not a few rival
teachers of medicine, some of whom favoured the
system he was about to condemn, he said : " Gentlemen, in my younger days anatomy was taught with
a view to medical practice and the development of
philosophical principles in zoology. The old authors,
however voluminous in their records, were cited by
our teachers and recommended for our perusal and
example. Alongside our practical studies in the dissecting rooms we were referred to works of this kind for
consultation "—holding up at the same time a huge
tome, which he carried around the area at arms' length.
" This, gentlemen, is a volume written by Vesalius, the
acknowledged father of our art. Look at its size, and
bear in mind that its thousand folio pages embrace only
a special part of the human anatomy." Then taking a

[1] About a week before the opening of this session he asked me what
should be the purport of his "introductory," "as now it was time to be
thinking of it." Some paper was brought for him to take notes, and he
wrote "Gentlemen" upon it. His conversation then turned on other
matters, and the single word received no additions ! His only preparation
was during his morning or evening walks.

stand centrally towards his class, he withdrew from his
waistcoat pocket the smallest of publications ever issued,
well named the " Pocket Anatomist." " Now, gentlemen, behold the advance of the age, the progress of our
science in these latter days ! Vesalius was the first and
greatest anatomist ; look at his work and contrast it with
this ignoble production, said to contain the whole of
your anatomy within the compass of three inches by
two!" As he held up the antipodes of Art to the gaze of
his class, cheers echoed from wall to wall ; and as these
subsided, Knox, with an air of reverence, deposited
Vesalius on the table, and then, with an expression of
thorough contempt, cast the Lilliputian to the floor.
The audience was electrified by this inimitable exposition of the difference between exalted Science and
debased Art. Vesalius, the founder and mighty pillar of
the past in anatomy, held up with the " Tom Thumb "
pocket vocabulary of the present day, was worthy of
Knox, and assuredly no man could have done it but
himself, and done it so admirably.

In listening to Knox as he swept across the chords of
his lyre, the historical men of the Georgian political
period—Burke, Sheridan, and Fox—crossed one's mental
vision ; not that his style was exactly like any of these
men, though his fiery vigour was equal to the best.
When he quoted a Ciceronian phrase you recalled the
denunciatory passages against Verres; and while your
eyes were riveted upon the moving figure in high gesture,
your mind would be instituting comparisons between
the modern Scot in his roofed apartment and the noble
Roman in the Forum at the base of the Capitol. Taking

his stand by the table, and resting his left hand upon it, whilst he raised his right somewhat semi-bent, and with his fingers oddly apart (as shown in his portrait), he personified a special and vigorous attitude that would have done admirably for the political leader of a constitutional assembly, or the graver-toned president of the higher Senate.

The portrait of Dr. Knox attached to this page was taken during the session 1834-35, by his chief artistic pupil, Edward Forbes, afterwards known to the world of science by his Natural History investigations. The sketch portrays the Doctor as he stood in his lecture-room addressing his class. Forbes' work admirably hits the salient features of the physiognomy, no less than the special attitude of the man: it bears the artist's well-known mark, "B.B." The portrait appeared among the Edinburgh celebrities in the *Students' Maga*, and naturally commanded a great sale of that monthly issue. It was accompanied by a few words of comment, also from the pen of the editorial Forbes, in which the Doctor is described as the great hater of humbug, and the leading anatomist of the age. To add to the fun in which my genial-hearted friend Forbes used to revel, he headed his remarks on his great master by a quotation from a Roman poet thus :—

> "———— Nox
> Semper."

And every student with a copy of the *Maga*—and who was without it ?—was ready to respond to the classical sentiment, and echo " Knox for ever !"

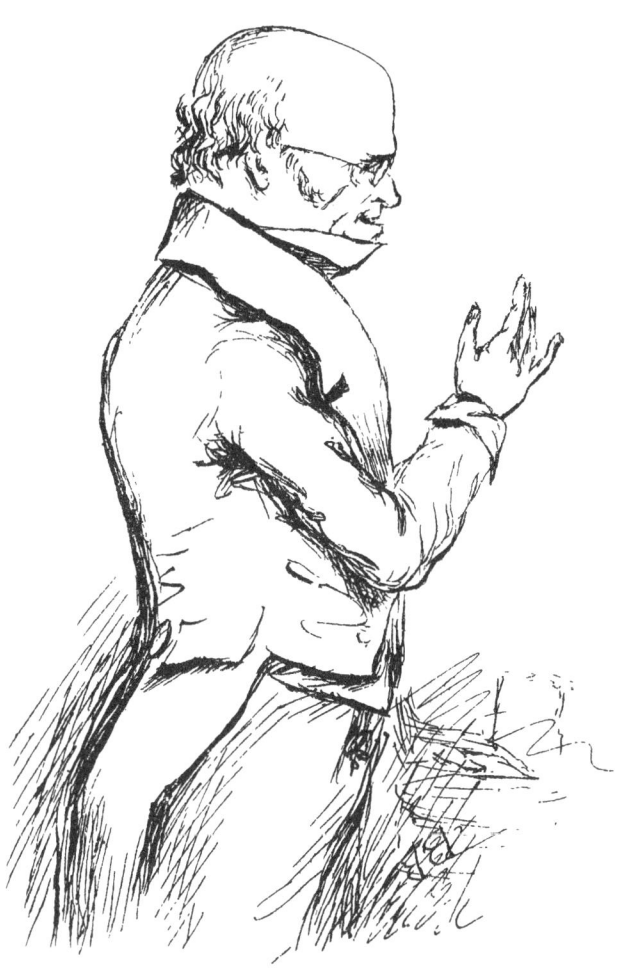

To face Page 140

He was much too classical to be ranked with the modern tribune, especially of these latter days. If the pose and uplifted arm claimed attention, how much more effective was the demonstration of the man when roused by a subject that conveyed historical warnings, and most of all when denouncing corporate monopolies, chicanery, and cliquism. Then his head was thrown back, his step was pronounced, his eye fixed, his arm swung from below upwards,—not only lending force to his utterances, but embracing the whole audience in its sweeping play. Woe betide the individual that came under Knox's censure, whether that censure was shown in a tone of derision or with the finger of scorn pointed to the offending mortal. Without naming he could hold up the foe to the mirror, and then with scathful and burning words cast him to the earth.

There was a philosophy in the very manner of his teaching, a freshness that caught and convinced everybody. With a rare suggestive faculty, he from day to day opened out new channels of inquiry to his students, and developed a broader basis of anatomical observation. Ready and copious in diction, he had the art of enlivening his class, now with historical opinions or current facts, now with narratives piquant, if not imaginative, but always with an eye to interest and instruct. Knox was never at a loss for words, and never had far to seek his illustrations. It was firmly believed that he could at a moment's notice lecture for an hour upon a piece of adipose tissue, by describing its character, uses, and position in man's body, and supplementing this by his natural history observations at the

Cape, or the equally telling episodes, always at command, derived from the pages of Bichat and Blumenbach, or the personal friendships of Baron Cuvier
and Geoffroy St. Hilaire. A single episode of Knox's
was of more worth than an entire lecture of many of his
rivals, and often proved as effective during the hour's
instruction as a bright patch of colour in an otherwise
sombre landscape.

If Knox was careful not to commit himself to a
doubtful opinion in theoretical medicine, he was pretty
affirmative in his views on pathology and practice. In
demonstrating the regional anatomy, say the muscles of
a limb, he passed with a light hand over the grouped
bundles *seriatim* and relationally; then interested his
audience by showing how muscular actions affected the
surgery of the part; and if the class seemed less *en
rapport* with him, he drew animating pictures, almost
tableaux vivants, of the powerful display of the athlete;
or if describing the muscles of the fore arm, exemplifying the fine touch and muscular power of the hand
from the fingers of Paganini.

CHAPTER VIII.

Comparative and General Anatomy.—Saturday Lectures.—The Caffre.—
Ciceronian displays.—The Pictorial School.—Educational Views.—
Training of Lads.—The Knox Triumvirate and Teachings.—The Master
and Idle Apprentices.—The Enthusiasm of his Class.

NOTWITHSTANDING the labours of John Hunter and the
Monros, England gave no signs of earnestness in zootomi-
cal science during the three first decades of the present
century. France had her Vicq d'Azyr, Daubenton,
Serres, Cuvier, St. Hilaire, and De Blainville, and Germany many men of promise; whilst England had scarcely
broken ground in the general field of zoology. Dr. John
Barclay, and his successor Dr. Robert Knox, were, as far
as I can learn, the first public teachers of comparative
anatomy in Britain. They had no English text-book
for their students, no special work to refer to but the
obsolete folios of Samuel Collins, published in London
in 1685. Professors Grant and Rymer Jones issued their
excellent works in 1840 and 1841, two years subsequently to the time (1839) when Knox made a memorandum now before me; "that for many years past—from
1829—the study of comparative anatomy was confined
to books and plates derived from the French." Herein
lies the credit due, first to Barclay, and notably to Knox,

for drawing the attention of the British medical inquirer
to the subject of zoology, and showing its great import
in the study of the higher anatomical science. It should
also be borne in mind that in 1826, when Knox delivered
his first course of lectures, human anatomy itself was
a superficial pursuit with the majority of students—a
three months' course of dissections sufficing for the medical boards of the United Kingdom—so that to incite a
further step anatomical-wards required no small energy
and skill on the part of the teacher. Nothing less than
the brilliancy of Knox's lecturing could have succeeded
forty-four years ago in investing the dry osteology of
the brute creation with such vast interest. To some
lecturers a bone was but a structure with certain physical
features, and nothing more. Knox made it assume an
historical position in the scale of organization ; its size
and form were patent enough, but he sought in the
osteogenesis and type and homologues to fix its place
in the general superstructure of the animal series : in
short, he gave not the mere description, but the philosophy
of the osseous form. Of Knox, in this special department
of his teaching as in many others, it could be truly said,
" *nil tetigit quod non ornavit.*"

He was in the habit of delivering a series of lectures
on Comparative and General Anatomy, and Ethnology,
on the Saturdays. These were the red-letter days in the
Knox calendar. Students, practitioners, and fellows
of the Royal Colleges used to assemble in great numbers
to enjoy the hour's treat of " Knox on a favourite subject." At one time a separate ticket was issued for these
lectures, the character or purport of which varied a good

deal each session. Whether zoology proper, or man in his Racial aspects or structural elements, formed the subject of his prelections, the lecturer showed a freshness of design and an amplitude of intellectual view that never failed to draw large audiences to Old Surgeons' Hall. Knox was in his happiest humour on Saturdays; the audience was of a more advanced character, and as a rule highly discriminative; the lectures were very much his own choice and capable of large historical treatment, and consequently better adapted to call forth a finer display of his faculties and genius.

On "General Anatomy" he professed to make "*Monsieur* Beclard" his guide, and an English translation (his own) of Beclard lay on the table as if for immediate use; rarely, however, were its pages referred to. Knox laboured under a curious difficulty,—he could not with any comfort to himself read to a class. To have his eye fixed upon a book, and so far out of the direct survey of the audience, was positively irksome to him. Yet he was quite an elocutionist. As he knew his theme, quotation could be done without, and the inspiration of his class served a far better purpose than either chapter or verse of "*Monsieur* Beclard." With an array of preparations on the green-baized table, and "fresh tissues" for the purpose of demonstration, Knox required no backing up, no authoritative aid; his chief reliance at all times rested with himself, and that self was never found wanting. He was lavish in his praise of Bichat[1]—"*ce Bichat que l'Europe envie à la France*"—for his Modern Philo-

---

[1] Knox perhaps attributed a little too much to Bichat, and would have endorsed Corvisart's opinion of his idolized countryman : " Personne, en si

sophy (1801), and Beclard for his later interpretation
of "L'Anatomie Générale,"[1] as he was of every distinguished name in science; but, after all, Knox appeared
very much his own oracle when describing what he
called "the history of the tissues."

Over the zoological domains of science Knox loved to
roam with the freedom that characterised his dashing
pace across the African prairies. He might consult the
compass and the provisional chart, but he had his own
horizoned beacon, his own track and goal, the gaining of
which by him apparently required but small effort. His
jaunty air of confidence impressed you with the belief
that he was as conversant with each walk in biology as
the farmer with the locality of his fields; on the other
hand, he practised a modesty that insinuated he was but
a pioneer breaking up the fallows of the science for his
pupils more successfully to till and fertilize. However
discursive he might appear in citing the ancient instances of Aristotle and Pliny, or the more modern
names of Linnæus and Buffon, the scientific purport of
his teachings was still kept in view; his discoursings
were never without their meaning and characteristic
relevancy. In picturing the author of the "Historia

peu de temps, n'a fait tant de choses, et aussi bien." Dr. Fletcher showed
that Bichat was preceded not only by the great anatomical authorities since
the time of Beranger and Vesalius, but by Aristotle and Galen. Haller,
Bonn, John Hunter, and Pinel, to come within the range of a century, no
doubt saw the leading characters of the tissues, and the pathological indications belonging to them; Bichat, however, deserved the palm of excellence,
by his transcendent abilities and originality.

[1] Elements of General Anatomy, translated from the last edition of the
French of P. A. Beclard, with Notes and Corrections by Dr. Knox. (Maclachlan and Stewart, 1830.)

Animalium" examining the marine fauna of the Bay of
Salamis, something of the classical halo might obtrude ;
it was only for the moment that he figured so grandly,
then he carried out the historical parallel by exhibiting
zoological specimens taken from the Firth of Forth,
upon which to indicate an Aristotelian analogue, or
possibly to amplify a generic illustration. Nothing could
well be more inciting to " ingenuous youth" than combining the historical and classical phases of his science
with the living and available resources of the adjacent
sea-board; such instructive lessons as these, coming from
so great a master as Knox, might well develop men of
the Goodsir, the John Reid, and Edward Forbes stamp.
With the works of the Greek and Roman sages Knox
showed a familiarity that was only surpassed by his
recounting in detail the last conversation he enjoyed
with his friend Baron Cuvier in the Jardin des Plantes.

His ingenuity in interweaving his own observations
with the experience of his great predecessors in the field
of anatomy, was not less remarkable than the felicitous
manner in which he presented all he knew to the recognition of his pupils. The text and context, the narrative
and the dialogue set forth by Knox, were uniformly clear
and inviting to every avenue of the understanding. Men
of culture—and there were many who sat on Knox's
benches—were rapt in admiration of the lecturer's display
of Esculapian lore, nay, an unfathomable fertility of literary and scientific resource. The historical prologue, the
array of data digested or otherwise, the nicely balanced
argument, the logical inference, and the "telling hit," and
all in happy sequence, were pronounced in faultless

language,[1] and garnished with a silvery tongue, whose measured accents fell like melody upon the ear. An hour with Knox glided away like a day dream; you never cast your eyes upon the dial, and could hardly be awakened from your half-entranced condition when the " To-morrow, gentlemen," and the graceful bow, showed the falling of the curtain. If the student could not be roused by Knox's teaching, he was past all mending ; or if he failed in the acceptance of principles so well enunciated, his lot could only be in the abode of the helpless, and among the dull and God-forgotten sons of men.

Recognized as singularly choice in his treatment of every anatomical question, Knox surpassed himself in his lectures on the Races of Men, The mode in which he took up a cranium bespoke the artist as well as the anatomist, and his demonstration of its special characters or conformation was done with a freedom that simulated the putting in of the fine touches of a drawing by a master hand ; then came the ethnological questionings and significance, and finally the grandiose and historical flourish. For truly he could speak " of all the learned and authentic fellows," from Aristotle to Cuvier, from Galen to Blumenbach. Taking the Caffre for his text on the African races, he dwelt upon the activity and prowess of the tribe, and contrasted these faculties with the sluggishness of the

---

[1] In one of his sly hits, drawn from the conventionalities of the would-be Malthusians of the age—principally French, it must be admitted—he bordered pretty closely upon the social proprieties. When describing a part of the human anatomy which terminated in a closed cavity, he added : "A *cul de sac*, gentlemen ; a form of structure, I may remark, by no means approved of by French ladies of gaiety." This Shandean episode, derived from " *les gands d'amour,*" was only caught by a very few of the knowing ones.

Dutch Boer. After noting a few historical data, he would address his class somewhat in this fashion:—"Gentlemen, I hold in my hand the cranium[1] of a Caffrarian chief, whom I saw on the hostile field, leading his undisciplined but brave tribes forth against British infantry; and for a time he maintained his position against fearful odds. His dauntless spirit, that could bear no curb, brought him within close range of our troops, and of course he fell under a rattling fire. I was fortunate enough to secure his body, and to bring this ethnological specimen home to England. Look at the development of this cranium, and compare it with the known Europeans presented in such numbers to your observation. View the African and European crania from every point, and tell me if you could fairly distinguish the Caffre from the so-called Anglo-Saxon. Are we to be told that the Caffre of this cerebral stamp is a savage because he lives in the 'wilde,' and that John Bull is the happy creature of civilization because he wears breeches, learns catechisms, and does his best to cheat his neighbours—always, of course, on Christian principles!" Such telling incidents, such exquisite satire, were, if possible, magnified in the eyes of the student by the dramatic personification

---

[1] Of the many wicked stories told by his enemies, one had reference to his possessing so many Caffre skulls in his museum. It was alleged that when one of his students inquired of the Doctor how he got them, he replied : "Why, sir, there was no difficulty in Caffraria; I had but to walk out of my tent and shoot as many Caffres as I wanted for scientific and ethnological purposes." This monstrous accusation had its believers. Knox was tender to a degree, wherever humanity was concerned ; he never approved of the Caffre war, and always extolled the Caffre man for his courageous conduct.

exhibited by the narrator.   On this and kindred subjects, *e.g.* life and organization, each step across the area, each swing of the right arm that stamped the Knox dictum, appeared to the pupil like another turn of the Knox kaleidoscope, revealing fresh colours and fresh facets of surprise.

Knox's feeling was commensurate with his words. These, however, did not flow out into long reaches of language, as was Edmund Burke's wont; his sentences were in easy compass, and each division had its increasing emphasis ; then came the connected rush, the characteristic gesture, and sweeping torrent.   Few men in this country were possessed of the mien that in Knox gave so much apparent sincerity to his words, and manliness and dignity to his pathos.   He personified and was truly himself; there was no counterfeit—indeed there could be none, for where was the previous instance ?   In his greater efforts he seldom had the chance of completing his peroration, for his words—*vires acquirit eundo*— gathered still faster the enthusiasm of his class, watching for the *crescendo* of the orator, as academic youths do, to give vent to their applause.   It was a grand spectacle to see Knox in his higher flights, startling, impetuous, and pronunciative.   Who could then doubt the Knox dogma ?   Who could argue with the inspired possessor of a platform ?   There he stood, before a body of educated men, earnest in attitude, confirmed in faith, and more and more convincing as he warmed in his discourse.   As his skill in words invested everything with a gloss, his vehement declarations came forth as the pervading spirit of the man, yet with the force of Jove,

that wrought his listeners into a state of high excitement, totally irreconcilable with the temperate behaviour
usually exhibited by the members of a scientific class. In
his sudden bursts of oratory, his sharp, pithy sentences,
which came like sparks from a furnace, and not always
evanescent, but igniting by their satire, created sad havoc
among doubtful medical reputations. A *mot* of Knox's
oft became the talk of the school ; a nickname or telling
sarcasm of his would circulate throughout Scotland. In
his great efforts he appeared, though on a different arena,
an Antony to more than Cleopatra :—

> "His rear'd arm
> Crested the world : his voice was propertied
> As all the tuned spheres, and that to friends;
> But when he meant to quail and shake the orb,
> He was as rattling thunder."

While his class seemed spell-bound under the operations of his rhetoric, the dull and bucolic-minded men, with
eyes and mouth agape, wondered at the light of their
neighbours' countenance, and then seemed to become
more or less infected with the enthusiasm of the intelligent members, who, getting excited with the rush of
oratory, started from their seats and vociferated as
lustily as an uproarious House of Commons on the
second reading of a Reform Bill. At one of his Saturday's
lectures, where Knox had been unusually eloquent and
humorous, quoting Shakespeare, "Tristram Shandy," or
a bit of Horace's spicy satire, and where he summed
up in a measured and lofty style that rivalled the best
examples of ancient or modern times, the crowded
audience stood up *en masse* as he bowed his exit, and

waved hats and handkerchiefs, and cried "Bravo! bravo! Knox for ever, and one cheer more!"

He seemed to live to lecture, and enjoyed it more as a recreation than anything else. No charm in rural life, not even the incense-breathing morn, was half so exhilarating to the mind of Knox as the air of his own amphitheatre, where a rapturous welcome hailed his presence. There the vexations of the world and the prickly thorns of his enemies found no place. As the folding doors closed in upon the anatomist in his enchanted circle, all external Satanic influence was put behind him; and with the passing hour all seemed serene in the lecturer's mind. Too often, however, the old leaven of the man himself would ferment and rise up in hasty judgment upon his compeers and the world at large. It cannot be gainsaid by his most fervent admirers, that Knox was at times highly injudicious in holding up society to the glare of his bull-eyed lantern, and construing the professed verities of English life into worldly shams and hypocrisies; and when disposed to be personal, stigmatizing men of public character as readily as he would issue a philippic against his private foe. His temper, generally placid, might well be tried by seeing how the merest pretensions to science could be tolerated, nay, sometimes encouraged, in high places; and how men of solid acquirements and original research fared worse than the mediocrities trailing along the road with no higher credentials than a well-timed orthodoxy. He saw littleness extolled far beyond its deserts, and his own experience too sadly proved that if you cannot be St. Paul to all men and in every walk of life, your brightest intellect affords no guarantee for success. Imbued with such feelings, he was apt to be incautious in hazarding comments on his contemporaries, and as often fell into trouble. Now and then he became bitter in his expressions, as if to say with Don John, "It better fits my blood to be disdainful of all, than to fashion a carriage to rob love from any;" and thus acted as if regardless of the retaliation of his foes.

Knox was eminently diverting when he aimed his satirical shafts at the "Pictorial-Anatomy School," as he designated certain anatomical teachers whose class-room walls were covered with huge diagrams and coloured illustrations. Several of his contemporaries showed a weakness for a kind of mural art, neither natural nor æsthetic; and artificial aids to, rather than the demonstration of the anatomy itself. The brothers John and Alexander Lizars were the chief sinners of the pictorial school. They were draughtsmen-anatomists, who favoured alphabetical mnemonics and puerilities of learning, and dealt uncommonly in gaudy colours and big pictures. Knox defined, and pretty fairly too, their pictorial helps to anatomy as "huge misrepresentations of nature" calculated to mislead the young anatomist, nay, to destroy all chance of his ever becoming a surgeon, or even a medical practitioner.

In describing the human heart, and speaking in his usual felicitous way of its anatomy, functions, and sympathies, Knox would add: "Study this beautiful piece of mechanism *in situ,* and trace the vessels passing to and from it, so as to become familiar with its structure; do not look for its anatomy upon the walls of a class-

room glaring with reds and yellows and blues, such
as exist in a sister institution, where the human heart and
aorta are depicted as large as the whale's. Why, bless
you, gentlemen, you might creep up such an aorta, and
thrust your arm along the corresponding subclavian !"

Other opportunities would occur to Knox during the
descriptive course of anatomy similar to the foregoing,
and such he did not let slip. A highly enlarged drawing
of a female *mamma*, with milk ducts the size of a finger,
used to be presented for the edification of the same pictorial, or, as he called it, the Infant School of Anatomy ;
and Knox would hold it up to ridicule by asking his
class if they had ever been to a country fair and seen
the "grand shows" attracting the bucolic multitude—the
picture of the "fat lady" and "other phenomenons,"
and then finish by saying: "I am told that a similar
picture is to be seen in town, in an establishment professedly scientific—but this can hardly be—or at least a
drawing of one of the *mammæ* of 'the fat lady,' not
only 'as large as life and quite as natural,' but out-
stripping humanity and all artistic conception."

From day to day he impressed upon his pupils the
import of appealing to nature for knowledge of structure, and the investigation of the human form not only
per se, but as a component part of the vertebrate system.
Theory and practice he viewed as twin supports to the
fabric of Practical Medicine. The dissecting-rooms and
hospital were his great levers in medical education, and
the pathological investigation after death the crucial test
of a man's fitness or unfitness for the practice of his art.
Books and lectures were of small weight compared with

the lessons obtained in hospitals ; hence his strong objection to the " coaching " system—a system so baneful in every way, emasculating the mind, and raising up a herd of conceited practitioners doing more harm than good in the world. It was in reference to such persons that he would speak of the practice of physic as being but a speculative art, and not worthy of the name of science : and probably some of the seniors of our profession would be disposed to endorse his opinions.

The views which Knox so strongly and repeatedly expressed on medical education, practical anatomy and hospital practice being the essential features in his scheme, are now pretty generally accepted in the profession. Theoretical medicine, chemistry, and the collateral sciences were so far well, but he looked upon these as subordinate to the practical knowledge that is to make a diagnostic physician and a successful surgeon. As far back as 1829 Knox contended against the constant inroads made upon the time of the student, withdrawing him from the *clinique,* and the dissecting-room, and the opportunities of seeing disease. It was easy to see that with the extension of the medical curriculum by the licensing bodies, and the larger introduction of Latin, Greek, and Physics, a system of cramming would arise calculated to affect the purport of a special calling or practical art. How was it possible for lads only escaping from their teens to carry themselves through a stiff classical and mathematical examination, and at the same time be practical surgeons, chemists, and pathologists ?[1]

---

[1] Sir J. Gray stated in Parliament (1869), that the heads of the Military and Naval Medical departments were so dissatisfied with the licensed

Could the physician's guinea honorarium be raised to the 50*l.* "refresher" of the Chancery barrister, time might be well bestowed in making the Esculapian class philosophical surgeons instead of general practitioners, men distinguished as linguists, physicists, learned in the arts and sciences, and fully equipped for all branches of medicine and surgery.

It is but justice to Dr. Knox and his eminent associates to state, that the reputation of Edinburgh as a school of medicine was mainly sustained at this time by the private schools clustered round the walls of the University. Foremost of all was Knox himself, after whom came Liston, Syme, Lizars, and McIntosh, and for a time Dr. Sharpey. The teaching of anatomy in the University had degenerated into a formalism, distasteful and repulsive to the student, while the flourishing condition of the extra-mural school testified to the energies of Knox and others at its head.

It was a saying of Knox, that if he could get lads of seventeen years old, of fair elementary training, he would make anatomists for every walk of professional life. This was no empty boast, for with his marvellous insight into human character he could almost at a glance perceive the working powers of "freshmen," and adapt his instruc-

surgeons and physicians who had presented themselves as candidates for public employment, that in three years (1865-68) they had to reject 150 persons : yet these men were entitled to practise every branch of the healing art in Great Britain. Thus it is shown that the theoretical learning and cramming for the occasions will not bear the true test of examination for medical and surgical practice. It may again be asked if Hoffman's precept, "*Fuge medicos, et eorum medicamenta, si vis esse salvus,*" does not contain a good deal of truth.

tion accordingly. If brain power existed in a pupil, Knox would infallibly develop it, and no greater pleasure could accrue to him than quarrying out the richer ores imbedded in youthful minds. From the very first he sought to establish classes of excellent men around him, from whose ranks he could choose serviceable coadjutors. He was among the earliest, if not the first, to have paid assistants in the rooms ; and these were aided by juniors glad to be enlisted as volunteers in the service of the popular teacher. The practical instruction was continued from 9 A.M. to 4 P.M. About the years 1829-30, Knox commissioned Mr. Fergusson to give demonstrations on surgical anatomy. This was quite a new feature in anatomical teaching ; and though the demonstrations were gratuitous contributions to his class, Knox aimed to make them worthy of his establishment. Special surgical regions were selected for these demonstrations, which were given three times a week ; and as the students sat around the table and saw the exposition of the parts, they derived great benefit. Mr. Fergusson was the chief demonstrator, and his penchant for surgery proved of material service to numbers of men. In January 1833, Dr. John Reid joined Dr. Knox and Mr. Fergusson in conducting the anatomical rooms. After paying 250*l.* to his colleagues, he enjoyed one-third share of the proceeds of the practical class. Each member of the copartnery seemed to exert himself for the common good, their diligence and supervision extended over the whole day, and the result was eminently successful in promoting the anatomical interests of large classes in Old Surgeons' Hall.

Such a triumvirate as Knox, the master, and William Fergusson and John Reid, apprenticed coadjutors, labouring together in one institution, could hardly be paralleled in the history of anatomical teaching. Whilst alike in setting forth the elementary instruction, each teacher had his higher walk, and assiduously cultivated it. If Mr. Fergusson, by his dexterity and thorough knowledge of anatomy, created a love for surgery, his colleague, Dr. John Reid, gave promise of high reward from the following of physiology : both men were highly prized by their pupils. Knox was not wanting in any direction, and his experience as an army surgeon, his indoctrination in the French school, and maturer mind, naturally gave an exalted character to his teachings. There was a " dash and go " in Knox that surpassed all men of his times, as it does all description here ; it lent a charm to everything he did ; his expositions were as visible centres of illumination brightening the wits of his class. With this trinity of teaching power prevailing, Knox's Rooms might well claim a character of their own that sufficed to bring together the aspiring youths of this country, and many from afar, even the most distant parts of civilization.

Dr. Knox took great pains to encourage neatness and order in dissecting,—the scalpel of the anatomist being upheld by him as the fittest cutting instrument to the surgeon. Mr. Fergusson, carrying out his master's wishes, made some choice arterial preparations, which, being set before a class, failed not to excite large emulation. Of those who followed suit, mention may be made of Robert T. Lightfoot, the distinguished surgeon of Newcastle-

upon-Tyne, than whom, as Knox used to say, no one
had better hands or sounder judgment; and James
Spence, now the well-known Professor of Surgery in the
University of Edinburgh. Some of the dissections made
by the advanced students were unexceptionably good,
whether as anatomical or æsthetical displays. No comparison could be instituted between the work done by
Knox's class and anything seen in the rooms of his
rivals. Those who saw the prize[1] dissections of 1836
can never forget their beauty and excellence.

Though he delivered two lectures daily, Knox gave a
fair share of attention to the practical department; and
when he sat down to instruct a pupil, it was in a masterly
fashion. No youth could well forget the lesson; he saw
the fine sweep of the scalpel, the line of precision, the
unfolding of tissues, and finally a clear demonstration,
whilst he listened to a fund of information—physiological,
surgical, and pathological. Five minutes of Knox were
equal to any man's half-hour, and the student must have
been stolid indeed who did not rise to a higher comprehension of the anatomy, and a fuller belief in its applicability to his art or science. He was always good-natured
with his students, and conveyed his criticism of any imperfect work very happily, and often facetiously. When
he saw the pupil slashing away at the muscles of a part,
he touched the young man's shoulder, and said : " Ah,

---

[1] Stephen Stanley was first prizeman : his "bend of the elbow" was a
picture of a dissection. My facetious friend Stanley became chief surgeon
of the ill-fated Franklin expedition; he was a fine fellow, who sank his
seniority to afford every facility to his assistant-surgeon, Harry Goodsir, the
famed and much-lamented naturalist.

sir! I see you are dissecting for the sake of the bones;
would it not be well to pick up a few facts as to the
attachments and uses of these muscles before you reach
the skeleton ?" To an Irishman removing the superficial veins and fasciæ of the arm at one fell sweep, he
would ask if venesection at the bend of the elbow had
been entirely abandoned in Tipperary—the county of
the young gentleman's birth—or if the doctors drew
blood from the heads of their patients in the shillelah
fashion of Donnybrook Fair? A word of Knox's struck
home, and his playful hints could not possibly offend
either the heavy Saxon or the susceptible Celt, or the
numerous representatives of foreign nations to be met
with in his motley class.

As sunlight waned, and the practical pupils got
wearied, Knox would occasionally take a position with
his back to the fire, and make the last half-hour of the
day exceedingly chatty and pleasant. It was no small
treat to listen to the master in his moments of relaxation, surrounded by his idle apprentices. There you
realized the freedom of a cheerful and social republic—
the incongruous elements of the assemblage being kept
well in hand by its loquacious Præses. Knox in his
humour, criticising the *on dits* of Edinburgh, or the
greater theological and scientific questions of the day,
might well become the focus of attraction; the students
never hesitated to throw down their instruments and
to cluster around him. How happily he could draw
out the leading traits in the characters of his admiring
listeners! He would speak of horses to the Yorkshire-
man, of Britannic prowess to the "Men of Kent," as if

Cæsar's landing-place and the last winner of the St. Leger were equally familiar to him. The Welshman was more than pleased when reminded by Knox of the ancient lineage of the Cymri, that scarcely stopped short of "the Flood." The Highlander had his blood warmed by reference being made to Ossian, and Napoleon's admiration for the grand poems; or by stories told of the Clans of the Macgregors levying black mail on the Southern Borders. The Irishman got such a fill of blarney about the historical Phœnicians and other Kings of Erin, that he used to vow by St. Patrick that Knox was no Scot "at all, at all," but of true Milesian blood.

There was a struggle to obtain good places in Knox's lecture-room each day at eleven o'clock. The first year's students attending Chemistry, and the second year's men attending Surgery, between the hours of ten and eleven, were the chief claimants for Knox's front seats. The University, from whose class-rooms the majority of Knox's men came to hear his morning lecture, was about three minutes' walk from Old Surgeons' Hall. The competitors in their flight down two stairs from Hope's Chemistry Rooms, their racing across the quadrangle of the University, their sweeping rush over every obstacle to gain Infirmary Street, offered an exciting spectacle. The race was neck and neck, and woe betide the folk who happened to come between the flushed medical student and the wind of his nobility. Old and young passers-by were thrown down in the *mêlée* caused by scores of agile-limbed fellows contending for the Knox goal. If a baker, carrying his big wooden tray of loaves, stood in the line of the im-

petuous current, he was sure to come to grief. As he
lost his balance and parted with his tray, the loaves
and rolls were scattered along the pavement, to the
great delight of his mortal enemy, the medical student.
"Knox's men" offered great fun to the shopkeepers
of the South Bridge, the street in which the University
stands, as they were seen running roughshod over
the citizens, or coming in personal collision with each
other: great was the huzzaing when ten or a dozen
strapping young fellows, in broadcloth and smart
attire, measured themselves on Mother Earth at
the corner of Infirmary Street—by no means a rare
occurrence on frosty days and on icy pavement. The
rare and intense enthusiasm that Knox created in
his class belongs to the past; no such high fervour is
manifested by the student of these latter days. The
reason is obvious: he who called it forth is gone, and
his counterpart is nowhere to be found; indeed, it is
more than doubtful if another Knox will ever appear
before a British audience. Old pupils of Knox, both
privately and publicly, still speak with sparkling eyes
of the grand excitement and rush for favoured seats
in his lecture-room.

Dr. Knox may have had some imitators, but he had
no real rivals in the schools of anatomy. From 1826
to 1835 there was but one temple worthy of the name
in Edinburgh, in which aspiring youths might worship
in the spirit of Galen, and sing the hymns that the
anatomico-theosophist delighted in; and that temple
was "Old Surgeons' Hall," where Robert Knox presided
as high priest, oracle, and philosopher.

CHAPTER IX.

DUGONG AND CETACEA.

Great Northern and Young Whalebone Whales.—Food of Whales.—*Balæna Mysticetus.*—Dolphins.—Soosoo.—Porpoises.—Dugong.—Teeth of the Cachelot.—Stomach of certain Cetacea.

THE Royal Society of Edinburgh would seem to have looked upon Dr. Knox as its chief anatomist, by consulting him on all zoological questions, and entrusting him with the dissection of animals obtained from abroad. In this way he came to have at his disposal a Dugong from the Indian seas; also the bones of another Dugong furnished him by Professor Jameson for comparison with the perfect animal. On December 21, 1829, and January 18, 1830, Knox read his "Observations to determine the Dentition of the Dugong;" to which are added, "Observations illustrating the Anatomical Structure and Natural History of certain of the Cetacea" (*Trans. Royal Soc. Edin.,* vol. xi. pp. 389—417).

Dr. Knox claimed to be the first to point out that the osteology of the Dugong, contained in the "Ossemens Fossiles," published in 1825, had been drawn up from an imperfect skeleton furnished by MM. Diard and Duvanceal. His observations led him to infer :—

1. No complete skeleton of the Dugong exists in any of the European museums, or, if it does, is not described.

2. The incisive teeth in the upper jaw, exclusive of the fang-like incisives, are thrown off or shed at an early period, and not replaced by others ; an extremely firm horny-looking substance seems to supply the place of the incisive teeth ; it encrusts that remarkable sloping portion of the upper jaw which, together with a corresponding and opposite one in the lower jaw (also encrusted with a dense horny covering), forms an extraordinary feature in the general appearance of the Dugong.

3. The incisive teeth in the lower maxillary bone remain imbedded in their sockets throughout life ; they are neither shed nor replaced ; and seem to be eight in number.

4. The teeth, termed milk-fangs by Sir E. Home, cannot be temporary teeth, because they are found in the head of an apparently adult specimen, and because there is not the slightest appearance of any approaching change in the form of the tooth, or indication of the approach of another or permanent tooth. Knox therefore looked upon them as *permanent teeth, not as temporary,* and, to reconcile these contradictory statements on the part of anatomists, supposed it not unlikely that the differences in the form of these tusks may originate, not in a difference of age, but in their belonging to distinct varieties or species of the Dugong.

Baron Cuvier's arranging the Dugong, Lamantin,

and the animal of Steller with the Cetacea, or rather the Herbivorous Cetacea, was objected to by Knox, who argued, on the form of the cranium of the Dugong, the structure of the molar teeth and tusks and general dentition, the structure of the stomach, position of *mammæ* of the female (so different from that of the Cetacea), that the Dugong would be more naturally grouped with the Walrus than with any of the whale tribe as yet described (1830).

In the Essay he describes the skeleton of the Narwal, the *Delphinus Phocæna*, and other specimens of the genus *Delphinus*, and draws attention to the great size of the fœtus of the Cetacea at the time of birth, the condition of the *symphysis pubis* previous to and during parturition : also the dentition and digestive organs of the Cetacea, and the microscopic examination of the mucous membranes. The Essay is full of anatomical interest.

Professor Owen has since shown that the dental differences pointed out by Knox related to age and sex, and not to species ; he therefore objects to the classification of the Dugong with the Walrus, and is of opinion that the Dugong and its congeners should form a group apart from both the Carnivora and Cetacea of Cuvier. This group he shows anatomically to be more nearly allied to Cuvier's Pachyderms, and he calls them "Apodal Pachyderms." The Dugongs, Rhytinas, and Manatees have since been accepted as forming a distinct order, called *Sirenia*. (See Owen "On the Anatomy of the Dugong," *Proc. Zool. Soc.* London, March 1838, in which Essay, p. 42, he does justice to "that able comparative anatomist Dr. Knox," for his original observations on the Dugong.)

On October 5, 1831, the carcase of a whale was observed floating off Dunbar at the mouth of the Firth of Forth, and was landed to the west of North Berwick. This whale was purchased by Dr. Knox and his brother Frederick for scientific purposes. On March 18, 1833, Dr. Knox read a paper to the Royal Society of Edinburgh (*Proceedings of the Society*, or *Edin. New Philos. Journ.*, vol. xvi. p. 111) : " Observations on the Anatomy of the Rorqual (Whalebone Whale of the largest magnitude), drawn up from the dissection of a specimen found dead off North Berwick." [1]   He

---

[1] The "monstrous fish," as the Rorqual was called by the public, attracted thousands of visitors.   How Jonah could find room "in the whale's belly" was now perfectly well understood ; and the preachers in the pulpits of the Lothians improved the occasion by dwelling upon "God's good providence" in sending so unexampled a proof of His creative wisdom to the shores of Scotland, when the cholera was raging and the country was in the throes of excitement about a Reform Bill.   The theologians did not wait or the description of the anatomist as to the gullet of the "big whale" only admitting of a man's closed fist, and the presence of a stomach relatively as small.   Jonah might have found space within the jaws of the whale, and made its tongue his bed—not so soft, or even in the Rorqual, as that of the Spermaceti Whale, which John Hunter likened to a feather bed—and the baleen his curtains.   He might also have amused himself in catching the shrimps and other "small fry" taken in by the devourer ; but how of his respiration in the maxillary chamber? for no mention is made of Jonah being provided with the gills of fishes during his aqueous sojourn ; and history is still silent as to the exhibition of any philanthropic endeavour by the zoophagous animals of the deep.   Blumenbach was witty upon the exegetists and the prophet Jonah ; and, according to Marx, "stood by the opinion of Hermann von der Hardt, in Helmstadt, who wrote a very nasty commentary on that man of God ; that he lodged in Nineveh at the Whale; that his cash ran out ; the landlord would give him no more credit—he was turned out of the club ; or—the Whale cast him out."

named the whale *Balæna maximus borealis*, or Great
Northern Whale, with integumentary folds ; and ranked
it with the *Balæna Rorqualus borealis* of Lacepede and
Desmoulins ; *Rorqualus Boops* of Cuvier.   An author of
eminence, Dr. J. E. Gray, refers it to the *Physalus
Antiquorum*, the Razor-back, the *Balæna antiquorum*
of Fischer, the *Rorqual de la Méditerranée* of Cuvier.[1]

The animal was a male.   The girth of its carcase
immediately behind its pectoral extremities was 52 feet.
Two cross lines were drawn on the sand, from the snout
and centre of tail, and the interspace gave a measure-
ment of 78 feet.   The tail, from tip to tip, measured
20 feet.   The blood-vessels were full of a dark, semi-fluid
blood.   The stomach contained only mucosity, the
intestines being partially filled with a yellow glairy
mucus.   The cause of death was not ascertained.

As reference has often been made to Knox's whale
by English and Continental writers, it is needful to
state for the sake of reference that three years were
occupied in the preparation of the skeleton of the Great
Rorqual ; it was exhibited to the public in the years
1834 and 1835, in the Royal Institution, Edinburgh,
and for a time in Glasgow.   On the suggestion of the
late Professor Jameson, the city of Edinburgh bought
the skeleton for the Natural History Museum.   After
being exhibited in North College Street, in 1839, by

[1] In the month of November, 1869, a large Balænoptera of the female
sex came ashore at Longniddry on the Firth of Forth, not more than ten
miles from the place where Knox's whale was stranded.   This whale was
anatomised by Professor Turner, who identified it as the *Balænoptera Sib-
baldii*, and by whom it is described in the Proc. Roy. Soc. Edinburgh,
December 1869.

Mr. Frederick Knox, it found a place in the Zoological Gardens, and when these were broken up it was transferred to the National Museum of Science and Art in Edinburgh, where it now constitutes the most noticeable object in the Natural History collection.

The most complete description of Dr. Knox's "Great Northern Whale" is to be found in a "Catalogue of Anatomical Preparations illustrative of the Whale," published in 1838, and professedly edited by Frederick John Knox; there is no doubt, however, that the best part of this 39-paged pamphlet was from the pen of Dr. Knox. This catalogue is so exceedingly scarce, that I am induced to quote the salient points in the anatomy of the Great Rorqual especially:

COMPOSITION OF SKELETON OF THE GREAT RORQUAL.

Cranium, lower jaw, and lingual apparatus.

Cervical vertebræ, 7. Dorsal, 15. Lumbar and caudal, 43. Total, 65. Ribs, 15 + 15 = 30.

Sternum, one flattened bone, articulated with the first pair of ribs.

V-shaped bones commencing at the intervertebral substance, between the 39th and 40th vertebræ; the largest of these peculiar bones is the second, which is about 15 inches long.

Pectoral extremities or arms, right and left, consisting of scapula, humerus, radius, ulna, carpal bones (3), metacarpal bones (4). Four fingers, the radial, or thumb, not developed in this species of whale.

Pelvis in a rudimentary state, consisting of two flattened bones (the pubic portions of the *ossa innominata*). Pelvic extremities not developed.

Length of base of cranium, 19 feet; of spinal column, 59 feet = 78 feet. Length of the lower jaw, 21 feet 4 inches.

Interspace between right and left rami of lower jaw, about half-way between symphysis and articulation, 11 feet.

Length of the sixth rib, 11 feet. Total length of pectoral extremity, 3 feet 11 inches.

Weight of cranium when first removed from the beach . . 7 tons.
Spine, ribs, and extremities . . . . 21 tons.

Total, 28 tons.

The whole surface of the palatal plates of the superior maxillary bone, each extending to 14 feet in length, was covered with a mass of what appeared to be well-teazed hair, of a clear and shining black. This was the whalebone, arranged in a most regular manner, and composed of many thousand plates. Of the baleen, or whalebone of commerce, there were 314 external or labial plates on each side ; towards each extremity these plates degenerate into bristles, and admit of being counted with difficulty. The baleen diminished gradually in depth towards the mesial line, giving the whole palatine surface an elegant arched form. For each external plate twelve (*internal*) smaller ones could be easily counted, so that the number of plates which could be counted, and not including the bristly terminations towards the snout, pharynx, and mesial line, stand thus :—

External or labial plates 314
Internal small plates corresponding to each external one . . . 12

Total number of baleen plates, 3,768

The longest plate of baleen measured 26 inches in length by 15 inches in breadth. The substance when recent is highly elastic and very heavy, the whole weighing nearly two tons in the *Balæna maximus*, and contains so much fluid in its composition as to lose fully half its weight and a third of its bulk in drying.

A section of the integuments revealed (1), the cuticle ; (2), the cutis, equalling 3½ inches in thickness, and containing the blubber of commerce ; (3), the *paniculus carnosis*, or cutaneous muscle.

The larynx, whilst totally unlike that of the dolphin and porpoise, resembled in part the anatomy of the *Balæna minimus borealis* and *Balæna mysticetus borealis*. The nostrils were filled with two enormous cartilaginous masses acted upon by muscles occupying the centre of the superior maxillary bones. When the animal breathes, they are withdrawn sideways to admit the passage of air. This structure appeared unique to Knox, and that it had not been previously noticed by any scientific observer.

The epiglottis was 14 inches long. The position and form of the arytenoid cartilages are very peculiar in the *Balæna maximus*, and by projecting into the pharynx in the manner of the epiglottis, make the upper opening of the larynx a sort of triangle. "The arytenoid cartilages, however, sent, each in addition, a lengthened prolongation down on the inner surface of the cricoid cartilage ; and these arytenoid prolongations passing across the interior of the larynx, assisted with the inferior margin of the thyroid cartilage in supporting a bag-shaped cavity.   This cavity extended fully half-way down on the inferior surface of the larynx ; its walls were muscular, and its interior lined with a prolongation of the common investing membrane of the larynx.   The same mechanism was found in the *Balæna minimus borealis* and in the *Balæna mysticetus borealis.*   The whale has evidently the power of closing and opening this bag, but its economy is evidently extremely obscure."

The measurements of the cerebral cavity were :—Vertical depth, 9½ inches ; antero-posterior diameter, 11 inches ; horizontal breadth, 18 inches.   This capacity of cranium implied, according to Sir W. Hamilton's method, 80 lb. of brain.   Fortunately for a more correct interpretation of the facts, the fresh cerebral contents of the *Balæna minimus borealis* came into Dr. Knox's hands, and showed the existence of a great mass or plexus of blood lying under the *dura mater*, and constituting one-half at least of the cranial contents.

Along with the skeleton of the Great Rorqual, Mr. F. Knox exhibited twenty-seven dissections illustrative of its anatomy, and twenty-six preparations obtained from the Piked Whale (*Balænoptera rostrata*), which Dr. Knox termed *Balæna minimus borealis,* and the specific difference of which from the Great Rorqual was satisfactorily established by his dissections ; also thirty preparations from the Greenland Whale, or *Balæna mysticetus,* and forty others illustrative of the genera *Delphinus, Phocæna, Soosoo,* and *Halicore.* Of this valuable collection the late Professor Goodsir purchased for the Anatomical Museum of the University of Edinburgh, in which they are now to be found, specimens marked in the Knox Catalogue as Nos. 17, 21, 23, 24, 28 (skeleton of the *Balæna minimus borealis*), 57, 84, 107 (skeleton of Dugong), and 116.   The remainder of the majority of the preparations were variously dispersed, to the detriment, it may be said, of the History of the Cetacea, which Dr. Knox undoubtedly meant to write, but in time found it necessary to abandon, on the ground that scientific labours were not appreciated, and comparative anatomy least of all, in England. For Knox's own fame it would have been desirable that he had issued a monograph on the Cetacea, and laid claim to his discoveries,—for instance, the laryngeal pouch, which Drs. Carte and Macalister (*Lond. Philos. Trans.*) afterwards observed in the Piked Whale, and Eschricht and Reinhardt in the Greenland Right-Whale in 1861 (translated from the Danish in the Transactions of the Ray Society, 1866), and Turner last year in the Longniddry Whale. The *rete mirabile* in the cranial cavity, and other anatomical points which he demonstrated for the first time in the Cetacea, have been much overlooked by authors in general.

On April 27, 1834, Knox read to the Royal Society of Edinburgh his account of the dissection of the Young Rorqual, or Short Whalebone Whale (*Balæna minimus borealis* of Knox, *Balæna rostrata* of Fabricius, Piked Whale of John Hunter), with a few observations on the anatomy of the fœtal Mysticetus (*Proc. Roy. Soc.*, or *Edin. New Philos. Journal*, vol. xviii. p. 197). Twenty-six preparations obtained from this whale have already been referred to in the Knox Catalogue : they embrace Nos. 28 to 53 inclusively.

This young Whalebone Whale was taken near Queensferry, in the Firth of Forth, in February of the same year.

Knox viewed it as quite distinct from the Great Rorqual.[1]
It was 9 feet 11 inches in length, 3 feet from snout to
ear, and 4 feet 8 inches in girth at the termination of the
plica and folds. The whalebone was about $2\frac{1}{2}$ inches—
the longest plate 4 inches—and varied from a pale rose
colour to a dull white : 614 large external plates were
counted towards each extremity ; these plates degenerate
into fine bristles, and these were not counted. According
to Knox, the proper functions of the baleen were clearly
illustrated by this specimen. The plates were observed
to hang perfectly parallel with each other, and from their
closeness and fringed lingual aspect, acted as a very
perfect filter in collecting the minute molluscous animals,
and at the same time they enabled the whale to reject
the water.

The food of the whale is still a disputed point. It is
now generally admitted that the Mysticetus lives only on
small medusæ, shrimps, &c., but that the other species of
whalebone whales devour inconceivable quantities of

---

[1] Composition of Skeleton of *Balæna minimus borealis*.

Cranium with lingual apparatus *in situ*.
Vertebræ : Cervical, 7 ; dorsal, 11 ; lumbar and caudal, 30 = 48.
Ribs, 11 + 11 = 22.
Sternum, one flattened bone articulated with the first pair of ribs.
V-shaped bones commencing between the 31st and 32nd vertebræ.
Scapula, humerus, radius, and ulna.
Carpus cartilaginous ; metacarpus, 5 bones ; fingers, 5 ; the thumb in
a rudimentary state. Pelvis rudimentary ; two small cylindrical-shaped bones
(the pubic portion of the *ossa innominata*) preserved, connected to the
vagina. The pelvic extremities or legs not developed.
The skeleton of the Young Rorqual is in the Anatomical Museum of the
University of Edinburgh.

various fishes. M. Desmoulins had been rash enough to state that "600 great cod and an immensity of pilchards" had been found in the stomach of a single Rorqual. Now the Messrs. Knox in the Great Rorqual (measuring 78 feet in length) saw no cavity in the course of the viscera which would have contained six cod of ordinary size. The stomach of the *Balæna minimus*, now under discussion, was empty, although the Firth of Forth abounds at all seasons with herrings and other fishes and their fry. "The *want of teeth* by no means renders it impossible that the Balæna with baleen can live on large fishes, but the extreme narrowness of the gullet (that of the Great Rorqual barely allowed of the passage of the closed human hand, and that of the *Balæna minimus* was certainly narrower than an ordinary-sized cow), added to the want of teeth and the want of proper authenticated information, are strong arguments in favour of the hypothesis that they do not." Mr. Knox and some students had a steak of this Young Rorqual done on a gridiron, but did not hesitate to express a decided preference for that of the West Highland beef.

There was no vestige of teeth, though Dr. Knox supposed they might exist in the fœtus as well as in that of the Mysticetus, as pointed out by G. St. Hilaire. The cranium, besides containing the brain and its membranes, enclosed a very large mass of a vascular substance—a vast plexus of arteries closely resembling erectile tissue.[1]

[1] The great plexus of arteries observed for the first time in the cranial cavity of the Young Rorqual, in 1834, by Dr. Knox, had been described in his quaint way by Tyson, in another part of the "Anatomy of the Porpesse," long ago. The same circumvolution of arteries, or blood reservoirs, or *rete mirabile*, had been seen and ably described by John Hunter in the thoracic

The same tissue filled three-fourths of the spinal canal and surrounded the spinal marrow and nerves, and was two inches in thickness in some places. The whole cerebral mass (nervous), comprising two inches of spinal cord, weighed 3½ pounds—the cerebrum alone 2¾ pounds : the cerebellum, pons, and two inches of the spinal cord weighed only three-quarters of a pound. The respiratory organs resembled the Great Rorqual.

Below the thyroid cartilage was found the remarkable pear-shaped bag or pouch peculiar to the Balænæ, or Whalebone Cetacea, and already noted in the description of the Great Rorqual. The cartilaginous rings of the trachea were observed deficient for a space corresponding to the size of the bag, which " is in fact nearly the whole length of the trachea."

The question as to the structure and functions of the abdominal glands of the Cetacea, so frequently discussed in the French Institute the year previously—some maintaining that the glands were mammiferous, and others, with St. Hilaire, that they were sexual, specific, and odoriferous—Knox was disposed to settle in favour of the former opinion; in other words, to consider the said glands to be true *mammæ*, as he saw in them what resembled the lactiferous glands of other mammalia in their structure.

In presenting his drawings of the Rorqual to the Royal

cavity and spinal canal of the whales (*Lond. Philos. Trans.* 1787), and by Dr. Barclay in 1815, in the spinal canal of the Beluga (*Werner. Soc. Trans.*). In the very year, 1834, that Dr. Knox saw and figured the arterial plexus of the cranial cavity, M. Breschet laid claim to the discovery of the intercostal plexus, evidently in ignorance of Tyson, Hunter, and Barclay's observations.

Society, Knox " begged leave to state that they were the only authentic drawings of their kind to be met with in Britain." Professor Traill, who believed himself to be a great authority on the Cetacea, as on most other subjects under heaven, asked in a petulant tone if the Society was to understand from Dr. Knox that the drawings he had just presented were the only ones trustworthy. Knox nodded assent. Traill then inquired, " Has Dr. Knox not seen mine of the same species of Rorqual, and are they not accurate and of scientific value ?" Knox rose very deliberately to meet this pointed question, and first looking at Traill, as if scanning the vaunted drawings through the draughtsman himself, and then turning to the chair occupied by Sir Thomas Brisbane, replied in a characteristic tone, " Very like a whale, Sir Thomas,—very ! "

The Messrs. Knox made thirty preparations from the fœtus of the Greenland Whale (*Balæna mysticetus borealis*, Knox Catalogue Nos. 54 to 83 inclusive). They found from sixty to seventy dentar pulps on each side of each jaw—260 to 300 in all. " Had these pulps been confined to the upper jaw, and corresponded to the number of baleen plates, it would have formed a strong analogy between the baleen and the teeth ; but the number of baleen plates in the whale greatly exceed the number of dentar pulps ; and the lower jaw, which contained an equal number of pulps with the upper, supports neither teeth nor baleen in the adult whale. When the baleen is removed from the palate in the adult whale, we observe no remains of the alveolar grooves: and upon a longitudinal section of the lower jaw (*Balæna maxi-*

mus), we found no vestige of dentar pulps or teeth. Their presence, therefore, in the fœtal Mysticetus forms one of the most beautiful illustrations of the unity of organization in the animal economy. The teeth in the Balæna never cut the gum, but become gradually re-absorbed into the system: the very cavity in which the germs were lodged disappear; while, to suit the purposes of nature, the integumentary system furnishes the baleen, which is evidently a modified form of hair and cuticle." No. 57 in the catalogue shows seven dentar pulps from the fœtal Mysticetus (Edin. University Mus.).

The genus *Delphinus* was illustrated by eight preparations (Knox Catal., Nos. 84 to 91). The skeleton of the *Delphinus tursio* or the White-sided Bottlenose, obtained from the Orkneys in May 1835, is here given :—

COMPOSITION OF SKELETON.

Cranium and lower jaw.   Teeth, $\frac{30}{30} + \frac{30}{30} = 120$.

Vertebræ : Cervical, 7 ; dorsal, 15 ; lumbar, sacral, and caudal, 59. Total, 81.

V-shaped bones commencing between the 40th and 41st vertebræ.

The pectoral extremities consisted of the usual larger bones ; the carpus had seven centres of ossification ; metacarpus five centres ; fingers five in number, the second or forefinger the longest, having seven centres of ossification developed.

Pelvis rudimentary, consisting of two cylindrical-shaped bones.

The animal was a female, and weighed 14 stone.

In the jaws of the *Delphinus Delphis* caught in the Bay of Biscay, wher the teeth had partially dropped out, the formula seems to have been $\frac{50}{47} + \frac{50}{47}$ = 194. "Length of dentar portion of upper jaw, 9 inches. Breadth of jaw at proximal end of dentar portion, $2\frac{1}{2}$ inches.

Thirteen preparations (Knox Catal. Nos. 92 to 104 inclusive) illustrate the genus *Phocæna*. One of the porpoises,[1] described by Messrs. Knox, was a female, in a gravid state, caught in the Firth of Forth, which measured 56 inches in length and 34 inches in circumference; the other was killed in the Thames, also a female, 74 inches long.[2] The fœtus of the former measured from snout to centre of tail 26 inches, circumference 16 inches. "Its great bulk, considering the size of the parent porpoise, is remarkable, and renders the supposition that the porpoise does not suckle her young extremely probable." No. 103 was the skeleton of a young porpoise caught in the Forth, only a few days old, as the teeth had not cut the gums. The osteogeny of the cranium seems to have been pretty clearly seen, but is not described.

The cranium and lower jaw of the Soosoo (*Platanista Gangetica*) of the Ganges, and its *ossicula auditus*, constitute Nos. 105 and 106 of Knox's Catalogue.

The genus *Halicore* was illustrated by twenty preparations (Knox's Catal. Nos. 107 to 126 inclusive), the

[1]   SKELETON OF *Phocæna communis*, OR COMMON PORPOISE.

Cranium and lower jaw.   Teeth $\frac{28}{26} + \frac{28}{26} = 102$.

Vertebræ: Cervical, 7; dorsal, 13; lumbar, sacral, and coccygeal, 45. Total, 65.

Ribs, 13 + 13 = 26.

V-shaped bones commencing between the 34th and 35th vertebræ.

Pectoral extremities as usual. Carpus and metacarpus, five centres of ossification. Digites, 5, the second or forefinger the longest, and with four centres of ossification. Pelvis rudimentary.

[2] The skeleton of the Thames porpoise presented "the remarkable appearance of coracoid clavicles." It differed from the Forth skeleton in having 12 ribs on each side, and in its lower vertebræ being more slender and delicate, whilst the transverse processes of the dorsal and lumbar were broader and stronger.

N

description of which is worthy the attention of naturalists. Whilst the chief points in the anatomy of the
Halicore Indicus or Dugong (popularly the mermaid,
sea-cow, &c.) are set forth, Dr. Knox gave special consideration to the osteology and teeth of the animal. As
to the relative position of the Dugong and Manatees
in the zoological scale, he felt, as others have done,
much difficulty. He held the bones of the Dugong to
be "extremely dense and of stony hardness;" that the
long bones, like the humerus, contained no medullary
cavity, but consisted of a texture nearly as close as
ivory, and capable of being polished. The extraordinary
weight of the skeleton of the Dugong, compared with
the dolphin, &c., he held to be peculiar.[1] After noting
the unusual form of the jaw in the Dugong, he described "a portion of the upper jaw bent in the cranium
as nearly four inches long, and the buccal surface presenting a rough reticulated appearance not unlike a
necrosed bone. The tusks traverse the centre of this
bent portion." He considered the tusks to be teeth

---

[1]   SKELETON OF THE DUGONG.

Cranium, with lower jaw. Tusks, 2, upper jaw. Molar, $\frac{4}{4} + \frac{4}{4} = 16$.
Vertebræ : Cervical, 7 ; dorsal, 19 ; lumbar, sacral, and coccygeal,
30 = 56.
Ribs, 19 + 19 = 38.
V-shaped bones commencing between the 32nd and 33rd vertebræ, and
continuing to the last intervertebral space, as in all the Cetacea.
Pectoral extremities : Scapula, humerus, radius, ulna, carpus (3 bones),
metacarpus (5 bones), 5 fingers, the radial or thumb rudimentary, only one
bone. The fourth finger the longest, having only 3 phalanges, however, as
in the human hand.
Pelvis in a rudimentary state, consisting, however, of four distinct portions, two on each side. Pelvic extremities or legs not developed.

connected with the lachrymal bone, and not developed in, but merely passing through, the intermaxillary bones. " The truncated extremity of the lower jaw is $3\frac{1}{2}$ inches long by $2\frac{1}{2}$ inches about the centre; it is traversed mesially by a suture, on each side of which the bone presents a remarkable worm-eaten appearance, and four distinct facets capable of admitting the point of a man's finger; in the third pair of facets, counting from the snout, will be observed two white cylindrical bodies about one inch in length by $\frac{1}{8}$th of an inch in diameter; these are rudimentary teeth, which, not being required in the Dugong, are never protruded through the gum. Both these remarkable and unique surfaces on the upper and lower jaw are covered in the recent state by a horny covering."

The tusk (right side) of the adult male Dugong measured $6\frac{1}{2}$ inches in length by $\frac{5}{8}$ths at root and $\frac{4}{8}$ths of an inch at point in breadth, and weighed 2 oz. 360 gr. Knox had some years previously shown to the Royal Society "that the tusks consisted of two substances, a cortical and a medullary: the cortical, though holding the situation of enamel, is similar to bone, and possesses none of the qualities of that peculiar substance; the medullary portion is extremely hard, of a dense texture and homogeneous appearance."

On May 2nd, 1836, Knox exhibited to the Royal Society of Edinburgh some specimens of the teeth of the Cachelot, divided longitudinally, and which presented a central and cortical substance. " The central substance resembles, and is no doubt analogous to, the ivory of other teeth; but the cortical exhibits not the slightest analogy to enamel. In texture it is softer than the ivory portion, and probably continues to grow or be deposited during the greater part of the life of the Cachelot, until it in fact at least completely encloses the central part, which can be nothing but an ossified pulp : it encloses the central portion in the manner that the ivory of the human tooth encloses the soft dentar pulp." Sections of a great variety of teeth of the Cetacea were shown to exhibit a similar structure.

Professor Goodsir, in his paper on Musket Bullets found in the Tusk of the Elephant, read to the same Society, on the 18th of January, 1841 (*Trans. Roy. Soc. Edin.*, vol. xv. p. 97), says : " The abnormal ivory in the elephant's tusk strongly resembles, if it be not identical with, the peculiar substance which fills the pulp-cavities of the tusks of the walrus and the teeth of the Cetacea, first announced as a distinct species of dentar tissue by Dr. Knox five years ago (1836), and since minutely described by Retzius, Owen, and Alexander Nasmyth. The species of dental tissue in the tusk of the walrus, which Cuvier compared to a pudding stone, Knox looked upon as a fourth substance, and being present in the formation of many teeth, in addition to the cement, enamel, and ivory. Thus in the teeth of certain fishes, this fourth substance, or a tissue closely allied to it, constituted a greater part of their mass, the other three elements having disappeared, or become greatly diminished in bulk or importance."

Knox had a " Notice regarding the Nature of a Peculiar Structure observed in the Second Stomach of certain Cetacea, generally considered as simply glandular, but seemingly analogous to the Electrical Organs of the Torpedo and Gymnotus," in *Brewster's Journal of Science* for 1830, New Series, vol. iii. He pointed out a perfectly smooth membrane, and this again closely invested by a series of fibres externally covered in by an extremely vascular and cellular tunic; that the fibres were not muscular, nor resembling any glandular structure, excepting perhaps the tubular part of the kidney. They were placed perpendicularly and close to each other, and stood out like a pile of velvet enclosed by thin laminæ or plates. To this stomach the greater part of the *nervi vagi* were distributed. Sir D. Brewster examined them under the microscope, and reported them a series of tubes perpendicular to the two membranes which enclosed them.

CHAPTER X.

DR. KNOX read his "Observations on the Natural History of the Salmon, Herring, and Vendace" to the Royal
Society of Edinburgh, on January 7th and 21st, 1833
(*Trans. Roy. Soc.*, vol. xii. pp. 462–518).[1] This paper, of
great length and illustrated by drawings, attracted a
good deal of attention as the production of a distinguished anatomist who relied for his facts on personal
observations. He spoke of "the true salmon, including
the grilse; the salmon-trout, merely an inferior kind
of salmon, and including the whitling of the Tay; the
herling,[2] abounding in the Solway Firth, and which some

---

[1] This long essay should be examined in detail by those interested in the
inquiry, as but a brief abstract is attempted in the text.

[2] "When herling first ascend a river, and are taken shortly after their
ascent, but within that part of the river influenced by the tide, they are
clear, silvery, and covered with scales, compared with what they become
after a short residence in fresh water above the influence of the tide. In
July and August, for example, herling taken in the stake-nets of the Solway,
or even in the Nith, as high or a little higher than the port of Kelton, are
in this prime state, and moreover have a redness of flesh, giving the fish a
general vermilion colour in certain positions; and an excellence of flesh as

naturalists had confounded with the salmon-trout or whitling." Two species of trout frequented our rivers and lakes—the Yellow Trout and the Parr-Trout. "The latter was often confounded with the Parr, Brindlin, Fingerling or Samlet, and the mistake has given rise to innumerable errors and endless disputation."

He held the vendace of Lochmaben, generally esteemed by naturalists as a *Corregonus*, to be closely allied to the salmon. He claimed the honour of discovering the food of the said vendace, and that it consisted of the microscopic entomostracous animals with which the lake abounds.[1] "Through the fish called *Corregonus*, of which the vendace of Lochmaben offers a good example, the *Salmonidæ* are allied to the *Clupeidæ*, or the salmon to the herring. This happens in our own country; in other countries there are perhaps some other fishes which more completely supply the link between those two most important tribes. Captain Franklin and his intrepid party, who twice visited the Arctic regions

an article of food in no shape inferior to the grilse. Their stomachs and intestines are empty, or contain only the peculiar salmon-food." Herling caught in the river Annan, twelve miles from the Solway, in the latter part of September, assumes the external appearance of the sea-trout; the spawning condition is then approaching; and the stomach contains minnow and the ordinary food of trout. He exhibited specimens of the *Caligus productus* and *Caligus curtus* from herlings taken in stake-nets near Annan.

[1] Lochmaben is a small town in Dumfriesshire. The presence of the vendace in the Castle Loch of Lochmaben has been traced to the times of Queen Mary, and even prior to her time. Knox thought that no precisely similar fish existed in Great Britain. He showed the food of the vendace, three different specimens taken in September and December 1832, and September 1833. Drawings of these Entomostraca accompany the essay, and are given on page 428 of the .volume referred to in the text. He also showed the viscera of the vendace at all seasons, and a skeleton of the fish.

of America, mention their subsisting mostly through the winter on a fish called the herring salmon of the Bear Lake."

The food of the true or *clean* salmon consisted of the *Asterias glacialis* or crossfish, and the ova or eggs of other Echinodermata and Crustacea.[1] The real habitat of the salmon is the shores and bays which most abound with this kind of food. The salmon-trout is by no means so nice in respect to its food ; for besides preying on the food of the true salmon, it takes very readily the sand-eels and herring fry ; and these it finds in more or less abundance in estuaries and at the mouths of rivers. The true feeding-ground for the salmon is strictly the ocean ; the breeding-ground is in the fresh-water streams, whether principal or tributary. The part of the river influenced by the tide is a kind of debatable ground in which he neither feeds nor breeds.

The parasitical animals which prey on the salmon in salt water, as the *Monoculus piscinus*, are disposed to leave him in the fresh water; also the tape-worm. And yet his sojourn in fresh water gives rise to other evils : the parasite *Lernæa* fastens on his gills; to these latter, sea water seems to prove a poison.

PART I.—THE SMOLT, FRY, OR YOUNG OF THE SALMON.

Two of the ordinary Tweed salmon, weighing from 14 lb. to 16 lb., were watched spawning in the river

---

[1] Knox exhibited the "food of the salmon whilst in the sea," and skeletons of the *Asterias glacialis* and *Asterias papposa*, to the Society, along with the ova of the salmon at various stages of incubation ; also smolts and their viscera, and the skeleton of a grilse.

Whitadder, on the 2nd of November. On the 25th of February, or 116 days subsequently, there was no visible alteration or change in the ova. The winter was one of the mildest ever observed. On the same day several trout were caught whose stomachs were full of small insects, beetles, larvæ of flies, and cod-bait generally, with which the gravel of the stream abounded. In the gravel-bed, which he described, the ova of salmon and trout lie safe from every living enemy, and in the midst of a profusion of food whose *habitat* is the same as their ova ; and whose progress of incubation and subsequent rise through the gravel is quite similar. On the 25th March, the spawning-bed was again opened ; nearly all the young fish had cast the outer shell, and this probably took place two days before, or in 142 days from the deposition of the ova. These young fry would not admit of transportation to Edinburgh. On their first bursting the shell, they are somewhat less than an inch in length ; on emerging from the gravel they continue to haunt the edges of the river in shallow places. The temperature of the gravel-bed was 41° Fahr. at 9 A.M., that of the water about two degrees higher. He fancied the temperature of these beds during winter to be 39°. "On the 20th April, the rivers (Tweed and Whitadder) were fished with fly, and were found full of salmon-smolts varying from 6 to 9 inches ; such being the rapidity of their growth in three weeks." Knox seems to have taken for granted that these smolts were his young ova of the 25th March ; if so, they exhibited a marvellous growth ! He could not preserve the smolt ; it died on handling or being carried. Of the further growth of the salmon-smolt to the size of the grilse, Knox maintained, "we really know nothing."

In reference to the "natural enemies of the salmon," he found vestiges of salmon-fry or smolt in the stomach of trout in rivers inhabited by the fry. In the stomachs of three kelts (spawned salmon) he found the usual food of trout; that is, beetles, aquatic insects of all kinds, and larvæ of flies or cod-bait. The spawning season, according to Knox, ceases in all rivers in or about the end of February, and in March, April, and May the kelts and smolts or fry descend towards the sea.

PART II.—THE HERRING AND VENDACE.

As the vendace or *Corregonus* was allied to the *Salmonidæ* and *Clupeidæ*, Knox thought if he could discover the food of the *Corregonus* he might be led to that of the herring. In fishing for the Lochmaben vendace, he only got one male fish to a dozen of females. Their food consisted exclusively of microscopic Entomostraca—about seven-twelfths of a line in length, and abounding in incredible numbers in the lake. To the nature of its food he attributed its great delicacy as a fish. He was anxious to see the vendace transferred to other lakes in Britain, and he believed their removal to be quite practicable. The vendace could not be taken by angling; the other kinds of fish, a family of the Daces of naturalists, in the lake were taken with the usual baits. The entomostracous food approached nearest the *Lynceus lamellatus*, and *Trigonatus* of Müller.

"The discovery of the food of vendace of Lochmaben

led immediately to that of the herring ; it became impossible to overlook the strong analogy subsisting between the species ; and although the one was marine and
the other lacustrine, we know their differences as to habitation to be but trifling in the great economy of nature."
Reasoning in this way, Knox found the food of the herring
to be the Entomostraca, but the characters of those under
his notice were so broken down by gastric juice, that a
tolerably perfect specimen was difficult to procure. He
figured only one of those microscopic animals. Knox
was not surprised at the ignorance of his predecessors in
the inquiry, from Fabricius to Rennie: they had not used
a microscope. The peculiar species of Entomostraca
which he found in the herring he was disposed to associate with the *Cyclops* of M. Dumeril, or that described
by Müller.[1]

In August 1837, Dr. Knox issued an octavo pamphlet
(pp. 26)—"Observations upon a Report by the Select
Committee on Salmon Fisheries, Scotland" (Adam and
Charles Black, Edinburgh). He prefaced his Essay by
a letter to Mr. William Murray, of Henderland, upon
whose estate, Castle Loch, Lochmaben, he had discovered
the food of the vendace. Some of these "observations"
are pretty similar to his "Opinions of Authors," in the
Appendix to Part II., "On the Natural History of the
Salmon, Herring, and Vendace" (*Trans. Roy. Soc.*,
vol. xii. pp. 512-18).

---

[1] Professor Tiedemann, dating Heidelberg, November 7, 1833, wrote
approvingly of Dr. Knox's inquiries, and offered to insert a notice of them
in his Physiological Journal.

He offered valuable suggestions for a further inquiry, and showed the unworthiness of much of the evidence gathered by H. Drummond's committee, and their remissness in not making out the food or the feeding-ground of the salmon, when he had decided both these facts in 1832. The true naturalist had never been examined by the Committee; hence a great amount of hypothesis and hearsay in their report.

Mr. Yarrell and Sir W. Jardine, it would appear, admitted Knox's claims to the discovery of the food of the vendace, but thought the salmon lived on grosser food than the minute Entomostraca. Knox notices the absurd opinions entertained by Sir H. Davy and others, as to the food of both herring and salmon. Davy conjectured from the emptiness of the stomach that the salmon, foreseeing his length of journey in ascending fresh-water streams, avoided food in order to lighten himself as much as possible; and Mr. Fraser, reasoning upon the same data, attributed the condition to a rapid digestion: his words are, " the digestive powers of the salmon's stomach are like a consuming fire." No wonder Knox wrote: "The less these persons know of the matter, the bolder uniformly are their assertions; and as they care not one farthing about scientific truths, they fearlessly affirm whatever seems best calculated to support their hypothesis ;" and "what they imagine to be true, that they believe to be true; and what they believe to be true, that they will swear to be true."

Knox could hardly feel otherwise than aggrieved to find his opinions on the food of the salmon and herring passed over by such men as Professor Rennie of King's

College, London, as late as 1834; and the evidence
adduced before a Parliamentary Committee devoid of
scientific character. The food of the herring he proved
in 1832, by examining considerable numbers of fine
herrings taken off the Isle of May, and in a subsequent
page further evidence, that of Harry Goodsir, confirms his
statements.

He believed that marine microscopic Entomostraca
formed the food of vast numbers of those fishes now fossilized in the limestone and other formations. On March
2nd, 1835, the Doctor read a paper to the Royal Society
on the Food of the Char (*Salmo alpinus*, Linné), and
produced specimens of the food of these fishes, viz. microscopic Entomostraca, and hazarded the opinion that if
the lake in which the char is found be changed, as by
draining, &c., so as to destroy the Entomostraca, the char
dies out.

He explained the fact of other food than what he
specified as *the* food being found in the stomachs of the
herring and salmon as being dependent on anomalous
conditions in their life. "The herring, when disordered by
the spawning condition, as well before as after the deposition of the milt and roe, will, *like all other animals, including even the human race,* take to other food than what
is natural to them." He applied the same remarks to
the salmon. It may be stated in the way of parenthesis,
that his views of the "closing time" correspond very
much with the views now adopted by the Legislature.

In concluding his essay, he desired that some public
body interested in fisheries would cause a minute and
searching inquiry into his facts and opinions, as he had

but one wish, namely, to extend the boundaries of science.

It should be noted that in 1833, or sooner, a marked change of feeling towards Knox came over the University section of the Royal Society. He who had been so popular, now received but the cold shoulder from those parties. Some said it arose from the West Port tragedy; this opinion, however, need not be entertained for a moment : it might probably have sprung from his tendency to spare neither friend nor foe who attempted to impose pseudo-science upon a learned body. Whatever his faults were, it was not sound policy to oppose the only anatomist in their ranks of real distinction in Edinburgh prior to John Goodsir, and whose papers were among the redeeming features of the Society's " Transactions " (182–333). In subsequent years the amiability of the anatomical professor met with only a shade more acknowledgment than the satire and heterodoxy of Robert Knox. Both the master (Knox) and the pupil (Goodsir) did their best to uphold the reputation of the Royal Society ; and both lived to know that the essays they had contributed to the "Transactions" were unread at home and almost unknown abroad.

Mr. John Stark, a printer in the city, and also a naturalist, wrote a reply to Dr. Knox's Essay on the Food of the Herring and Salmon, which he communicated to the Royal Society, December 4, 1837. As it got rumoured by Dr. Knox's enemies that Mr. Stark's paper would contain an exposure of the Doctor's plagiarism and recklessness of statement, the Hall of the Society was crowded beyond precedent. Sir Thomas

Brisbane was in the chair. Mr. Stark held that there was no analogy between the vendace and the herring, seeing that they lived in different mediums, one in salt, the other in fresh water; and that they were of different natural families. His historical notes were looked upon with greater interest as affecting Knox's claims to precedence; for Stark maintained that Leeuwenhoeck had figured the identical animal found in the stomach of the vendace in 1833 by Knox, more than 130 years before; that the food of the herring was described from personal examination by Neucrantz previous to the year 1654, by Leeuwenhoeck in 1696, by Fabricius in 1781, by Müller and Block about 1785, by Lacipede and Latreille in 1798, by the Rev. Dr. Scoresby in 1820, and by Pennant and other writers who had treated of the natural history of fishes.

As if in no wise discomfited by the Stark indictment against his literary reputation, Knox rose up quite calm and collected ; and turning at his then triumphant enemies like a lion at bay, began his reply by saying: " Is it necessary for me, Sir Thomas, the friend and companion of Baron Cuvier, to defend myself in the society of my compeers against the base and personal scurrilities of a mere dabbler in science ? " And in this strain, avoiding the merits of the question at issue, he continued to pour out in the most fervent style the vials of his wrath on Mr. Stark. His speech came like a flood of invective and wit; the big stones heaped up by his enemies to stem the Knox current were swept away by force of eloquence and pointed satire, such as had never been heard within the walls of the Society. An almost

breathless stillness prevailed whilst the Doctor continued
to unveil the tactics of the opposition, and each pause in
his speech was filled up by a round of applause.   By
and by he turned upon the Rev. Dr. John Fleming, a
noted naturalist, who had written on the same subject,
and took his notions to pieces ; then suddenly reverting
to Mr. Stark, he denounced him for allowing himself to
be made "the catspaw of a party"—words which he
took care to repeat so as to indicate the persons behind
the scenes.   At this point Knox was interrupted by
Professor Traill, who thought that he was still speaking
of Dr. Fleming, and who in great wrath declared he
would not allow any one in the Royal Society to call a
minister of the Church of Scotland "the catspaw of a
party." Mr. Stark, taken suddenly aback, and wishing
to correct the Professor's mistake, called out, "It's me,
he means, Sir Thomas ; it's me." "Yes!" said Knox,
with ready wit and infinite point; "it is *you:* he knows
himself, Sir Thomas ; he knows himself to be the catspaw of a party, and that he has come forward at the
instigation of a clique." Up started another Professor
(Christison), quite as indignant as Traill, who could not
bear to have it stated that there existed anything of the
nature of a clique in the Royal Society.   "He is one of
them," calmly replied Knox, "and naturally feels a little
sore on the subject ; you observe, Sir Thomas." He
was now left alone to finish what sounded like a triumphant retort upon the reader of the paper, and was
received throughout with roars of laughter and applause,
When Knox sat down, a third Professor (Syme), believing that he had an arrow in his quiver which would

hit the Doctor effectively, rose and asked why Dr. Knox
ridiculed Sir H. Davy for telling his readers that a whale
was not a fish. " Did Dr. Knox think a whale was a
fish ; or, if he did not, why cast ridicule upon Sir Hum-
phry for saying it was not ?" " Sir Thomas," said the
doctor, in reply, "the scientific character of any naturalist who would think it necessary to tell his readers
that a whale is not a fish, and the scientific character of
any one who would ask whether the whale was a fish or
not, require no comment !" Thus ended a grand passage at arms between Robert Knox and the " professorial
clique" of the Royal Society. The anatomist, armed
with his own weapons—a polished satire more keen and
incisive than any Damascus blade in Saracen's hands—
cut right and left, smiting his enemies hip and thigh.
No such laughing interlude occupied the boards of the
Theatre Royal in Edinburgh, and no such tiptoe excitement prevailed amongst the "gallery gods" of the Hall
of Comedy, as was witnessed that night within the walls
of a learned society.

Dr. Knox's views as to the food of the herring received
full confirmation at the hands of his distinguished pupil,
Harry Goodsir, whose opinions, conveyed in a letter
dated Anstruther, 15th June, 1843, are worth quoting
He wrote :—

" 1. The Entomostraca are at certain seasons the
almost exclusive food of the herring. There can be no
doubt either that they follow shoals of these Crustacea
to prey upon them, for it is only when the latter make
their appearance on this coast that the former are seen,
and when this food is most plentiful the herrings are in

O

best condition. It is during the summer months also that we find the larvæ of the more common species of Decapoda along with those of Balani, and occasionally a minute shellfish among the contents of the stomach.

" 2. It appears to be chiefly during the winter and spring months that the herring takes other kinds of food than the Entomostraca; during these months, however, we find the stomach oftener empty, and only occasionally filled with the larger Crustacea, such as the shrimps, &c.; in other cases with Entomostraca.

" 3. As to the Entomostraca being the partial or exclusive food of other fish besides the herring. There can be no doubt that during the summer months, when the shoals of Entomostraca, or what our fishermen term Maidre,[1] are in great abundance, they form the food of a great number of other animals besides the herring.

" It appears to me also that the shoals of Cetacea which make their appearance in the Forth during the herring season are in pursuit of the Maidre, and not of the herring, as is most generally thought to be the case."

[1] Mr. H. Goodsir, in frequent excursions to the Isle of May (Firth of Forth) in 1842, found that the Maidre consisted of one immense continuous body of minute animals belonging to the Cirripeds, Crustaceans, and Acalepha. The Crustaceans existed in the greatest numbers; partly Amphipoda, but chiefly Entomostraca. The spoils of the Maidre were shared in by other animals besides the herring, *e.g.* dolphins, porpoises, and the Great Rorquals which he had seen coursing round and round the island. He corroborated Knox's views as to the food of the Cetacea. He said he had examined several, and never seen anything resembling the remains of herrings or fish of any other kind in the stomach, although the former were very abundant at the time in the Firth of Forth. He naturally inferred that the Cetacea only accompany the herring in pursuit of their common food, viz. Entomostraca and Acalepha. (*Edinburgh New Philos. Journal* for July 1843).

Knox lectured on Comparative Anatomy for several summers, and then, it would appear, he abandoned the subject. In January 1833 a number of his senior students signed a requisition, soliciting him to give a course of lectures on Comparative Anatomy and Physiology, on the ground that "this important branch of medical science had not received the attention it merited in Edinburgh."

Knox planned a great deal more than he ever accomplished. From time to time I made several dissections of regional or surgical anatomy for his special consideration ; and in my third year he asked me to join him in issuing a work on the Ligaments. Mitchell's engravings of the ligaments had long been called " Knox's plates," and he wished to have a more complete edition. A commencement was made, but with my health giving way and his engagements multiplying, nothing came of the proposal ; indeed, it is only mentioned here to show one of Knox's weak points—his inability to cope with his resolves.

Changes of import were made in Dr. Knox's establishment in 1836–37. Mr. Fergusson's increasing practice and hospital duties lessened his opportunities of attending the practical rooms ; and Dr. John Reid having succeeded Dr. Fletcher as Lecturer on Physiology in Argyle Square, left his demonstratorship altogether. Knox now engaged his brother Frederick as assistant, and benefited also by the services of some of his senior students. With these changes there was a falling off in the number of his class ; the tide was on the ebb, and the growing animosities of his contemporaries rendered that ebb more and more apparent.

O 2

The medical school of Edinburgh, to the fame of which Knox had contributed so largely, began to show signs of falling off in numbers about 1835, and went on declining for many subsequent years. Several circumstances helped to bring this about : 1. The want of anatomical *matériel.* 2. The advancing character of the London and Dublin schools. 3. The springing up of provincial medical institutions. 4. The occupation of certain chairs in the University of Edinburgh by senile professors. 5. An extended curriculum of study attended by greater expense and difficulties; and, 6. The glut in the medical market. All these causes were more or less operative, but the first told most severely upon the prosperity of Edinburgh. The imperfect supply of bodies became a matter of public animadversion in the shape of meetings of the students in 1834-35-36,[1] followed by remonstrances to the authorities. Warburton's Act did not work well in the North ; the Whigs and " Little John " Russell were passive upon all matters but holding place ; and no impress could be made upon the town authorities—the fussy Beadledom and fuddling Bailliedom of the ancient city. The consequence was obvious : numbers of students went to Glasgow and Dublin, where greater facilities were offered them. Knox bestirred himself in the business,

[1] The largest grievance meeting of students ever seen in Edinburgh was held in the Argyle Square Rooms, where the suicidal policy of the parochial and other authorities was shown up, and much indignation cast upon the University monopoly. Lord John Russell and other Cabinet Ministers were also memorialized on the subject. I have much reason to remember this stormy meeting, over which I presided before the expiration of my teens, as it brought me more publicity than favour with the medical professors.

and so did his students, but all to no avail. The University enjoyed a monopoly that was deemed the more intolerable outside the walls, that it recalled too truly the fable of the dog in the manger.

In 1837, Dr. Knox brought out "The Edinburgh Dissector," a manual for the use of students in the dissecting rooms. His name did not appear on the title-page, only that of "A Fellow of the Royal College of Surgeons in Edinburgh." This was a mistake, for no name in the college was equal to his own in anatomical repute, and none was likely to be so attractive to the medical student. If the "Dissector" was of real value, he might as well claim the honours; if, on the other hand, he had misgivings as to his own handiwork and wished to shelter himself from the criticism of his enemies, he had not the art of maintaining his *incognito*. The first page of his text showed the author as unequivocally as a line engraving of his physiognomy, for who in Edinburgh could mistake the following as the production of any man but Robert Knox? "Schools of anatomy are of two kinds: 1. Those taught by *medical men*. 2. Those taught by persons who merely know details of human structure; and who, having never applied the art to any practical purposes, *i.e.* having never practised as physician or surgeon, repeat in a dull and formal manner, often with much pomposity and in a Quixotic style, the opinions of others," &c. "They are in fact mere grinding schools of anatomy; and although now a little hackneyed, and the trick is somewhat stale, they still succeed incredibly with the inexperienced student, who seldom reflects on the astounding fact that the

lecturer may not only be a worse-educated person than
himself, but actually totally ignorant of the arts of surgery and physic."

"The Edinburgh Dissector" was too much based on
Cloquet and Meckel to be welcomed by the majority of
students, who did not like its apparently dry and elabo-
rate construction. Knox was led to expect that his
manual would displace "The Dublin Dissector," then so
much in vogue in the dissecting rooms of Edinburgh, but
it never vied with the popularity of Dr. Harrison's
volume, and fell more into the shade as the illustrated
Manuals of Anatomy by Erasmus Wilson and others
were issued from the London press.

In the report of contributions presented to the museum
at Fort Pitt, Chatham, July 16, 1827, it is recorded that
certain skeletons of birds, mammals, and preparations
showing the anatomy of the eye, arterial injections,
lymphatics, &c., contributed by Dr. Knox, are "very
valuable preparations, beautifully prepared and in good
condition." From the year 1827 to 1839, Knox sent
various donations to the Army Medical Department, of
morbid preparations and natural history specimens, for
the museum at Chatham; also his own pamphlets
and other works, *e.g.* Scarpa's anatomical plates for the
library; and he had the pleasure of receiving more than
a formal acknowledgment of their acceptance, in the
shape of hearty and well-expressed thanks from Sir J.
McGregor and other officials. On the 12th June, 1835,
Dr. John Davy, authorized by Sir James, wrote to Knox
to say how glad the Army Medical Department would
be to receive his specimens (105 in number) of organic

remains from the limestone quarry of Burdie House, Edinburgh, as such a contribution would be particularly valuable, and would claim a favourable place in the museum. Examples of the torpedo brought from the Mediterranean by Dr. Davy were offered Knox in return for his presents. In 1839 he sent the specimens of fossil shells, and received very flattering thanks for his " handsome support to the Chatham institution."

Here it may be appropriately mentioned that Sir James McGregor was a great correspondent of Knox's, and formed the highest opinion of him. As early as June 1827, Sir James wrote Knox :— " You know I never doubted your success as a teacher. I rejoice to hear that it has been so complete." Again he assures Knox that the whole Army Medical Department feel grateful to him for his handsome donations to the museum, adding : " What you have so kindly bestowed on us will form a nucleus, and likewise direct us to what we will be ambitious to follow." Sir James frequently honoured Knox by obtaining commissions for his pupils, and did it in so pleasing and hearty a way as greatly to enhance the value of the compliment conferred. The late Director-General, Dr. Alexander, is only one of many examples that might be cited of young army surgeons being promoted through the kind interest of Knox with his friend Sir James.

CHAPTER XI.

ON the 6th July, 1837, Dr. Knox, having learned that
Dr. John Thomson was about to resign his professorship, offered himself as a candidate for the vacant chair of
General Pathology.   In his letter addressed to the Lord
Provost and Town Council of Edinburgh, the Patrons of
the University, he appealed to the success of his teaching
as an anatomist, his surgical experience in Flanders,
in English military hospitals, and abroad in the colonies,
and at La Charité, in Paris, his facilities for pathological
inquiry in Edinburgh, his formation of the College of
Surgeons' Museum, &c.   He introduced his election as
corresponding member of the French Academy of
Medicine as a proof of his scientific status abroad, and
added that " the determined opposition and hostility of
numerous individuals, and even of associated public and
corporate bodies in my own country, present the best
proofs which those acquainted with the world can
require, that the individual so strongly opposed must at
least have attainments and a status in science, which

could not with safety be entirely overlooked." He explained his objections to so many chairs being made imperative upon the medical student, who, he held, should be free to obtain his education "*where and how he liked.*"

Dr. John Thomson had been Professor of Surgery to the Royal College of Surgeons, and afterwards of Military Surgery and Pathology in the University, which led Knox to designate him "the old chair-maker," also the "Medical Commissioner of the Whigs." Dr. Thomson was an able man, and his works on inflammation and varioloid diseases are historical. If Sir H. Davy's greatest discovery was Michael Faraday the bookbinder, Professor Thomson deserved the credit of eliciting the great talents of James Y. Simpson, who became his amanuensis and *alter ego* in conducting the Pathology chair, and is now the most distinguished Esculapian of his epoch. [Alas that I should have to alter this statement in going through the press, and to record the death, on the 6th May, 1870, of Sir J. Y. Simpson, Bart., whose intimate friendship I had the honour of enjoying for so many years, and whose name now ranks among the historical and truly immortal!]

Knox addressed a second letter to the Town Council on the 15th July, with the view, in which he succeeded, of upsetting a proposal made to them by Professors Alison, Christison, Syme, and Sir Charles Bell, who recommended the abolition of the chair of Pathology, and at the same time offered to give a course of lectures that would realize a retiring pension of 150*l.* a year to Dr. Thomson. Knox looked upon this as putting the chair of Pathology into commission, and as a curious make-shift of

the "Pathological Commissioners," whose views upon
most points of doctrine differed so widely that they
would flatly contradict each other and puzzle the student. He called the formation of the chair of Clinical
Surgery "an odious job," and the making so many chairs
imperative and *exclusive* as harassing to the student by
reducing his whole acquaintance of medical matters to
that condition happily and best expressed by the phrase
"Diffusion of useless knowledge." Both letters were
specially stinging, and created a sensation ; the truths
contained in them, though highly unpalatable, did
good, but assuredly the writer benefited nothing by his
exposure of University jobs and "thoroughbred critics."

Knox seems to have contributed to every periodical
that appeared on medicine and the collateral sciences—
no doubt owing to his being solicited to do so, to
give *éclat* to the early numbers. The *London Medical
Gazette,* established in December 1827, contained
(March 8, 1828) his paper on the "Altered condition
of that portion of the tendon of the biceps, *Flexor
Cubiti,* which passes into the shoulder joint."

In the *Edin. Med. and Surg. Journ.* vol. xlvi. p. 76,
will be found Knox's "Observations on the Statistics
of Hernia and on the anatomical causes which determine its production." (Read to the Medico-Chirurgical Society, session 1835–36). Three plates of the
pelvis accompanied the essay. He was afraid that the
statements of medical writers on the frequency of hernia
would hardly bear strict scrutiny: that Dr. Monro's
opinion of 7 per cent. of the population being ruptured
was not consistent with the facts, the Professor had

himself recorded from the experience of Dr. Verstrum, who had examined 40,460 young German recruits; nor did it agree with the official records furnished the French Academy of Surgery.

Knox had never observed a case of hernia "in any unmixed dark-coloured savage race," though he had seen thousands of individuals whom necessity drove "to extraordinary efforts, as in the chase, which efforts they seemed to meet with perfect impunity." On the other hand, he was well aware that hernia frequently attacks mulattoes. The inhabitants of the Cape, known for their indolence, according to Knox, are liable to hernia; he acted for nine months as surgeon to a corps of yeomanry 900 strong, composed almost exclusively of Dutch farmers and their sons, and of all ages, and common repute was strongly in favour of their being so affected. Was it owing to their corpulency, or to too much horseback exercise?

The anatomical structure predisposing to hernia was "greath width of pelvis, and consequent increase in the measurements of this cavity, whether male or female." He discountenanced the idea of femoral hernia in the female being attributable to the comparative smallness of Gimbernaut's ligament, as the said ligament is often larger in females than in males. It was not the use of the right arm and side that caused the numerical disproportion between right and left ruptures, but the larger capacity of the right side of the pelvis as compared with the left; yet Mr. Marshall's statistics on the subject of hernia pointed to a greater laxity or enlargement of the inguinal ring on the left side.

Knox believed in the reduction of hernia by the
taxis in most instances, and, failing this, early operations;
in support of which he cited various surgical authorities.
The records of the Rupture Society of London, from
1805 to 1835, showed that 31,400 cases had been relieved by the Society, and that one in fifteen at least
(of both sexes) are affected with this complaint, and
among such as are exposed to great bodily exertions
the average is one in eight or nine. Knox did not
place faith in these averages, as he held that there are
whole classes of society nearly exempt from hernia;
the *very rich*, for example, and also the *mendicant
by trade.*

"Remarks on the lately discovered Microscopic Entozoa infesting the Muscles of the Human Body, with
some Observations on a similar Animal found beneath
the Intestinal Mucous Membrane of the Horse," were
read to the Royal Society in 1836, and published in
the *Edin. Med. and Surg. Journ.* vol. xlvi. p. 89 (1836).
His opinions coincided pretty much with those expressed by Hilton, Paget, Owen, and Farre, recorded
in the *Medical Gazette* of the previous winter. The
person from whose body Knox took his Entozoa was
a female, aged 65 years, neither cleanly in habit nor
nice as to food, and in fact rather gluttonous. She
showed no signs of debility, and laboured under no constitutional disease. The muscles of voluntary motion
were affected; also the diaphragm, intercostals, levator
ani, and constrictors of the pharynx, or rather the cellular
tissue surrounding them. The worm, cylindrical and
filiform, resembled the *Vibrio Tritici* represented by

Mr. Bauer in the *Philosophical Transactions.*   Knox gave seven drawings of the human entozoon.

Professor Dick had furnished Knox with portions of the large intestines of a horse, upon the mucous membrane of which were a number of dark spots : these proved to be parasitical worms rolled up in a spiral manner, and similar to the human entozoon described above. " *They have no cysts,* and vary from one-tenth of an inch to a length of at least seven-tenths ; they have a digestive tube divided into numerous compartments and sacculated ; a mouth unarmed.   There appeared a cephalic ganglion and collar and two nervous filaments proceeding from these."   The entozoon had been found in several horses and at different stages of their growth, from the size of a pin point to that of $1\frac{1}{2}$ inches in length. A bad form of diarrhœa accompanied their presence. Unwholesome food was supposed to give rise to the parasite.   Five drawings were given of the animal.

Dr. Knox favoured the Medico-Chirurgical Society of Edinburgh with a " Case of Painful Crepitation in the course of the Radial Extensor Muscles of the Carpus," arising in a muscular adult after a hard day's fishing with a heavy rod.   Admitting M. Boyer's discovery and the value of MM. Velpeau and Poulain's supplementary observations, Knox differed in part from his French predecessors, in contending for a wider area than the interior of " real synovial capsules " for the generation of air.   He drew attention to the filamentous tissue surrounding the radial extensors and extensors of the thumb where they cross and play over each other, differing from the vaginiform synovial *bursæ*

and *bursæ mucosæ;* he marked its distribution throughout the body wherever great friction usually or occasionally takes place, and believed that in this intermediate structure air is generated pathologically, and
indeed more frequently than in the well-marked synovial
capsules.

To the above-named Society (in March 1836) he read
his "Observations on the Muscularity of the Hepatic
and Cystic Ducts, as explanatory of the production
of Jaundice by Moral Causes." He had been led to
this inquiry by some papers of Dr. A. T. Thomson,
and a curious case that had come under his own observation in La Charité as far back as 1821. He maintained the muscularity of the hepatic ducts and cystic
duct and gall-bladder; and parenthetically stated that
he found the ureters of the whale (*Balæna rostrata*)
distinctly muscular. With these anatomical facts before
him, Knox had no difficulty in believing in the occurrence of jaundice in a seemingly healthful person during
the course of a single night and from a moral cause. The
case of the Frenchman in La Charité who suddenly
and unexpectedly came upon a sentinel, and finding
his chest ruffled with the soldier's bayonet, became
jaundiced the following morning, was cited by Knox as
a pretty clear instance of jaundice from fright. Pathologists of late years have advanced facts strongly
corroborative of Knox's view.

In the same volume (*Edin. Med. and Surg. Journ.*
p. 404), Knox gave a short paper "On the Hemorrhagic
Hepatization of the Lungs, occasionally mistaken
for Pulmonary Apoplexy, and on the Origin of the

soft pulpy Tubercle of Baillie." He had seen but two cases, one in Brussels in 1815, the other in the museum of the College of Surgeons, Edinburgh; this latter was probably the one described by Dr. Baillie. A drawing of Knox's preparation accompanied the paper.

After twenty-two years Knox again took up the first of his many medical inquiries—the human pulse—and contributed " Physiological Observations on the Pulsations of the Heart, and on its diurnal Revolutions and Excitability," to the Royal Society in Edinburgh (*Edin. Med. and Surg. Journ.* vol. xlvii. p. 353). He showed that the results he obtained in 1815 were confirmed by Dr. Graves, of Dublin, in 1830; and that the Irish physician had reproduced nearly word for word of his, and even some of his conjectures. He gave Dr. Bryan Robinson the credit of having discovered the " differential pulse in man " a hundred years ago. He compared the labours of his predecessors with what he had done himself on this interesting subject ; and cited various curious experiments, or rather observations, made on the members of his class ; the effects of standing or other changes of posture, and all other circumstances calculated to affect the condition of the pulse. Nor did he omit M. Quetelet's extensive data, and the law of relation between the inspirations and pulsation of the heart. His conclusions differ but little from those he had expressed in 1815 ; nevertheless the paper is deservedly worthy the attention of those who wish to be informed on the nature of the human pulse.

Again, in 1838 (*Lond. Med. Gazette,* June 23) he is

combating the views of M. Lisle, also those of MM.
Levret and Mativie, regarding the nature of the pulse,
and repeating his old doctrines, of a diurnal revolution in
the *frequency* and *excitability* of the pulse, commencing
in the early part of the day, gradually attaining its
maximum about mid-day, and then declining until some
time after midnight.

Knox exhibited to the Royal Society, on January 15,
1838, specimens of the *Cysticercus Cellulosæ*, and maintained that the structure of the enclosing cyst or
capsule is an essential part of the worm, and that it is
not formed out of the surrounding cellular tissue ; and
that the disc of hooks served other purposes than
enabling the animal to attach itself, and probably were
connected more with the generative than the digestive
system ; as near the base of each hook he had seen
rounded or oval bodies which, he conjectured, were
young *Cysticerci.*

Sir Astley Cooper paid Edinburgh a visit in 1838,
and along with a courteous hospitality was shown everything of surgical interest, and what he had long dis-
believed, two well-authenticated cases of united fracture
of the neck of the *os femoris.* He spent an hour or two
in Knox's museum, but did not impress the Doctor with
the profundity of his remarks ; indeed, the Doctor was
peculiarly diverted by Sir Astley's comments upon
various professional matters, and his saying, "Ah ! we
do so and so at Guy's," or "We did so and so at St.
Thomas's ;" as if Cockaigne was the only atmosphere
that reflected British surgery and pathology.

Dr. John Reid, the famous physiologist, in examining two sharks, found no vestige of brain, or cerebral ganglia, or spinal cord in the upper part of the spinal canal. Being perplexed as to how the animals lived without the most important part of the cerebro-spinal system, he sent for Knox and others to look at them. On asking the Doctor what he thought of the anomaly, he replied : " My dear Reid, don't say anything about it ; nobody will believe you." On Dr. Reid pushing his interrogations further, and saying, was it not extraordinary ?—" Not the least extraordinary," replied Dr. Knox ; " if you go over to the Parliament House " (the Law Courts) "any morning, you will see a great number of live sharks walking about without any brains whatever."

In his short paper " On the Wild Ox of Scotland " (*Roy. Soc. Proc.*, April 2, 1838), Knox could offer no historical account of the animal, and believed that the white cattle of Britain did not constitute a distinct species of the bovine tribe : that is, distinct from any known species or variety of the domestic ox. He was disposed to associate the White Ox of Hamilton with the Galloway breed ; and believed they differed from the fossil specimens seen in museums, or which had been delineated by Cuvier.

In his article " On the Glands of Cowper in the Female " (*Lond. Med. Gazette*, January 19, 1839) he refers to his Essay on Hermaphrodite Structure, read to the Royal Society in 1828,[1] in which he maintained that the

---

[1] The Essay alluded to appeared in the *Medical Gazette*, 1843–44. He had " Observations on the Anatomy of the Human Fœtus, presenting several remarkable Congenital Deformities," in the *Edin. Journ. Med.*

"type of the generative systems of organs, both in the male and female, is hermaphrodite;" that is, in every individual embryo, all the organs which afterwards in an especial way characterise each sex of the human species are present. He was of opinion that—

1. The Glands of Cowper were present in both sexes, and *equally developed* in both.

2. That *both sets of organs* existed, as well normally as abnormally, in the full-grown individual—a view completely subversive of the French doctrine of transformation of organs.

3. That the doctrine of analogies could not be applied to the generative system in the sense that French and German authors had done, since the strictly *female* organs, instead of being analogous to the *male*, were precisely and in all respects the opposite and contrary.

He then gave a tabular view of the organs.

1. The embryo of the Mammalia is at first hermaphrodite.

2. The cause of the determination of the sex, and the precise period of the operation of this cause, is unknown.

3. If it fails, both sets of organs remain more or less perfect throughout life, and thus constitutes hermaphrodism to a greater or less extent.

4. The essential male organs, the testes, &c.

5. The essential female organs, the ovaria, &c.; yet

Science. In this fœtus the parietes of the abdomen were wanting, and the placenta was attached to the peritoneum. The genito-urinary organs opened into a large cavity connected with what appeared the termination of the intestinal canal. Other peculiarities existed.

these two sets of male and female organs, instead of being analogous to each other, are directly opposed.

6. The organs fully developed, but common to both sexes, are Cowper's Glands.

7. The rudimentary organs, whose presence in the adult is in accordance with the great law of formation, but which are of no physiological use to the individual.

He expressed his surprise that St. Hilaire should have described the remains more or less perfect of the *Vasa Deferentia* of the Ruminants and Pachydermatous animals, known under the names of the Ducts of Malpighi and of Gaertner, as "peritoneal tubes," when he had a long time ago shown them to be the remains of the *Vasa Deferentia of the male*, remaining in the rudimentary and consequently imperfect condition in the cow and pig. He described carefully the Glands of Cowper in the female—holding them to be as much developed as in the male, and the duct of the said glands as opening into the vulva, and not the vagina, as some had described ; he looked upon their functions as connected with the sexual desire. He highly approved of the dissections of De Graaff, Cowper, Morgagni, and others.

In a memorandum in Knox's own handwriting, made in January 1839, relative to his museum, he states that of a sum of 257*l.* 13*s.*, received for lectures on comparative anatomy (1825–26, I suppose), he got 190*l.* 3*s.*, and paid the remainder to Dr. Barclay, and then continues : "To support these lectures in a becoming manner, worthy of the country and myself, a museum was formed at an expense of about 2,000*l.* I have never used it since 1829, about which time it became unfashionable to study comparative anatomy, otherwise than from books and plates." Of the sum of 2,000*l.* invested by Knox in establishing his private museum, no doubt can be entertained by those who know the history of its formation ; but when he refers to the decadence of the study of comparative anatomy, he seems to have overlooked the fact of his having given special lectures on the subject to large classes long after 1829. His summer courses in 1825, 1826, and 1827 were well attended, and thoroughly appreciated in the school. Lying before me is the original document or requisition, signed by numerous of his advanced students, asking Knox to deliver a course of lectures on comparative anatomy in the session 1833, and to this request he at once acceded. The memorandum given above was made at a time when he began to despair of the Edinburgh School of Medicine.

Of the character and extent of the museum, and the wish of the owner to develop it still further, the reader may judge from the fact that in the year 1828 Knox paid a salary of 195*l.* a year to a conservator—a sum considerably more than the College of Surgeons, a chartered public body, paid their conservator. The Great Whale, he used to say, cost him nearly 500*l.*; probably he included all the Cetacea he had through his hands.

He bought every modern work that would elucidate his science, even the most costly illustrated ones from the continental press ; in short, he spared no means to render his anatomical teaching of the utmost possible service. While he did not spend 300*l.* a year on himself and family, he devoted the remaining large profits of his class to his museum and the advancement of science.

John Frederick Knox, generally known by the students as "Brother Fred," was a great concern, pecuniarily and otherwise, to Dr. Knox; indeed many adjudged him to be the Doctor's greatest plague in life. As conservator of the Knox Museum, and a great stickler for order and "maintenance intact," "Fred" had a horror of seeing anatomical preparations handled by the pupils of the class. Now, the Doctor viewed things more liberally, and the consequence was that the osteological department, if I may say it, afforded vastly too many bones of contention to the two brothers; in short, Fred's wilfulness and petty tyrannies cost the Doctor much temper. "Fred," it ought to be said, was the handsomer brother of the two, and seemed to pride himself upon this outward distinction—call it good luck. This hasty glance at the relations of the Brothers Knox will enable the reader more fully to appreciate the gist of the following paragraph.

A feeling of rivalry was often exhibited between the students attending Professor Monro and Dr. Knox, of which many proofs might be offered. It was repeatedly said by Knox's pupils "that nothing in the world could put him out;" that he could meet any *contretemps*, or the most alarming and unexpected contingency, with perfect composure and *sangfroid*. One of Monro's pupils would lay a heavy wager that he could disconcert Knox, or "put him out of his presence of mind;" and assuredly he made an impertinent, if not disgraceful, effort to win his bet. Watching his opportunity, he met Knox on his way home, and, planting himself immediately in his front and eyeing him steadily from head to foot, at length said : "Well, by Jove, Dr. Knox, you are the ugliest fellow I ever saw in my life !" "Ah," rejoined the Doctor, while he quietly patted the shoulder of the insolent intruder; "then you cannot have seen my brother Fred;" and then passed on his way as composedly as if he had been exchanging the ordinary civilities of the day with a passing acquaintance,—not the less rejoicing in his own imperturbable readiness and repartee, and at the grand revenge he had had for the moment by the hit at his worst grievance, "Brother Fred." How Knox could meet so unexpected an enemy in his walk, and in a moment cast the reproach of ugliness upon his "Brother Fred," almost baffles belief.

The *Lancet* of May 11, 1839, contains Knox's "Observations on the Structure and Physiology of the Eye and its Appendages." The operation for strabismus had become fashionable, and the discussion as to the action of the muscles of the eyeball had become invested with great interest; indeed so much so that surgeons from distant parts of the country repaired to the anatomical schools to rub up their knowledge of the said muscles, and, where practicable, to experiment on living monkeys; in short the "squint mania" prevailed, and very extensively, in Northern England. Knox's experiments induced him to state—

1. The Superior Oblique turned the pupil downwards and inwards, and drew the eyeball forwards, and if the

muscle was more strongly acted on, it turned the eye outwards.

2. The Inferior Oblique, when acted on *alone*, directed the pupil outwards and upwards, bringing the eyeball itself *forwards*.

3. When both Obliques were acted on, or shortened together, they pulled the eyeball forwards, and directed the pupil downwards and inwards.

4. When the Recti as well as the Obliques were acted on at the same moment so as to imitate their combined action during life, then the eyeball became fixed, and the pupil looked straight forwards.

Knox had, all his life, a natural horror [1] to experiments on living animals, and enjoyed the opportunity of showing that the experiments of Bransby Cooper and Sir C. Bell, on the monkey, had led these gentlemen to arrive at exactly opposite conclusions regarding the action of the muscles of the eyeball.

He objected to the opinion that the Recti were voluntary and the Obliqui involuntary muscles, and did not believe in the commonly received notion that when persons go to sleep the eyeball is under the guidance of the oblique muscles alone; nor did he believe in the eye being turned upwards and inwards during sleep or on the approach of death. On this latter point he was the more satisfied, as he had looked upon hundreds of brave men dying in hospitals. It was

---

[1] Words can hardly convey Knox's feelings towards the experimental physiologists—Magendie, Hall, Reid, and others—of his day. He shuddered as he depicted the barbarity of such proceedings, and spoke of Magendie and his school in no measured terms.

only in a few nervous and hysterical women, and in a few children, that he had observed such a phenomenon as the eye turned upwards and inwards.

On October 26th, 1839, the *Lancet* commenced the publication of Professor De Blainville's Lectures on Comparative Osteology, edited from the French, and additionally illustrated with numerous notes, observations, and drawings, by Dr. Knox. It was very praiseworthy on the part of the *Lancet* to introduce the historical and highly philosophical lectures of De Blainville to the English reader, and no one could have been found so well prepared to do justice to the translation and exposition of the Parisian Professor as Dr. Knox. The footnotes so frequently attached are very characteristic of Knox, and helped greatly to render the perusal of the text facile and interesting, and possibly more practical; moreover, the twenty lectures being well illustrated, and conveying the opinions of two such distinguished osteographers as De Blainville and Knox, helped the cause of biological science among the great body of English medical practitioners.

In April 1839 Knox asked John Goodsir, then a surgeon at Anstruther, Fife, to join him in the lectureship on anatomy, or, if he could not leave his father's practice, to persuade his brother Harry to take a share in the Practical Rooms. He urged upon the Goodsirs, that his "Brother Fred" was about to leave for New Zealand, and that they were wasting their time, energies, and abilities in the small burgh of Anstruther. For reasons explained in my Life of Goodsir, neither of the brothers could comply with Knox's wish. In the same month he applied to myself, and urged the very same reasons that he had offered my Fife friends. Feeling afraid of such a responsibility, I declined ; but after repeated solicitations extending over a year, and coun-selled by others, I consented to join Knox as his de-monstrator and partner, in May 1840.

Owing to Mr. Alexander Lizars gaining the Professor-ship of Anatomy in Aberdeen, Dr. Knox was induced to vacate Old Surgeons' Hall, where he had enjoyed such popularity and fame ten years previously, and join the Argyle Square Medical School, and of course as anato-mical lecturer. The same session, 1839-40, the Extra-mural Lecturers associated themselves under one institu-tion, which they termed " Queen's College of Edinburgh," in the hope of exercising a stronger rivalry against the University, which still rejoiced in certain monopolies by no means conducive to the welfare of the medical school at large, or its own special interests as a University with chartered privileges.

In the *Medical Gazette* Oct. 12 and Nov. 1, 1839, appeared "Contributions to Descriptive Anatomy,— The Pancreas," by Knox, who appended drawings and gave historical notes of the organ described.

The *Lancet* of May 9, 1840, contains the first part of Knox's "Contributions to the History of the Corpus Luteum, Human and Comparative." The second part does not seem to have appeared, nor is there in his paper any distinct solution of a question then undergoing much discussion both at home and abroad.

On the 16th May, or the next issue of the *Lancet*, his " Memoir on the Gibbon *Varié*, with a Critical Examina-

tion of Professor De Blainville's Account of the Gibbon,"
appeared. Knox possessed two authentic specimens of
the Gibbon, and evidently doubted the character of the
skeletons from which De Blainville drew his descriptions.
Here is a characteristic bit of Knox:—"We are quite
aware that the greater number of skeletons to be found
in museums are precisely of the nature of our author's
(De Blainville's) Gibbon ; that is, *composed or made up*
of a variety of *different animals*, in many cases differing
not only in species, but sometimes in genera. Thus we
have ourselves seen the trunk of an *elk* standing on the
limbs and supplied with the pelvis of a *common cow !*
We have seen the jaws of a young *dugong* filled with the
teeth of a *horse !*"

Knox gave a description of his two specimens of the
Gibbon, the skeletons of which had been prepared by
his brother Frederick ; the measurements in full, and all
the specially distinctive osteology of the animals.

On the following week (*Lancet*, May 23, 1840),
appeared his "Inquiry into the Present State of our
Knowledge respecting the Orang-Outang and Chimpanzee." Looking upon De Blainville's account of the
Orang-Outang and Chimpanzee as scanty and far from
authentic, he wished to show that the natural and
anatomical history of the adult of these two species of
most interesting Simiæ had not as yet been laid before
the public. Knox goes on to prove this by quoting
largely from Professor Owen's papers in the first volume
of the "Transactions of the Zoological Society," which
he criticised for their want of precision.

A few years previously he had some "Remarks on

the Structure of the Gibbons," in *Brewster's Edinburgh Journal of Science*, New Series, vol. i. p. 155. He had two specimens brought from Assam in spirits : they corresponded to the *Pithecus leuciscus* of Schreber and St. Hilaire. Whilst the cranial circumference of the male human adult was $21\frac{1}{2}$ inches, and the female $20\frac{1}{8}$ inches, the female Gibbon was only $9\frac{3}{4}$ inches. The height of the man was 69, of the woman $63\frac{1}{2}$, and the Gibbon (female) 32 inches.

In the *Medical Gazette* of Oct. 30, 1840, Knox had " Some Remarks on the Placental Tufts described by Weber : and on their Distribution and supposed Functions." This paper gave rise to a hot controversy in Edinburgh. Dr. John Reid, the physiologist, wrote a reply, which appeared in the *extra limites* of the *Medical Gazette* of Nov. 10, in which he accused Knox of having set forth certain anatomical facts which he had shown him upon a preparation of his own that was afterwards exhibited to the British Association Meeting at Glasgow in September of the same year. In proof of his severe animadversions upon Knox, Reid gave a history of his preparation, its examination by Knox in the presence of others, and his apparent acknowledgment of the novelty of the structures offered to his notice. On the other hand, Knox communicated to his class, in March 1839, what he considered new views of the anatomy of the placental tufts, and spoke much of Weber. Unfortunately, however, for his cause, the leading features of the anatomy had been got from Reid's preparation ; indeed, he admitted this much in his communication to the *Gazette*, and praised his former colleague for his great

courtesy in describing the parts. But why should Knox
have waited till October 1840 before he announced his
views, and one month at least after Reid had made
pretty nearly the same facts known to the British Association ? The evidence produced by Reid satisfied the
medical profession of Edinburgh that Knox was in the
wrong. The only remark that can be made in extenua-
tion of Knox was his marvellous power of vision, that
enabled him to penetrate far deeper into the minute
anatomy than his neighbours ; but even granting this,
his making public use of Reid's work and description
admits of no satisfactory explanation.

Knox felt much chagrined by the manifestation of
public opinion against him, and for a time avoided all recognition of his old anatomical friends. Even the amiable
John Goodsir was passed by in the street. He wished,
as he often told me, to remain isolated from those who
had joined the Reid standard, indeed from all connected
with the medical school ; and when I ventured to remark
that it would be sad to see him narrowing his circle of
friends, he replied, with bitter feeling, "My dear Doctor,
it is better to have no friends than doubtful ones."
After some weeks I got Knox to meet Goodsir under
my roof, and to forget the annoyances of the Reid
controversy.

The Lectureship on Anatomy to the art students of
the Scottish Academy being vacant in 1841, I was
induced by Lord Cockburn to become a candidate. On
soliciting Knox's aid he showed surprise, but said
nothing of himself either then or afterwards. Learning
from Sir Thomas Dick Lauder that Knox was at work

on his own behoof, I at once offered to withdraw my
application, out of respect to my old master and his
vastly superior claims. " You need not," said Sir Thomas,
" as poor Knox has not a vote, whilst your claims are
favourably received by the trustees of the Board." Mr.
James Miller, who on the following year was made
Professor of Surgery, and Mr. James Spence, now his
successor in the chair, were also candidates. Knox
was unquestionably the fittest man, yet he would not
have had a vote. Mr. Miller, seeing the chances of
success against him, played no less a game than the
"artful dodger," by offering his services gratuitously!
The temptation was too great for a Scottish Board,
proverbially poor, to pass by. What followed may be
surmised ; Mr. Miller's patriotism cooled down in the
course of the year, and then he asked for his predecessor's salary, and got it ! Knox's failure recalls Sir
Charles Bell's metropolitan experience. No one need be
told that Sir Charles was the greatest artistic anatomist
of the day, but he failed twice, if not thrice, in his application for the Professorship of Anatomy to the Royal
Academy in London.

CHAPTER XII.

Life at Home.—Prince of Talkers.—Ugly yet charming.—Historical
Contrasts.—The Actor and Story-teller.—Rural Enjoyments.—Dark
lines in the Portrait.—Trenchant Critic.—Tender-hearted and charitable.—The Bible and "Don Quixote."—Domestic Sorrows.

DR. KNOX'S acknowledged residence was 4, Newington-
place, on the south side of the city ; there his sister,
Miss Mary Knox, performed the part of hostess. He
gave dinners and evening parties in excellent style,
and with good musical accompaniments. Few men
knew more of music and musicians than Knox, who
was fond of contrasting the lofty feeling possessed
by the Germans and Italians with the slender attainments of the English : in the continental mind he read
the genius of music ; in the Britisher, but an evoking
of strains meet only for the Scotch bagpipes. He
used to say that his countrymen had never risen above
"Nancy Dawson" and "hum-drum ;" while, from
abroad, the glorious "Messiah" and the Dead March
in "Saul" had come to touch the chords of the human
heart, and to raise man to the contemplation of
the heavenly and glorious. It was a thorough treat
to see Knox responding to the music of Schubert and
Rossini when developed by skilful hands ; and if the

taste of the hour was in favour of a dance, he would readily join in an Irish jig, or the more welcome Scottish strathspey. His semi-pirouetting and graceful bowing, while he snapped his fingers consonantly with the emphatic notes, used to recall David Wilkie's picture of the Scotch merry-making, where fun and life are so strikingly portrayed. Everybody was made happy at Knox's fireside. The intellectual and the humorous could not fail to be pleased with mine host's talk and joke that always set the table in a roar. Knox at home was Knox triumphant; his cheery words and affable manner were as exhilarating as draughts of champagne. There was little need of the Falernian cup for prandial pleasantry if Knox fell upon a suitable theme for the display of his powers; nay, eating and drinking were unworthy of the hour sparkling with his wit and repartee.[1] My personal knowledge of De Quincey [2] was too limited to enable me to institute any comparison between his talking powers and those of Knox but others assure me, who met both these noted men in society, that the anatomist was fully entitled to the palm of distinction.

---

[1] A gentleman meeting Knox for the first time at dinner, at my lodgings in Edinburgh, was so charmed with his conversation that he begged for a weekly repetition—offering at the same time to furnish the symposium with Tokay or Johannisberg, suited to elicit the higher inspirations of the unrivalled conversationalist.

[2] De Quincey went to spend a night with Professor Wilson, and remained his guest a twelvemonth and a day. During this period "Christopher North" had many jovial parties, and when he wished for De Quincey's best talk, he reminded the philosopher of the exact hour for his display. The opium-eater took his dose accordingly, and then laid down on the hearth-rug till the dinner-bell rang. When his tongue got loose o'er the walnuts

Music had a great charm for Knox. He used to
invite me to accompany him in his visits to a lady
pianist, and on our way would purchase a basket of
fruit for her acceptance—an act of graciousness not
without its meaning. It was as natural to him to be
kind and sympathizing with women, whom he held to
be influential actors in the social world, as to stand with
convincing front before his public class, and there de-
nounce the tendencies of the age to imperfect methods
of learning. How he would have received the woman's
rights question of to-day is difficult to say ; but woman,
in her own circle, he considered as predominant as
man could be in his : the limitation or boundary line
of the sexes he, however, held to be clearly established
in modern society. As a classical scholar, a man of
refined taste and accomplishments, Knox was admirably adapted for society ; in his knowledge of the
world, and eagerness in scanning the men and women
playing upon its stages, few could rival him. His
originality of thought, his faculty of dressing up everything in striking freshness, and his remarkable fluency
of speech, showed him to be a man of rare attributes.
Possessing a happy diplomacy that could enable him
to reconcile the conflicting differences of a strongly-
argued question—and the spirit of disputation was not

and the wine, he would talk for hours on Greek plays and philosophy,
Egyptian mysteries, political economy, Shakespeare and Schiller, poets,
philanthropists, and beggars, and "*de omnibus et quibusdem aliis.*" People
listened to him as a Delphic oracle, and wondered at the unfailing source of
his ideas. Knox possessed the same charms, and with a greater coherency
than the opium-eater, left a larger and more lasting impression upon his
hearers.

uncommon in the polite circles of Edinburgh—Knox, by
his fresh interpretation of the argument, or persuasiveness,
was oft acknowledged as a desirable guest. He could
adapt himself to the conventionalisms of the world as
readily as take part in the intellectual arena with the
best men of his epoch, and in the most varied walks
of science. He was more English than Scottish in
character, and his urbanity savoured of French extraction : his graceful courtesy found its true place amid
the amenities of elegant society.

Neat in his attire, fashionable, or rather *distingué*, in
dress, he omitted nothing in the way of adornment to
secure attention ; but the richest costume would hardly
have availed had not the silvery tongue been brought
into play, which ever proved victorious. Dr. Macdonald,
now Professor of Natural History at St. Andrews, was
one day unexpectedly ushered into Dr. Knox's dining-
room, and there discovered the great anatomist subject-
ing the few locks of brown hair on his occiput to the
curling-tongs of his sister Mary. "Ah ! ah !" ejaculated
Macdonald ; "I see—the modern Apollo attired by the
Graces !" This successful impromptu was a bit of hard
hitting; nor was the anatomist far behind his friend
in the adroit way in which he got out of the dilemma ;
indeed, any amount of affectedness that might be manifested by Knox was redeemed at once by his superior
mind, so antipodal to what is met with in the mere
dandy. A calm in conversation was Knox's opportunity, and when obtained, the night was all his own.
Men, and especially women, were beguiled to listen to
him, and to listen was to believe in all they heard

from his lips, whether the narrative were simple,
historical, or fictional.

> " Hear him debate of Commonwealth affairs,
> You would say,—it hath been all-in-all his study ;
> List his discourse of war, and you shall hear
> A fearful battle render'd you in music :
> Turn him to any cause of policy,
> The Gordian Knot of it he will unloose,
> Familiar as his garter."

Seen in the social circle, Knox presented a figure in
marked contrast to his public gladiatorship. His graceful attitudes, his " at home " feeling and happy style
of converse, which so soon placed him *en rapport* with
others, could not fail to enlist a circle of admirers
around him ; and that circle always widened in the
drawing-room till it sometimes included the whole
assembly. Knox gloried in this kind of tribute that
placed him in the focus of attraction, and singled him
out as the oracular man of the party. Neither his name
nor his physiognomy were altogether in good favour
out of doors ; the same feeling prevailed on his first
entering a reception-room ; but as curiosity was drawn
towards the notability of the medical school, his discussion of the absorbing topics of the day, his *suaviter
in modo* recognition of the fair representatives of the
social gathering, in time dispelled the shadowy clouds
surrounding his repute ; and Knox at length came to
be pronounced " a delightful " or " a charming person "
by the prettiest of women.

The excellent portraits of Knox in this volume
convey a capital idea of the man in life and action ;
yet it might be said of him what Chauveau Lagarde,

the advocate of Charlotte Corday, said of his historical client : that her portrait might be tolerably
shown on canvas, but could not possibly reflect " *sa
grande âme, respirant toute entière dans sa physio-
nomie.*" Whilst Mirabeauan in force and oratorical
display, Knox's face somewhat resembled that of the
coarse and ugly revolutionist ; the fire of genius irra-
diated the visages of both men. Like John Wilkes the
demagogue, in being ugly yet attractive, like him also
Knox was scrupulously attentive to dress, and could be
equally successful in affairs of gallantry. Both men
were disposed to joke [1] on their ill-favoured looks ; so
did Fouché in the studio of David the painter. As
Othello's colour proved no hindrance to the love of
Desdemona, who ran from " her guardage to the sooty
bosom," so Wilkes and Knox found no impediments in
their looks to various conquests of the heart. It is said
that women shunned

"The wealthy, curled, darlings of the nation,"

to converse with the rabid politician of George III.'s
reign : the same feeling prevailed towards *our* anatomist. Knox had an advantage over men, whether of
the intellectual or the ugly school, in being able to tell
the stories of his life,

"Of moving accidents by flood and field,"

in the choicest Italian, and with a gentleness of manner

---

[1] Knox one day called my attention to a Manx student with red hair,
freckled face, wry features, and lean and lank frame, and said · " Doctor, do
you see that person at the other end of the dissecting-room—he of the scare-
crow looks ? Well, I always thought myself very plain-visaged ; but by all
that's precious, I am fairly beaten out of the field of ugliness by that fellow."

directed towards his fair hearers that made them part-
ners in his descriptions; no wonder his narratives, spiced
with the sensational, wrought as "mixtures powerful o'er
the blood" of women. They hung upon his sweet and
honeyed sentences as if he had been the prophet of a
new Mormonic faith, in the mysteries of which they
might hope to share, either as spiritual wives or minister-
ing angels.

Ripe in ideas and in the knowledge of men and manners, and not less ripe in utterances bespeaking a cultured
mind, Knox was admirably equipped for his position.
Well might youths nurtured in the isolated glens of
Perthshire or the retired dales of Westmoreland, and
brought for the first time within reach of Knox, seem
spell-bound, when those of mature age and worldly wisdom could not withstand his inspiriting manner and
plausible speech. How readily he could adapt himself
to the thoughts of the passing hour! Was it a piece of
gossip? he solved its character in a word. Was it a
social *faux pas?* he would urge Uncle Toby's advice on
such matters, or laugh it out of court. Was it a scientific
dispute? he would condemn the *ipse dixits* of partisans,
and call for an appeal to facts. Was it a Government
blunder or a job? he would produce a tabulated series of
such, and drown them in a flood of invective. Whig
commissions, Tory shams, scientific coteries and nepo-
tisms, Town Council "worthies," professorial intrigues,
medical shopocracy, *et hoc genus omne,* were favourable
targets for his well-aimed shafts of ridicule; and his
shots, if not always "bull's-eyes," were rarely outside the
white circle. "Ah, ah!" quoth Knox, in a smiling

humour, whilst addressing an old friend ; "have you heard the latest news ? " This was but a prelude to his description of some medical schemers whose rehearsals and parts he could prefigure so well ; indeed, as he talked you saw the *dramatis personæ* crossing the stage, and could hear the prompters at the side wings, and be *en rapport* with the varied scenes of the play, throughout its five or more acts, to its moral, or more probably its immoral, *dénouement.* But why speak of the simulated drama, when Knox's rhetorical figures, fancies, and sentiments *au naturel* constituted the richest of all entertainments, and, as such, far beyond all price ? What were " London *artistes*" or " provincial stars " in full choir, compared with Knox in his every-day mood, on his own platform —casting a dozen parts in the hour, each a happy coun- terfeit of nature's players ? Who could so pointedly set forth the manner of Hamlet, or so ably play on the pipe that discoursed such eloquent music ?

Everybody who has moved in what is called genteel society must have come across persons deemed "highly agreeable men," or " charming women," whose conversa- tion lay in an inflated or embellished style. Such persons are not without their use in the many dull and vapid circles of English life now-a-days termed *réunions :* their talk gives a piquancy to domestic narrative, and a brighter blue to gossip and garrulity. " Our hero" had this kind of thing in full measure. If his sails were fairly set to the wind, were they not filled with the Southern zephyrs redolent of Eastern glow and spicy fragrance ? And who could resist the temptation of a voyage with such a pilot, especially if the prows of

the ship were pointed to that haven of bliss, the Knox-
Arcadia ? Privileged as the traveller of fifty years ago
naturally was, when African explorers were few and far
between, he exercised all the claims granted to such a
position, and not unfrequently astonished his own countrymen as effectively as if their skulls had been tre-
panned for the reception of his wit.[1] Knox was a Defoe
in story-telling ; you saw the footprints on the sand,
even to the impress of the toe-nails of "Friday," and
all the wider surroundings of Robinson Crusoe : in short,
his narrative was as refreshing as a clear and limpid
stream to a dusty, fatigued pedestrian.

He used to tell with great animation the story of the
Caffre whose anatomical knowledge proved so fatal to
a band of British soldiers. In attempting to cross a
ravine, it became needful to go single file down a bank
thickly set with brushwood ; several soldiers passed out
of sight, but gave no signs of having reached the bottom.
The Captain got anxious, and despatched some of his
company by a circuitous route ; and, behold, they found
their comrades lying in their own gore. As the soldiers
stepped down, a Caffre stealthily plunged a knife into the
vessels at the lowest part of the neck of each man : so

---

[1] The Doctor should not for a moment be ranked with the class of vulgar
boasters such as the gallant Major "just returned to town after a delightful
visit to a noble country mansion, situated amid extensive parks and picturesque scenery, with loveable gardens and sculpture, all of the highest and
most *recherché* character ;" when the simple description, the unvarnished tale,
would have shown only a suburban villa with "picturesque" support from
a neighbour's gable wall, a dusty road, and duck-pond ; and instead of the
Versailles style of gardens, two small beds of Tom Thumb geraniums,
relieved, not by Greek sculpture, but the humbler forms of Staffordshire
pottery.

expert was the wild denizen in stabbing the vital part, that the Britisher fell at once, and never uttered a groan.

When dining at Bathgate with Dr. Reid's friends, Knox gave an account of a military expedition against the Caffres; of 500 British rank and file engaged, the precise number that fell by the way at the hands of the enemy, or from *coup de soleil*, the entire force at last dwindling down to some units; of his galloping among the vanguard across the plain; of the fine instinct of the horses hastening to the solitary palm or bush that marked a watering-place in the desert; the rush of steeds and their riders to drink the muddy water as if it had been a mountain stream, &c. Whilst Knox was fascinating all listeners by his graphic narrative, a West Lothian laird, rejoicing in his knowledge of "Cocker," asked what became of the 357 soldiers of whom no account had been given, and at the same time expressed his surprise at so marvellously small a remnant of the Britishers being left. Knox was imperturbable to even the repetition of such questions; but when the interrogator hung by his coat-tails and would not be shaken off, he would reply, "My dear sir, sheep require shepherds to count them, but armies don't carry arithmeticians and markers into the field." With this turning of the tables, followed by uproarious laughter, the bucolic matter-of-fact person found it best to appeal to his "whisky toddy," and leave the African story-teller to pursue his own course.

Like all anatomists, Knox specially enjoyed an excursion to the country; and a few days at Anstruther, the home of the Goodsirs, or amid friends whom he esteemed, gladdened his heart, and gave fresh tone to his mind·

His pleasantest holiday was spent on the banks of the Tay, or by Tweed-side, with rod in hand, and a companion to his liking, such as his hearty friend Dr. Stuart, of Kelso. His enjoyment of angling was only limited by the Borders, for in every Scottish river he cast his fly and filled his basket. After taking up his residence in London he tried the southern waters, but his old love was constant for the picturesque streams and heathery mountains of his native land.

Knox advocated temperance, early rising, and frequent change of linen. He maintained that thirst was unnatural to a man in a healthy state ; that he himself was never *water*-thirsty, though more than occasionally *wine*-thirsty. He was moderate in his cups under the most tempting allurements of Bacchus presented in silver jugs and clearest crystal. He naturally enjoyed the sumptuous dinners of his friend the Marquis of Breadalbane, in the Royal Palace of Holyrood. This rich nobleman had been a pupil of Knox's, and never forgot the attractive lectures of his distinguished teacher ; nor was the Marchioness less kind, so that on their annual visit to Holyrood they received Knox regularly. Though broad and sympathetic in his relations, and ready to do justice to a simple repast with a friend who welcomed him and gave willing ear to his converse, Knox liked high breeding and princely feasts. Whilst holding himself a true Saxon or born democrat, he dearly loved the attentions of a lord of ancestral name and in the possession of rich perquisites. Democracy with Knox, as with many others, was very well in the abstract ; it claimed for itself a lofty disinterestedness that sounded of Spartan patriotism ; but then it demanded a rigid self-denial, and a lowering of the social and intellectual standard, irre-concilable with Knox's aspirations after the ideal and realistic enjoyments of English life.

As a portrait of the anatomist without its shadows and sinuous lines would be no portrait at all, it is need-ful to mention that on matters of business involving a *bonâ fide* principle, Knox was prone to be evasive ; whilst on matters of fact he was not always considered trust-worthy. His prevarication at times was without any ostensible ground ; at other times it seemed dictated by selfish motives ; but under no circumstances whatever could it be held excusable : it bore upon personalities more than worldly affairs ; but, oddly enough, looseness of statement was not manifested by him in his scientific walk. In that direction, to the best of my knowledge, he sought after truth, and was ever anxious to render justice to the labours of his contemporaries in every department of science. When strangers to the quarrels of the profession in Edinburgh asked why such virulent opposition was shown towards Knox, they were told of his want of candour, his egotism, and marked disparagement of other people's characters ; all which faults were recog-nizable enough ; but unfortunately there was no *audi alteram partem* to mitigate the seeming severity of a man trying to repel his enemies by paying them back in their own coin. He would not conform to general usages or assent to the conventional and official dicta of either colleges or churches ; to have done so would have been a tacit submission of his own judgment to the enfeebling opinions of others. The line he took was too clearly innovating and independent; and to call a spade a spade forty years ago as now, was held to be offensive to etiquette, and incompatible with the safe working of established institutions. Knox was not free from the casuistry of the schools that hunted with the hare and held with the hounds; but he erred oftener in being too bold and explicit in his views, whether right or wrong; and left nothing to be inferred that was capable of interpretation against his enemies. He had a way of his own, and that not always discreet. Who, however, could expect to see the analytic, penetrating, and transmutative powers of such a man tied down to ancient or modern precedent, to academic lines, or scholastic dogmas? Who of those who knew his powerful mental grasp could expect him, a Samson in science, to be tamely submissive to the shears of the conventional Delilah of the period?

It was well said by Emerson, that in England the keeping of the proprieties is as indispensable as clean linen; that no merit can countervail the want of this, whilst it sometimes stands in lieu of all. Knox had no regard for our "Gibraltar of propriety," where "mediocrity gets intrenched and consolidated and founded on adamant." Saxon that he was, he saw vastly too much of the adamant and stubbornness of his race, their impatience of genius, and their disposition to cavil with any boldness of expression or sallies of thought calculated to interfere with the even, amiable tenor of society, or their own natural instincts.

Robert Knox the anatomist, as a trenchant critic and damaging opponent of both men and institutions, gave the best proof of his descent from John Knox the sweeping Radical Reformer, who spared neither Popes nor Queens. On the side of the Reformer, public opinion was ripe for the demolition of a system that ill accorded with the growing ascendency of human thought. In the limited sphere traversed by the anatomist of these latter days, it was a single-handed effort against large professional odds : both men had their opinions, and fought strenuously to uphold them. As in the sixteenth, so in the nineteenth century, who dared to oppose *the* Knox of Edinburgh—so ready in fence, so incisive in stroke, that not even the simile of the Damascus blade could set forth the worth of his steel? He was a bold knight who entered the lists against either of the Knoxes. The cynicism of the anatomist drew upon him lots of enemies, but no one dared to meet him in the open field. Yes, there was one exception to the ambush mode of attack, when Knox defended his views on the *Salmonidæ* before the Royal Society, already described in page 192. The parties who acted in concert on that memorable occasion levelled shaft after shaft against Knox, who withstood all complacently; and when the last shot had fallen upon his impenetrable armour, he advanced to the front, and speedily his enemies were swept from the field like stubble before the wind.

Knox did not deal in rubbishing paste ornaments; he had his cameos and precious stones, and these he surrounded with a true Tuscan setting. Such adornment was displeasing to plain matter-of-fact men, who, being unable to rival the Knox workmanship, cried it down as obtrusive and gaudy. Science used to be recorded in very

formal lines or propositions or heads of guidance, and
terribly dry-as-dust—reminding you of the *nineteenthly*
and not always *finally*, of the long-winded sermons of
the Scotch preachers. Such a farrago of professional
writing was distasteful to Knox, and should have been
to others of lesser fame : his eschewing all the old
paths, the dull and dreary and monotonous, and enlivening his statements with a flowing diction, instead
of being welcomed for its pleasantness and novelty, was
cited as a proof of his words being a colouring of events,
a varnished tale rather than the statement of a scientific
argument.

If disposed to be censorious of public institutions, or
to pick a hole in his neighbour's coat, Knox was not
without a kind and sympathizing nature. He combined
in his own person the extremes of courage and of tenderness ; and merited in part the compliment paid to
Sir J. Franklin by Sir J. Parry—"that he never turned
his back on a danger, yet was of that tenderness that
he would not brush away a mosquito." He was humane,
compassionate, and kind-hearted. People of limited and
vulgar thought are apt to look upon the anatomist in no
higher light than the butcher ; and the Law itself has
done no better in its refusing to accept both members of
the community as jurymen in our courts of justice. Of
the hydra-headed popular fallacies prevalent in nineteenth-century England, notwithstanding her churches,
her missionaries, and Reformed Parliaments, none is
greater than the supposition of the anatomist's familiarity
with the dead impairing or destroying his respect for the
living. Without wishing to obtrude a personal sensitive-

ness to human suffering, I can safely claim for a large majority of my anatomical friends the possession of the highest regard and delicacy for their species in every relation of life. Knox was the very antipodes of the Irish satirist, Dean Swift, and could well afford to laugh at the sentimentality of Laurence Sterne weeping over the dead donkey. Of his sympathies, both broad and special, many instances might be cited. I shall be content with one furnished me by my friend Dr. James Adams, of Glasgow.

At a meeting of the Glasgow Medico-Chirurgical Society (1844), Dr. Knox was present when a case of fearful mutilation was being exhibited by one of the surgeons. After the poor fellow had undergone the examination of the meeting, a subscription for his benefit was spontaneously taken up, and a hat was sent round, in which "a shower of sixpences was soon collected." Dr. Adams, sitting beside Dr. Knox, observed him very stealthily slip a crown-piece into the hat. Soon after leaving the meeting, Knox went into a baker's shop and purchased a penny roll and asked for a glass of water. The roll he ate in portions from his pocket, during a strolling perambulation of the street with his friends Drs. A. and J. Adams, who, on comparing notes, found that Knox had had no dinner that day; that he was low in pecuniary means, and that his only meal since breakfast was the penny roll and glass of water.

Knox's heart was as readily touched as most men's, when the sympathies of our common humanity were fairly put to the test. I have known him almost in tears on seeing cases of disease attended by acute or prolonged suffering. He had a kind word also for animals, and could not bear to see them harshly dealt with ; whilst his repugnance to vivisection amounted to something like horror. He admitted the great advantages gained for physiology by Sir Charles Bell's experiments on living animals, leading to important discoveries in the whole field of Neurology, but he maintained that Sir Charles's experiments were of limited extent, and afforded no justification for the aimless probings and torturings practised by Magendie and his disciples. The expression of detestation Knox used to manifest towards the French experimental physiologists was by no means lessened in force when their English imitators came to be animadverted upon. Unquestionably he had a fine sensibility in relation to physical suffering in either man or brute, and would have done anything for its relief ; the same generous feeling, in all probability, had to do with his aversion to oppression in every shape affecting man's moral or political nature. Reflecting on his large sympathies and special sensibility, how grossly vile must appear the vituperation heaped upon his head after the West Port disclosures ! He would not have caused pain to the lowest of living creatures, much less touch the lives of innocent men, yet he was repeatedly spoken of as if he had inherited the worst feelings that could be found in the most savage barbarian.

At all times and seasons, he was alike consistent in enjoining that pain should be relieved at whatever cost in treating disease—the same with the brute. Looking one day at the Carnivora in the Edinburgh Zoological Gardens, he observed a large swelling upon the fore-paw of a lion, and drew the keeper's attention to it. No one would venture to approach the animal to see what was wrong. After careful watching of the lion's movements, he diagnosed the presence of an abscess, and fixing a lancet to the end of a long stick, succeeded in puncturing the swelling and relieving the afflicted monarch of the woods. He always expressed his regret that some effort had not been made to treat the jaguar—"Carter's great tiger"—that died of pleurisy in Edinburgh, and noticed in another page of this volume.

Walking arm in arm along the public street with Dr. James Adams, and while in the full flow of animated conversation, Dr. Knox suddenly left his side, and retracing a few steps, picked up a large crust of bread lying on the pavement. A few minutes afterwards he placed the crust conspicuously on the parapet of a railing. Being asked for an explanation, Knox said he had from his youth never seen a wasted piece of food without a painful visage becoming immediately present in his mind of some wretch in the pangs of hunger, and that he was quite unable to pass by a piece of food exposed to waste. Not unfrequently he had set aside a crust of bread, as on the present occasion, and then loitered about until gratified by seeing it "pounced upon eagerly by some picturesque specimen of our common humanity."

Knox was like the Mahometan in regard to the saving of every crumb of bread; in his eyes nothing should be wasted that could be applied to the service of man. These anecdotes show the kindly disposition of the anatomist. His own wants were few, and happily so, as his deprivations were many after the year 1842, when the

tide was ebbing strongly, and his domestic life had become
so changed. The world was vastly less kind to him than
he was to the Glasgow cripple ; had it shown a tithe of
the bounteous charity that could unpocket a crown-piece
for the help of a proletariat, and reserve only a penny
roll for his own dinner, Knox would have been well off.

He used to say that two books were always to be
found on the table of his dressing-room, the Bible and
"Don Quixote," whom he used to style the *beau idéal* of an
accomplished gentleman ; their positions might be incongruous, and to some it would appear profane or immoral
to associate them : he could not help it ; there they were
for his reading and instruction. Now, whatever benefit
he might derive from the Bible must remain untold,
but undoubtedly he could quote its pages as readily as
any ancient divine. On one occasion, when the noble
part performed by the Covenanters was under discussion,
Knox warmed with his subject, and spoke vehemently
of the heroism of his countrymen, in whose ranks he
would above all things have wished to be enrolled ; and
as he pictured some of his forefathers in the conflict, he
quoted the strongest passages of the Psalmist, and with
uplifted arms and reddened visage seemed little less than
inspired with biblical mindedness. Under such circumstances, he would claim his descent from " the Reformer,"
who " truly deserved that name ; the man to whom Scotland owes her liberty, freedom of conscience, exemption
from tithes and bishops, popery and prelacy, alike abhorred by Scot." In recalling these struggles for liberty
of thought, in which the ancestral blood had mingled,
his own democratic feeling was roused to its highest

pitch ; and had the times demanded a platform for its display, Knox the anatomist would have called forth more national fervour and more devoted heroism than the Reformer himself accomplished two centuries previously.

Dr. Knox having lost a favourite child from scarlatina, asked me to accompany him to the interment in Newington Cemetery, a few hundred yards from his residence. He and myself constituted the entire following to the grave-side. Going along, he spoke with pain of the custom of day-interments, of the tried feelings of parents harassed by witnessing the procession and other steps of the funeral, and of being exposed to the morbid curiosity of the people in the streets. He extolled the practice of the Roman and of modern Catholic countries, where the burial of the dead took place in the shadow of night. *Inter alia* he cited Daniel O'Connell's remarks on Lord Brougham's mad behaviour at the grave-side of his daughter ; and so beguiled the way to and from the cemetery : and this helped to soften the anguish of his last farewell of a child he had loved so affectionately. His anxiety to restrain the sorrowful emotions of his heart was an effort that must have cost him dear ; for no man had deeper affections, or could feel the touching sympathy of a friend more truly, than Knox.

When his wife died, in 1841, after puerperal fever, he sought me early the following morning to tell me of his loss. The effort to appear gracious as he approached could not be sustained ; his face and eyes betrayed what he had passed through, and all he could say on clasping my hands in his own was—" She is gone, she is gone ! "

Of the six children she bore to him, five died before himself. His son Edward is the only survivor. He was advised to withdraw from the rooms for a week, but the day after the funeral he returned to his ordinary pursuits, feeling, as thousands of suffering hearts have done, that occupation and duty are the only chances of lessening present griefs and diverting the thoughts till that great arbiter, Time, spreads his softening wings over the sorrows of the soul. Poor Knox, though wanting in many things, was sound to the core when love and affection stood face to face with the sufferings of mortality.

CHAPTER XIII.

The Philosophy of Anatomy.—Newton, Goethe, St. Hilaire, Serres. &c.
—Wings of the Angels!—Supra-Condyloid Process.—Hip Joint.—
Surgical Opinions.—Monkey and Man.—Lectures in Glasgow.—The
sad Fall.

THE idea of a general unity or type in the animal
structure had been pregnant to Aristotle and the leading
minds of Natural History and Philosophy in ages long
gone by. William Lawrence, the most philosophic of English surgeons of this century, spoke of Aristotle's classification of animals as based on the theory of analogies in
organs, and constituting a "vast and luminous plan to
which none of his successors had approached." Sir Isaac
Newton, who thought deeply about the Cosmic atoms
and the nature of organisms, as well as Physics, had
evidently got a ray of light on this subject when he
wrote, "*Similiter posita omnia in omnibus fere ani-
malibus,*" and this unity was by him referred to laws
similar to those which regulate the economy of the
universe. The theory of analogies, however, as Dr.
Fletcher records, or the idea that to certain corresponding organs of all animals there is a

"" Facies non omnibus uña,
Nec diversa tamen,"

R 2

only acquired scientific import in the hands of Geoffroy
St. Hilaire. Now Knox appears to have been among
the foremost to make St. Hilaire's doctrines on the unity
of organic structure known to large classes of British
students. His lectures on osteology were all the more
attractive that he indicated to the pupils the structural
elements or essential parts of each bone in man, the
developmental relations these bore to other vertebrated
animals, the borrowing of elements, so to speak, here,
the imparting of elements there ; or what St. Hilaire
called *balancement des organes*, and, as he further
expressed, "*l'atrophie d'un organe tourne toujours au profit
d'un autre.*" Knox used to speak of a presumed unity
as rather that of structural elements or primitive types
than that of whole organs ; and here he showed his
scientific caution, as it was more frequently the structural elements alone, and not the organs, which could
with propriety be said to be repeated.

Bearing upon the unity and history of organic structures, Knox gave much attention to the laws of development as illustrative of the general argument, and as
valuable contributions to a more philosophic anatomy.
With a good teaching museum, rich in osteology, he had
ample opportunities of setting forth his views, and imparting a large amount of physiological and surgical
information. Having also numerous preparations exemplifying organogenesy, he would trace with great skill
the individual organs in their progressive evolution
through the foetal state, and seek to extend the theories
of Serres as to embryonic forms in the higher tribes
repeating the permanent form of the lower orders of

beings. Following out his own pertinent and unique mode of instruction, he would hold up to his class a small phial containing the *Cysticercus cellulosus*, and another with the first trace of the human ovum (found in the Fallopian tube), and then remark: " Gentlemen, there is no appreciable difference, as far as you can observe, in the bodies floating in these two phials; but what do you suppose would be their future history if placed in their proper habitat and furnished with nutrition ? The one—the *Cysticercus*—will remain *in statu quo*, microscopic in the world of life, yet marvellously mischievous in its way in human tissues ; the other, teeming with force or the *vis genetrix naturæ*,

> " To ascend
> From small beginnings to a glorious end,"

would make a long journey of progression, and, after passing through many phases towards his *ultimatum*, eventually become what the poet termed the paragon of animals—Man himself! The opportunity of contrasting the *homicida* with the *homunculus*, the parasite with his prey, was great for Knox ; and on such a peg he could hang philosophy and moral reflections, pathology and Hudibrastic satire, to your heart's content.

Looking to a prototype of form or type upon which all organized bodies were based—the fungus and the polype being but epitomized emblems of the lofty pine and reasoning man—the observant anatomist might be disposed to sanction the doctrine of Pascal, that " animated beings were, in their commencement, nothing but formless and ambiguous individuals, whose constitution was originally decided by the permanent circumstances in the midst of which they lived ; "[1] or the modified view entertained by Lamarck, and more largely dwelt upon by St. Hilaire in his *"Philosophie Zoologique."* Knox believed in all nature's work being admirably wrought out ; in other words, a perfection in creation; and that to each individual in the scale of being the lot of physical enjoyment fell in accordance with its organization.

In the hands of the author of the " New Heloise," the great sentimentalist of his epoch, Phytology subserved a new philosophical idea that Goethe, without previous concert, but rather in a flashed moment of inspiration, extended to the highest mammal ; a doctrine which came to be unfolded by the labours of J. P. Franks, Oken, A. Meckel, Spix, Carus, Bojanus, Burdach, and others in Germany ; by Geoffroy St. Hilaire, Burdin, Dumeril, and others in France. Knox imbibed the Germanic, or transcendental anatomy, as it was called, from St. Hilaire, and preached the new doctrines from his earliest career as a lecturer. While he spoke of the similarity of constitution traceable in the osseous formation of the vertebræ and cranium, the English student, fond of matter-of-fact principles, was disposed to smile at the " Transcendentalists." Knox rode no hobby in this matter, but gave a cautious exposition of both the data and the doctrines—the best precursor to further

---

[1] Pascal seems to have anticipated by two centuries at least the protoplasmic theory which Huxley gets considerable credit for having originated less than two years ago. It is not too much to say that the same views had long been pregnant to other minds in this country.

inquiry among men whose minds had to be prepared for a further insight into the Continental philosophy. It is probable that his own opinions were in accordance with those expressed by M. Serres (*Anatom. Comp. du Cerveau,* 1824, p. 21) in reference to this subject : " *Quelques lustres se sont à peine écoulés, et déjà cette idée, devenue classique, a changé la face de la Science, et a fait naître une partie toute nouvelle, celle des Homologues.*"[1] Considering his natural acumen, marked individuality, and enlarged views, it is somewhat singular that Knox did so little in Morphology—a walk so captivating and fairly claimant of his higher study. Hazarding little of his own, he rested content with being the chief exponent of his master, St. Hilaire's views ; and as Sir C. Bell and others in authority either did not see or would not listen to the morphological argument, there

[1] Knox was eloquent on the science of transcendental or philosophic anatomy, " whose object it was to explain in a connected chain the pheno- mena of the living material world ; to connect the history of living plants and animals with those which now lie entombed in the strata of the crust of the globe ; to explain the mysterious metamorphoses which occur in the growth of animals and plants from their embryonic state to their maturity of growth and final decay ; to trace a plan of creation, and to guess at that plan,—these are the objects of transcendental anatomy. To the South German, to the mixed race of Slavonian and German origin, we owe this doctrine of transcendental anatomy ; to that imaginative race to whom we owe all that is imaginative, romantic, and transcendental in the so-called German language and German people. In a vertebra the matter-of-fact Saxon mind sees merely a vertebra ; beyond this it seldom proceeds— uninventive, unimaginative. Nor is the Celtic mind very peculiarly gifted in this respect: the doctrines of Goethe and of Spix, of Oken and of Geoffroy, were resisted to the last by Cuvier and by the Academy over which he held sway. Sir Charles Bell could never comprehend the import of the transcendental doctrine ; he stood by the coarse utilitarianism of Paley, which with him was the *ne plus ultra.*"

was but small encouragement to pursue the subject beyond the wants of his class. In time, however, matters greatly changed, and his pupils, Owen and Goodsir, came boldly to the front, and gained high historical position in the ranks of philosophical anatomy.

He wished anatomy to be regarded, not as a heap of ultimate facts more or less isolated and detached, but as a consistent and rational science, each instance of which has an obvious relation to every other in the series. Marking the rapid strides towards the perfection of his science, he was in hopes that, in due season, Nature's great organic laws, in all their harmony and simplicity, would be revealed to the earnest searcher after truth.

In the meantime, Morphology had to wait for further interpretation. Disposed as Knox was to accord tolerable latitude to novelty of doctrine, he never could give countenance to the supermundane hypotheses of his friend Professor W. Macdonald, whose anatomical inquiries led him far beyond and above the human form to the contemplation of that diviner sort of beings called angels, and to a special structure—the wing, morphologically termed "a limb"—always associated with their supposed corporeity. The physical structure of man had ever been looked upon as enough for man to understand. Not so, thought the Scottish Professor, when he occupied the attention of the Royal Physical Society of Edinburgh (in 1841?) with an essay "On the Physical Structure of the Angels."[1]

[1] Benjamin Disraeli, M.P., it can hardly be forgotten, in addressing a large gathering of "bucolics" in Buckingham three years ago, said he

Dr. Knox made several communications to the Anatomical and Physiological Society in Edinburgh; perhaps none of his papers claimed so much interest as that "On the Occasional Presence of a Supra-Con-dyloid Process in the Human Humerus" (*Edin. Med. and Surg. Journ.* vol. lvi. p. 125). The history of the paper was altogether a curious one. Whilst Dr. Knox and myself were arranging a series of humeri for the morning lecture, my finger was caught by a sharp spicula of bone on the inner side of an adult humerus; and further examination revealed a process or eminence of bone along the inner ridge of other specimens. It was quite new to Knox, and, at first sight, difficult of interpretation. Reflecting, however, on the comparative anatomy of the arm, Knox, with his usual acumen and readiness to grasp any anatomical difficulty, said: " This is a rudimentary structure, Dr. Lonsdale, and rest assured you will some day find in man a supra-con-dyloid foramen transmitting the brachial vessels and median nerve as you see in the Carnivora." [1] A few

"would go in strongly for the angels." The lawn-sleeves of the "Upper House" fluttered at the sentiment, and "the Commons," knowing the new candidate for angelic honours, considered the ascent "pretty cheeky" even for the son of a Jew! Had Disraeli read and been converted by the Mac-donald philosophy? If so, the conversion is the best Jewish one extant, and highly flattering to science. If the study of the wing of the angels, viewed morphologically, carried Disraeli's imagination to the seraphic longings, well might his colleague, Secretary Walpole, show lachrymation under the personal spell of Radical Beales!

[1] The structure is well seen in the Tiger, Lion, Aye-Aye, Cat, Otter, Racoon, Seal, Wombat, Ant-Eater, and Opossum. The Royal College of Surgeons' Museum, London, contains a beautiful series of preparations illustrating the supra-condyloid foramen in different animals. It is to be

weeks elapsed and he showed the specimens to the Anatomical Society, and called attention to two ridges and a groove [1] proceeding from the process of bone towards the inner condyle for the lodgment, as he believed, of the humeral nerve and vessels. " It happened by a singular coincidence," writes Dr. Knox, " that within two days after this communication was made to the Society, a case actually occurred to bring the opinion to the test." The left arm of a stout muscular middle-aged man was being dissected, and " the *pronator teres* muscle was observed to have an unusually high origin ; and on looking attentively at the structure, my assistant immediately called my attention to an anomaly corresponding strictly with what I had predicted two nights previously to the Anatomical Society, viz. the presence of a supra-condyloid process : its connection with the inner condyle of the humerus by means of a ligament or aponeurotic expansion, *and the consequent deviation of the main artery and median nerve from their usual course, in order to pass behind this process in the groove, half osseous, half ligamentous, thus formed,* afterwards to return, a little lower down, so as rapidly to regain their usual relative

regretted that there is no specimen of the human semi-osseous form in the collection.

[1] Dr. F. J. Julius Willbrand, of Giessen, found on the humerus of the Carnivora the depressions and ridge described by Knox upon the human humerus, similarly situated as to the vessels and median nerve. Curiously enough, Willbrand saw something analogous on the femur among the *Edentata, Rodentia,* and *Pachydermata,* and, as if the analogy should be found higher in the scale, also in man. Later observations, however, do not sanction Willbrand's views—the point of bone he described being held in the light of an exostosis or slight thickening of the bone.

position in the bend of the elbow; in short, the precise anatomy of the arm of the Jaguar,[1] with this difference merely, that in the latter the supra-condyloid canal is entirely osseous, whilst in man it is only partly so, the process not extending so as to unite itself by bone with the condyle." Knox looked upon this arrangement of parts as a "startling proof of the strength of the analogies subsisting occasionally between man and the lower animals, and an undeniable argument of the existence of a general scheme or plan embracing the whole range of the animal kingdom, even to a minuteness of detail quite inconceivable by those who adopt the views and the physiology of the Bridgewater Treatises." Drawings accompanied the paper.

A happier generalization than that of Knox's just described can hardly be found in the whole range of biological science. He was mightily pleased with the manner in which his discovery was received by the profession in Edinburgh. It should be noted that Dr. Barclay possessed arterial preparations where a supra-condyloid process existed, yet they had been overlooked by himself, Knox, and others through whose hands they must have passed before and after they were placed in the College of Surgeons' Museum.

[1] Knox's Rooms, early in 1841, attracted numerous visitors, and not without reason. The fine Jaguar, or American Panther, of the famous Mr. Carter, lay on one table, with its perfect supra-condyloid foramen; monkeys lay on another, which had been obtained from a travelling menagerie, some with and others without the carnivorous type of humerus; whilst on a third table was the anomalous human arm described in the text—by far the most interesting of the group.

Tiedemann seems to have been the first to notice, in 1822, the process of bone now known as the human "supra-condyloid," but he considered it a disease or exostosis—"*Excrescentia ossis humeri insolita.*" A. W. Otto, in 1839,[1] with greater discrimination, is said to have recognized it as the analogue of the supra-condyloid process in the Mammalia. Within eighteen months of Knox's discovery three examples of the same process came under my own observation in Surgeons' Square, but as my old teacher had so clearly established the history of the supra-condyloid process in the human arm, I did not deem it necessary to publish them.[2] Willbrand saw the same arrangement of parts in 1843, Quain in 1844, and Tiedemann in 1846, after which year this anatomical form or curious anomaly lost much of its novelty. Professer Wenzel Gruber had collected up to 1859, partly from his own observations and from the works of previous writers (my three not being published

[1] Otto's thesis came into Knox's hands after his discovery. I have not been able to see it, and cannot at this moment say whether Otto described a case such as Knox's, or only inferred its existence from comparative anatomy. Assuredly Knox had no help to his bold deduction, though he talked of Magendie having seen the supra-condyloid foramen in the yellow races of Africa.

[2] In one of the three instances that fell under my observation, the radial artery arose from the lowest part of the axillary, continued its course downwards, and after parting with the brachial, when seeking a direction to reach the semi-osseous "supra-condyloid" foramen, crossed over the larger trunk towards the bend of the elbow. In no case was the foramen strictly osseous. In the arm of a seal, which I dissected in 1842, the median nerve passed through the foramen, while the brachial artery ran over the bony arch and joined the nerve below the foramen. Such a case would indicate that osseous protection was needed for the nerve only.

were not included), sixty-two cases. Other examples have since been met with.

The discussion arising from time to time among the better-educated pupils of his class often led Knox to give a larger elucidation of some parts of the anatomy than could be found in the best text-books extant. Let him have a subject that interested his surgical penchant, Knox would be sure to unravel its history. Induced by some pertinent questions, he sat alongside a Newcastle student to help in the dissection of the hip-joint, and to give him his latest views of the uses of the round ligament. To Knox's great surprise there was no round ligament in the subject! The joint was healthy in other respects. This was the first time (and he believed he had seen 500 hip-joints opened) that he had noted the absence of this marked structure. His "Observations on the probable Use of the Round Ligament of the Thigh-bone in Man" were read to the Anatomical and Physiological Society : they are of interest anatomically and surgically (*Edin. Med. and Surg. Journ.* vol. lvi. p. 128). As the laws of deformation seemed to Knox to be nearly as regular as the laws of formation, he knew " no reason why occasionally that arrangement, which we find constantly in the elephant and some other mammals, should not occasionally occur in man." He alluded to the contradictory statements respecting the uses of the round ligament of the hip-joint in man, the errors of Boyer, Meckel, Cooper, Gerdy, and Cruveilhier on this subject ; his own views apparently coincided in part with those expressed by Mr. Mayo. He held that rotation of the thigh, either outwards or inwards, can be carried only to the extent allowed by the round ligament; whilst "all attempts to combine to any great extent the *element of rotation* with the other movements of which the joint is capable, receive a complete *check* from the presence of the said ligament; and more especially the motion of *adduction*, which cannot be performed at all when the limb is *at the same time rotated outwards* or *inwards*." He thought it by no means improbable that, as the round ligament may vary in length in different persons, a congenital comparative shortness of this ligament may contribute to the production of the deformity of "*in-toes*." He remarked upon the congenital laxity of the round ligament in some persons either *per se* or as forming a part of a general laxity of all the ligaments and fibro-cartilaginous structures throughout the body.

His comments "On Fracture of the Radius Bone near its carpal extremity, with and without complication" (*Edin. Med. and Surg. Journ.* vol. lvi. p. 330), are worthy of attention. His views, though chiefly drawn from the dissecting-room and museums, bore the practical character that experience drawn from the living subject only can confer. He suggested that many cases of supposed dislocations of the ulna, and even of the wrist-joint, refer merely to a fracture of the radius close to its distal extremity, accompanied by a displacement of the lower fragment of fractured bone, set partially free by a rupture or laceration of the inarticular cartilage of Weitbrecht. To this latter condition, along with a dislocation of the carpal end of the bone, he attributed the remarkable shortening of the radius after certain fractures. His paper, as usual, was illustrated by drawings.

Few people were aware of Knox's strong penchant for surgery, and his great ability in that direction. It was impossible to look at his examination of a limb without being struck with the method of his manipulation, so elegant and yet so effective, whether as testing the finer movements, what the mechanicians would term the sweetness of the adjusting surfaces; or in eliciting the greater actions, say of forcible abduction, rotation, &c., of the joint. In handling injured and diseased limbs he reminded me most of Sir C. Bell among his compeers; whilst he stood in striking contrast to Velpeau and Breschet, and other continental surgeons. Had his surgical aim been cultivated, Knox would have risen to great eminence. He disliked the knife, that opprobrium of the art betraying the butcher rather than the surgeon; in short, he was an advocate of true Conservative Surgery. When one of his pupils in the North of Scotland showed him a diseased knee-joint that others beside himself had condemned for amputation, Knox advised his friend to put the limb in splints, to assuage suffering, and attend to the general health of his patient for two months longer, and see the effects. The limb was thereby saved, and his intelligent pupil speaks of the case till this day as exemplifying Dr. Knox's surgical acumen and diagnosis.

In the early spring of 1841, numbers of monkeys that had died of phthisis in a travelling menagerie in Edinburgh were obtained for the practical rooms. Impressed with the apparently close approximation of the Simian to the Human type, I solicited Dr. Knox's attention to several points in their respective anatomies, and to the brain in particular, assigning my reason that the time was at hand when zoological questions bearing on man's development would render such inquiries of vast interest; and who so likely as himself to anticipate the discussion? Though admitting a part of my argument, he stoutly maintained that there was a wide gap between the lowest man and the highest ape. Having shown him the chimpanzee in curious juxtaposition with the body of a lad of Scoto-Hibernian features of the animal type, and also some dissections of the two forms for further comparison, he remarked : "True, they are like, painfully like—caricatures if you will ; but man is man, after all." John Goodsir came purposely to see these comparative anatomizations, and endorsed his master's views. It has been said, but no proof is adduced, that Knox subsequently modified his opinions. Goodsir unquestionably stood by the high dignity of man and his moral and psychological attributes, and viewed these as isolating man entirely from the rest of the animal creation (Memoirs, vol. i. p. 182). If Knox accepted the Roman poet's dictum,—

> "——— cœlumque tueri
> Jussus,"

it must have been in a theological sense, for with the rest of the quotation, "*et erectos ad sidera tollere vultus*," he used to fence, or rather attack the arguments of the "Bridgewater School" in regard to man's characteristic biped form and head erect, or his privilege of looking to the heavens. "These writers," he used to say, "could never have been in a farm-yard, or they would have seen the *biped* bantam cock, with head erect, strutting along with star-like gaze, and crowing to the very echo."

During the spring and summer of 1841, Dr. Knox was superintending and editing for Messrs. Chambers, the spirited publishers of Edinburgh, Quetelet's work on Man (*"Sur l'Homme et le Développement de ses Facultés."* M. A. Quetelet, Secrétaire perpetuel de l'Académie Royale de Bruxelles). The name of Knox was a passport to a work but little known in this country (it had been published in Paris in 1835), and Messrs. Chambers had much reason to be pleased with the success of the work, which has long been out of print.

Regardless of both legal and moral obligations, he commenced lecturing on anatomy in Edinburgh, in November 1842, but got no class. He attempted a course of physiology in the following session with as little success; and, what must have been more degrading, had to march through Coventry with men of inferior stamp as colleagues.[1] Being thwarted in Edinburgh, he looked in various directions for an opportunity of lecturing, but could find no vacancy in Scotland. To a man of his powers, what could be more trying or more sickening than compulsory inertia and seclusion? He had voluntarily disposed of his interests in Edinburgh, in the expectation, it is fully believed, of emigrating to more favoured shores; but when the day of decision came, possibly he felt like Danton, that as he could not carry the soil of Scotland under his feet, he had better bear the ills of life at home. It is not unlikely that his

---

[1] One of his colleagues was in the habit of designating himself A. H. Esquire, F.R.C.S. Ed.; and of the character of this person, when his opinion was asked, Knox said: " In everything pertaining to himself, A. H. has all the sagacity of a poodle-dog."

children weighed very much in his decision. Whatever may have been his guiding circumstance, he committed a great mistake in staying upon the course when the race had been run : there could be no chance of a second heat in his case, and all probability of regaining public confidence was lost.

Had he gone to the United States of America, where his fame had preceded him, he would there have found the very platform for his abilities, and undoubtedly succeeded in establishing his fame as the anatomist of the Far West. His democratic penchant, his scientific acquirements, his originality both as teacher and thinker, and his grand rhetorical displays, so suited to the atmosphere of a republic, would all have told in his favour, and gained him the *éclat* so freely awarded to intellectual vigour and special excellence.

Knox delivered the introductory lecture to the Portland Street School of Medicine in Glasgow—Session 1844-45. He was associated with Dr. Macdonald and Mr. Lyon, now the eminent consulting surgeon of Glasgow. Having to contend with the old-established University and the Andersonian Institution, his class was small. As usual, he delighted his audiences ; and to-day Dr. Weir speaks of his lecturing as a fascination beyond reading " Robinson Crusoe " in his youth ; that of all the lecturers he ever heard, Knox was *facile princeps* in richness and abundance of illustration. One evening, Knox came late to lecture, the class was highly impatient, and, what was worse, no subject had been prepared for him. He caught up a humerus, and, as if nothing disconcerted, stepped gracefully into the class-room ; what that bone became in the hands of a master was soon evident in the intense attention that rapidly stole over the audience, and in the vivid impress it stamped so indelibly on the mind of Dr. Weir, who relates the story.

His objection to the use of diagrams has been dwelt upon. One night in Glasgow, owing to deficient *matériel*, he attempted a sketch with white chalk on a black board; the gas went out at the moment, and with the darkness there was uproar in the class. The light being restored, Knox was seen standing in the same attitude as before the *contretemps ;* he, however, went no further with his drawing, but reverted to his anatomy. He looked upon the gas going out as a judgment upon his attempting an illegitimate mode of instruction; and in speaking of it, continued—

> "It saved a world of talk
> To resort to board and chalk,—

a stupid enough doggrel, but very applicable to the fact.'

In Glasgow he gained some friends and admirers, but no bread and butter. So small was his class, that he returned his fees to his pupils before November was out. The city of big chimneys, bigger piety, and biggest of all in the use of alcoholic liquors in Scotland, was not for Robert Knox, the heterodox man of science and the claimant of individual right. Where—so obviously seen in Glasgow—material interests, shopocracy, and a fervid Calvinism overshadowed all other considerations, could hardly be the place for a man of genius. As no University would appoint him to a Chair, and no medical school would open its gates in Scotland, he was no better than an ostracized citizen ; at an age, too (for he had passed his meridian) when the best place in the anatomical world should have been at his feet. Accomplished in every department of his profession, he nevertheless could get no employment and no countenance. Either the world was hard to please, or he had lost caste. In early life he was held of repute in the army. He had taught anatomy to some thousands. He had obtained French honours, and could appeal to original works in the Transactions of the Royal and other Societies. He had associated with the great of the land—men of judicial, scientific, and medical fame, and made himself known to the world of letters ; yet all these qualifications seemed of no weight in the balance of opinions that tested his adaptability to office by another standard than intellectual force, namely, the moral and the Christian. It is painful to look back upon this *descensus Averni* of a great man, and Knox's fall was little less than that which the phrase indicates. He who had risen to the highest top, been surrounded with so many admiring, nay, idolizing students, was now without a class at all—a history, indeed, upon which to point the moral and adorn the tale ; but it is needful to pass on to another page.

CHAPTER XIV.

The Edinburgh Physiology Chair.—The Historic Man.—His Onslaught on Institutions.—The Chivalrous Knight.—The Orator.—Hero Worship. —Introductory Lectures.—Distinguished Pupils.—Name talismanic.— No Home.

PROFESSOR ALISON of Edinburgh retired from the Chair of Physiology in 1841,[1] to take the more onerous one of Practice of Physic, and Dr. Knox offered himself for the vacancy. In setting forth his claims, he adverted to the decline of the University, and the danger of *untried lecturers;* that if he were appointed to the Chair of Physiology public confidence might be restored, seeing that his success as a Professor could not for a moment be doubted. In despite of every effort to crush him, he retained the good opinion of thousands of his professional brethren, whose support could not fail to be serviceable to the University. He condemned the mode of bolstering

[1] Chronologically the contest for the Physiology Chair should have been noted in the last chapter ; in other respects it fits better here. The letter to the Town Council, of which the text contains but a brief abstract, is one of the grandest specimens of Knox-art on record. Its biting, sarcastic tone implied that the writer had fully meant to leave Edinburgh, and wished to cast his heaviest stone of indignation at the door of the Council Chamber of the city. His criticism of the opposing candidates was not less stinging. No one attempted a reply to his letter.

up artificial reputations by testimonials wrung from polite foreigners, and added : " I will not, my lord, sanction, in so far as regards myself, one of the most infamous impostures of modern times—I mean the ' Testimonial System,' by putting forth any such disgraceful documents, stalking-horses under covert of which the foulest jobs have been perpetrated." He was most unsparing in his comments upon the rival candidates : one, Dr. Allen Thomson, an " *ex-professo* physiologist, that is, *he was nothing else,* neither a comparative anatomist, human anatomist, nor even a medical practitioner, who, after three attempts to obtain a class, disappeared about mid-winter and was pensioned on a noble English duke ; another, Dr. John Reid, equally unsuccessful as a lecturer, had taken refuge in the Endowment Scheme of the country ; and a third, Dr. W. B. Carpenter, whom he styled 'an old dog at physiology,' distinguished for his failures as a lecturer, his plagiarisms, and his powers of mystification."

" Nothing throughout this whole business," continued Knox, " has surprised me so much as the resemblance between the three candidates ; their repeated and extraordinary failures, their bolstered up reputations, their total want of all originality, their unpopularity with the student or the taught ; their powers of mystifying the plainest facts. They must unquestionably have all studied in one school, and that school I could name ; but, be this as it may, there is a resemblance clearly amounting to an identity in character ; the possibility of which identity *in metaphysicis* and individuality *in physicis* I beg leave to throw out as a hint to this gentleman (Dr. Carpenter),

which, if carefully studied, may be the humble means
through grace and faith, of removing certain conscientious
scruples exceedingly dangerous in character when held by
anatomists (supposing him to be one, though he be not)
and by physiologists ; perilous moreover to their temporal
and eternal welfare : he failed in Edinburgh as a lecturer,
causing a heavy loss to a popular institution here, and
he failed in Liverpool, reducing his audience in ten days
from 1,000 to ten ! . . . . Admitting, for argument's
sake, that these opinions of mine were mere prejudices,
they would still be entitled to respect, seeing that they
come from one who may without vanity lay claim to a
greater amount of experience in the practical education
of the medical student than has fallen to the lot of
any person now alive. A reference to the number of
distinguished physicians and surgeons whom I have
educated *practically* would, I am persuaded, surprise
your lordship and the Council." He then gave the following list of names, as he said, "quoted hastily and from
memory," to satisfy the Town Council on this point :—
"R. Boyd, W. Fergusson, T. W. Jones, John Goodsir,
Harry Goodsir, Henry Lonsdale, John Reid, J. W.
Balfour, James Duncan, Douglas Maclagan, Patrick
Newbigging, John H. Bennett, &c."

Every sentence of Knox's letter conveyed a home-
thrust at private individuals or corporate bodies. He
spoke of the Chairs of the University as having "fallen
much below the income of a steady-going retail grocery
or bakery," and as much sunk in public estimation ;
and feels sure that the Provost and Town Council will
merely see in all this the straightforward opinion of a

fellow-citizen. If the decay of the medical school went
much further, " the most prudent course," thought Knox,
" would be to follow rapidly the steps of the Listons
and Fergussons, the Turners and Grahams, and seek in
the metropolis of the empire that return for exertion
and hard-earned reputation denied us here." He mentioned that between 1838 and 1841 the number of the
medical classes had declined from 556 to 356, being a
total loss in these few years of 200 students ; which decline he attributed to three causes: viz. " the overloading
of the curriculum, the absence from the University of all
men of originality and of European reputation, and the
baneful effects of a monopoly exercised by the University,
whose sure result, like all other monopolies, is first to
ruin itself and afterwards its neighbours."

Knox called on Mr. Adam Black, the well-known
publisher and influential citizen, with the view of sound-
ing him as to the impending election and obtaining his
vote. Mr. Black observed : " Of your remarkable abilities, Doctor, and your fitness for the Chair, I have no
doubt ; but you know that our Town Council have strong
religious scruples." "Well," replied Knox, "? am I not
as good a Christian as Baillie ———, or any of my
neighbours?" " It may be," said the publisher ; " had
you only been an Elder of the Kirk, Doctor!" " Ah,
ah, I see," rejoined Knox ; "the Calvinistic credentials
are wanting." Then both joined in a hearty laugh.

The candidate of "remarkable abilities and fitness for
the Chair" had not a vote. Dr. Allen Thomson was
elected, and Dr. John Reid was a good second in the
contest.

Such instances of want of favour, arising out of circumstances foreign to the teaching of science, might well provoke the anatomist to cast ridicule upon his opponents, and in doing so he would quote Scriptural texts, or the authority of high divines : this was wormwood of the bitterest kind. For what could equal in galling influence the satire of a man without religious profession using Bible passages to crush his enemies with?

His irony used to crop up in various ways. At one of the medical societies, the case of a boy was described, whose chest had been injured by the explosion of a small cannon mounted on a piece of wood. A few weeks afterwards the boy died, and on examination the right ventricle of the heart was found distended by a piece of stick stretched across its interior. How had it got there? There was no cicatrix or wound of the heart, a small cicatrix only on the surface of the chest. After making some suitable remarks, Dr. Knox quietly said that he "thought this case must have occurred in England; hence the origin of the phrase, gentlemen, ' Hearts of oak! Hearts of oak!'"

The real historic interest of the man Knox is centred in himself; it derives nothing from his medical and social fraternizations, and nowhere reflects the influences of other men's companionship and counsel. Self-made, and resting on no ancillary support, he achieved a remarkable position as an anatomical teacher; and it should be always borne in mind that this was truly his forte and grand distinctive merit. His work in science (I am speaking of his Edinburgh history up to 1842) was pretty nearly buried in the archives of the Royal Society and the little-read pages of the *Edinburgh Medical and Surgical Journal.*

His citizenship, his public position, and high popularity belong to the place of his birth, so that before tracing his immigration southwards it may be well here to complete the chapter of his Edinburgh life—a life of unequalled prosperity and almost unequalled reverse. Medical history could hardly furnish so brilliant an advance as Knox obtained in the third year of his anatomical lectureship. A world of fame lay before him, and he marched in Alexandrian fashion to the conquest; and that conquest would have been complete had not circumstances inconceivable in civilized life, the slightest connivance with which was as thoroughly alien to Knox's nature as to any man's on earth, arisen to mar the historical figure and deface its best proportions. There was, it is true, something in the figure itself not free from blemish, and that blemish became heightened in the focus of a Scottish inquisitorial microscope. The personal flaw, however, was trifling compared with the advent of affairs of the most untoward character associated with the carrying on of his establishment, in casting the beam against the anatomist. Society, standing aghast, was in no mood to listen to evidence, either of the Chief Justiciary Court, or of a committee of inquiry composed of the best citizens of Edinburgh, much less to reason dispassionately and soberly on the events. The guilty culprit Burke met his fate at the gallows of the Lawnmarket; but the brunt of a lasting and national reproach fell upon the head of the innocent

Robert Knox.   And so deep-rooted is prejudice, that it is doubtful if these pages, compiled from authentic data and personal experience, and with a view to sustain the entire truth, will altogether eradicate forty years of unfounded aspersion and perverted feeling.

Like all men who venture upon excursions into fresh realms of thought, or seek to divert the human mind from ancient precedents and the cherished dogmas which senility is apt to hug so closely, Knox came in for a large share of detraction.   He who would found new principles of action or culture, should calculate the cost —the creation of jealousy in mediocre minds, and, not infrequently, the operations of a worse malignity.   Knox dwelt upon the shortcomings of medical education and the inefficiency of the public boards entrusted with the keys of the gates of the profession ; he sought to infuse fresh blood into the "time-honoured," or rather the somewhat time-worn, institutions of the country.   His attempt was a bold one, and, as his words were bolder, they roused a swelling indignation and hate.   He was one of the free spirits of the age ; if he saw an abuse he showed it up.   Now, any encroachment upon the old stage-work, any enlargement of the proscenium or shifting of the players, was sure to give rise to clamour behind the scenes : our "privileges," our "established precedents," our "vested rights," came forth in deep-mouthed barkings against the champion for progressive science.   Knox saw in most corporations a prevailing fogeyism, coteries, and nepotism, and a want of vigour and non-recognition of the higher aspirations of the school.   He sought for a greater expansion of the legislative and executive functions in the medical institutions, and to make the places of honour therein subservient to mental superiority and promise. All such ideas as these were looked upon as rank heresy forty years ago in Edinburgh. There were Beatons in the medical corporations as strongly opposed to Robert Knox of the nineteenth as the persecuting Cardinal had been to John Knox of the sixteenth century; and quite as readily disposed to banish or to burn at the stake the anatomical innovator.

To attack the traditional doctrines and the social and religious standards in their stronghold of infallibility, as Knox did so poignantly, by asking their *raison d'être*, was sure to bring down upon him the epithets "atheist" and "infidel," — familiar terms among the would-be saintly in their charitable construction of other men's opinions. If you have no case, abuse the plaintiff's attorney; if you fail in argument, you can at least throw dirt, and some of it is sure to stick, especially if it be taken from the heaps of the *Record* and *Scottish Banner*. The Doctor might have understood this, yet for long he laboured under the impression that the path which he saw so clearly could be pointed out to others; and that the inexorable logic of events must in time convince his opponents. He seemed blind to the cravened ignorance of the masses and the uncultured thought of the higher ranks even of the profession itself; and that gods and men fight in vain against inborn stupidity and superstition.

If he cannot be said to have commanded the stronger virtues, many of his comments upon the men and the

events of his epoch rested more with the fit of his humour
and outspokenness than a tendency to *malice prepense.*
Had he been less critical, less candid, and more truthful,
he would have been in happier relations with his contemporaries, several of whom, feeling his stinging remarks,
railed at him in return, and must have verified—

> " The gods are just, and of our pleasant vices
> Make instruments to scourge us. "

Instead of a tongue that speaketh no evil, and the soft
word that turneth away wrath, he showed an almost
habitual disregard for prudent reticence. Yet at all
times his bark was worse than his bite. His touches of
irony, or ridicule, if you will, breathed less of sarcastic
and evil thoughts than many supposed. Persons on the
qui vive for Knox's utterances oft mistook the emphasis
and bold avowal of opinion for fierceness of assault ;
and the repetition of his words from mouth to ear
necessarily gave rise to much misrepresentation, till at
length that which might have been a playful retort
came to be construed into personal enmity and the
worst form of ill-nature. A hardy personality, marked
by unmistakeable courage, a cynicism, and a kind of
neo-platonism, were perhaps too demonstrative in Knox's
public character, and these unfortunately obscured the
tenderer qualities of the heart manifested in his social
and private life.

Knox had a fair amount of egotism in his constitution ;
then he had also great powers of mind to sustain it. In
acumen, in scholarship, and in his own science, few men
of the day were more highly credited ; and *pari passu*

with his exaltation arose the carping jealousy of his less favoured compeers, ready at all times and seasons to depreciate his worth.   Attacked on many sides, he unhesitatingly cast the glove of defiance against all comers, and as certainly as he combated he unhorsed the foe. To compare Knox with his assailants in the Edinburgh medical tournament—a life of antagonism *ab initio usque ad finem*—would be to lower the Cœur de Lion of a chivalrous age to the buckram and fustian of the nineteenth century, marked by the huckstering of medical degrees and the elevation of fifth-rate men to College presidential chairs.[1]   The anatomist was not of the order of knights-errant, but a constant champion of interests more ennobling than the "white ensign" of "*our* St. George," that bacon-curing and not too clean-handed Cappadocian whom England, unwittingly it is presumed, elevated to the position of a nation's patron saint! Knox fought for his own individualism and faith in science,

---

[1] This train of thought recalls a conversation with Knox in the library of the Royal Society of Edinburgh in 1841, on my asking his opinion as to the propriety of joining the Society.   He called my attention to the list of Fellows hanging on the wall, and after pointing to the names of Sir D. Brewster, Sir C. Bell, and a few others, swept his hand across the rest as "nobodies."   "There," said he, "is a pupil of mine—excellent fingers, but," raising his finger to his forehead, "nothing here."   Another "never could comprehend the meaning of the word 'generalization,'" &c.   "Why would you throw money away upon a Society rapidly hastening to the guidance of banker's clerks, fifth-rate medical practitioners, and the like? You gain nothing of science, and as little honour."   He then animadverted upon the two Royal Colleges of Surgeons and Physicians, whose professional dignity he considered to be on the wane: he augured their coalition for their own ends and gains, their granting of diplomas and degrees for the £. s. d. consideration, and the coming time when mediocrity would prevail over medical interests and scientific emulation.

and for a time with great success ; for who can be said
to have held higher ground than the noted naturalist of
the North, the anatomical teacher with 500 pupils under
one roof ; the bold exponent of biological doctrines based
on facts—consonant or not as they might be with Hebraic
signs, traditions, and belief? Among his contemporaries
he stood as pre-eminent as the pyramid of Cheops amid
the smaller and ruder constructions of the Gheezeh group
on the edge of the desert ; or, as some would have him
to be, the Sphinx at the base, struggling with the drifting
sand—anomalistic yet attractive, mythic yet historical.

Not a few of his contemporaries, whilst admitting his
oratorical grandeur, would have it that he was too much
of an actor in his public appearances. Now, almost all
oratory, be it of the pulpit, or plebeian, or parliamentary,
is full of arts, if not of tricks ; and the style of oratory
that does not disdain to be artificial at times is often
winning and effective. Guided possibly by what Demos-
thenes held to be an essential element in public speaking
—" action " and again " action "—Knox enjoyed the rare
accomplishment of gaining the entire attention of his
audiences. He possessed grace, and tact, and supple-
ness, and these most valuable adjuncts to his public
efforts were often made visible in his apt diversions, and
equal readiness to cope with any difficulty that might
untowardly arise. Opportunities for eloquence are rarely
afforded the anatomist, whose work is full of details and
descriptions, so that the fact of any one earning distinction in that line is all the more remarkable. If Knox
could invest the osteology with an historical meaning,
and revive the geological past, or make arteries and

muscles reflect the laws of natural philosophy and the
visibly living action, what might he not do with his
thoughts engaged on a more fitting and popular theme ?
If the component parts of a dead organism sufficed
for the exhibition of a rare descriptive power that
could clothe them in motory action and real life, what
greatness might he not achieve on the political platform, pointing out the proverbial blunders of the War
Office, the red-tapeism of officials, and the " organized
hypocrisy " of Governments ! The great impression prevailing among those who had studied and knew his
character thoroughly, was Knox's fitness to meet any
emergency, or to accomplish anything within the range
of human intellect, or in the more exciting arena of
medical debate.

The crucial test is wanting, but the inference is sufficiently strong to warrant the belief that Knox might
have cut a great figure in public life ; nay, more, had he
taken to the tribune, would hardly have been matched by
John Bright, M.P., George Dawson of Birmingham, and
Henry Vincent[1] of London, the three men who during
the last twenty years have obtained most largely the con-
fidential approval of democratic England. As political
agitator, Knox would have been a pungent thorn in the
side of any Government that failed to respect popular
rights. The careless grace which he would at one time
exhibit as to his own individuality and importance, then

---

[1] The doctor asked me to accompany him to a lecture by Henry Vincent
one night in Edinburgh, and his remark on coming out was : " Well,
Lonsdale, with four such men as H. Vincent I would undertake to revolu-
tionize England in less than six months."

the lively egotism of another hour, charmed by their contrast ; and these were varied again by the display of a grand trenchant style, the effects of which in discomfiting the opposition surpassed all belief. No prepared philippic of Bright's could ever reach the height and force of Knox's impromptus. Take the instance of the mob surrounding his lecture-room, when his life was in peril, or the attack of the "professorial clique" in the Royal Society. There might be a singular combination of tendencies, of great defects and of greater faculties, but as a man for a tribune, to rouse the popular feeling and to carry the popular voice, Knox could hardly have been surpassed. Having listened to every noted public speaker in the British Isles, to the Ministers and Opposition of Louis Philippe's *régime*, and the greater celebrities of the French Institute ; also to the leading men of the revolutionary epoch of 1848, I am disposed to think that with the exception of Louis Kossuth's historical efforts, beyond all comparison the grandest of their kind, Knox would have measured well with the best men of his day at home or abroad. Assuredly he eclipsed all anatomical and medical teachers in Britain and France. Most orators show their full strength on every public occasion ; now, whatever effort Knox made, you felt that he had a *corps de réserve* that could be brought to the front when needful to bear upon special points, and with sweeping effect upon his enemy's lines.

From long observation of his character, Knox was led to designate the medical student "a most curious and troublesome person to deal with," often flying off at tangents, or soliciting a royal road to learning. Yet

T

no lecturer could boast of so warm an attachment to his person, amounting almost to a devotional feeling, as Knox had from the vast majority of his pupils. Of Bibliolatry, Scotland knows enough, and of Mariolatry the world is daily getting more informed ; but neither of these affecting theological interests only could vie with the demonstration of Knoxolatry of anatomical Edinburgh from 1826 to 1836. Within the collegiate precincts, in the Halls where medical fraternities met for discussion, or amid the social gatherings of students, one name figured superlatively, and that name was Robert Knox. Various classical and historical cognomens were applied to the anatomist, often, too, in significant portraiture of some of his characteristics as well as his grander parts on the world's stage. It was highly amusing to read the various interpretations of the man—Knox, and to listen to the comments made upon him by his motley class. The reader of the " Iliad " saw Knox amid the Trojan warriors ; the Manxman tracing the historic Mona, found a parallel to the daring Norse Sea-kings in the bold Scot, and named him accordingly ; the student who had the night previous witnessed Vandenhoff, the tragedian, in his fine portrayal of Coriolanus, next morning verified the noble Roman on the boards of Surgeons' Hall ! When the anatomist was in his high philosophic moods, he was likened to Socrates the ugly husband of Xantippe ; if warmly enthusiastic, to Vesalius ; if satirical, to Juvenal, or, as the Irishman would have it, Dean Swift ; if highly eloquent, worthy to occupy the Bema and lead the Athenians, or to rival Cicero in frustrating conspiracies against the Republic. A clever pupil of Knox's (R. M. Glover) named him "Old Cyclops :" many knew him by his Christian name only, and spoke of him familiarly as Robert—so far objectionable, however, that the enemy took advantage and added—*le Diable.* Known by a host of *aliases*, but always invested with the highest attributes—

> " In all this world ne was there none him like
> To speak of physic and of surgery,"—

and what a delightful companion he would have been in the pilgrimage to Canterbury, as the Doctor of Physic, the story-teller, and beguiler of time's dreary hours.

Knox had numbers of graduation theses, " Probationary Essays," and poetical effusions of students dedicated to him. The present distinguished Professor Sharpey, though not a pupil of the Doctor's, acknowledged his regard for the great teacher in this way ; and Sir W. Fergusson, on joining the Royal College of Surgeons, naturally offered homage to his master. A youthful poet dedicated a poem to " Dr. Knox, the first lecturer on anatomy," &c. Here is a specimen of his preface in the form of a sonnet :—

> " Immortal genius ! may thy brow for ever
> Be bound with laurels—verdant, fresh, and green ;
> Scorn back the paltry minions who endeavour
> To wound thy fame—so fair—with envious spleen.
> I cannot laud thee more than say—Be what thou'st been."

Knox had more substantial offerings in the way of fish, fruit, and the dainties of the country forwarded to him during the season ; indeed the specialities of each county's produce were regular offerings on the part of students to the man they loved.

Here was hero-worship filling the Knox cup and running over, and due entirely to the recognition of the talents of a great master. His reputation was in no way fictitious, but rested on intellectual strength, and a native vigour and force of character that swept past ordinary obstacles in the struggle for life and life's ennobling rewards. The spirit of the man was visible in every action ; he was restless and impetuous, ever on the forward march to reach the goal of success. His exhortations to self-reliance, conveyed in the most inviting way, had the happiest effect upon his class. Seeing in him the exaltation of merit, they would drink of the same Pierian spring that had refreshed their master's soul, crediting themselves with the hope of imbibing part of his enthusiasm and noble emulation.

Knox passionately loved the approbation of his class, and faithfully tried to earn it. The cheers that greeted his appearance, or arose during the hour in hearty appreciation of his sentiments, were to him ample guerdon for all his pains and study and labour. He never stooped to commonplace, to weak platitudes and washy colouring, much less to vulgar parlance ; his forte lay in smart epigram and classical similes, the logical definition and historical parallel, or the zoological generalization of impressive interest.

Over the portals of Old Surgeons' Hall, a standard inscribed in bold letters *Excelsior* might have waved with significance in honour of Knox, the grand chief, his lieutenants, Fergusson and Reid, and the rank and file of some thousands of good men and true. Many worthy Esculapii, the Monros, Bells, and others, had passed through these portals since 1697 ; but at no time perhaps in the Collegiate history of the building in which Knox lectured, had there been such marked anatomical zeal in the aspirants for surgical honours, such public ardour and success in a teacher, and such high promise for the future of the Edinburgh school, as was displayed by Robert Knox and his pupils. If the sun had set upon the habitation of the old chirurgeons, its setting was rendered glorious by Knox, its last representative, of whom there had been no prototype in the history of the College. If each of the anatomists from the days of James IV. of Scotland had had a pillar erected to his memory in the great hall, Knox would have been entitled to a noble design—the fluted column, with the spiral ornates and emblem crowning capital, as significant and distinctive as the famous Apprentices' Pillar in the chapels of Roslin and Melrose.

Country practitioners thought nothing of riding to Edinburgh from a distance of twenty miles and upwards to hear "Knox's Introductory," and expressed themselves amply repaid for their journey, were it made through November frost or sleet. A previous perusal of the reports of the London opening session enabled them the better to appreciate the anatomist of another atmosphere ; for no more marked contrast could be met with in the range of medical thought and expression thirty-five years ago than the Metropolitan prefatory lectures and Knox's oral Introductory. The Southern, as a general rule, was formal and stereotyped, beginning with the definition of ἀνα-τέμνω, then traversing the alphabet of osteologies and myologies, and ending with the paternal counsel of " Be good boys, and you will get diplomas." Knox, on the other hand, was always fresh, free, and flowing : he offered no hard lines, no repulsive detail, and no sermonising. Without a note, and with no further preparation than "thinking of it" in his walks a day or two previously, every November Introductory appeared like a new coinage from a new dye. Having on one occasion ventured to speak to him of the memoranda he meant to make for his " Introductory," he said that if he took notes he might be tempted to read them, and if he read a dozen lines he would assuredly spoil his lecture.

There was point and significance in all his remarks, which told upon his juniors and seniors alike ; then the vigour, the confidence, and hopefulness of his strain, his winning, impressive, and elevating manner, stood antipodal to the flat, stale, and unprofitable so common in the schools. He naturally kept the divisions of his course in view, but in his prefatory lecture he cared less for definition and classification, and more for the opportunity of coaxing the student within the laboratory of his art, and giving him a direction sciencewards. The historical allusion based on a trite example, the distinction between true and pseudo-science, and the high aim of the surgeon, were graphically delineated ; indeed, his lectures were like panoramas of varied interest. So far from painting a leaden surface and pluviose sky, sheep on the moor, and a shepherd with his conventional crook and " collie," the ruminants

and the "plaided" bucolic being much akin to the
students and teachers of certain anatomical schools,
Knox furnished a glowing landscape with colour in the
foreground reflected in the pebbly stream, human figures
in human attitudes, a columnar edifice seen through
pensile foliage—the Temple of Esculapius, if you will ;
the distant vale, the cloud-capt hills and azure vault ;
and all in harmony and good taste. His pencil was
of the ready sort, his tones were light and warm, and
his work, if at times sketchy, was ever pleasing and
effective.

Too much is apt to be assigned to the influence of
the teacher upon the taught, and many an incompetent
lecturer, marking the success of one of his pupils, has
mounted the stilts of the pedant, and exclaimed, " See
what my instructions have done," when the young
gentleman spoken of had advanced *himself,* and shown
his greatest advance in escaping from the bonds of his
master's tuition. In the majority of instances self-
reliance and Saxon industry carry the day with English
lads; in others, again, an impetus is essential to the start.
The Doctor hesitated not to claim a good deal of personal influence over his pupils, and it must be admitted
that he seldom over-rated his powers in that direction.
The student saw in him a high fervour, and love of
science, and became persuaded of the value of his work
and its adaptability to the interests of humanity. The
persuasive force of his example and rhetoric upon
others was like a transfusion of healthy blood to the
semi-collapsed veins of a choleraic or hæmorrhagic
patient; there was a response at the student's heart to

every stroke of the Knox piston propelling the flow of the invigorating stimulus to the brain.[1]

My intercourse with Knox's pupils has been considerable, and I cannot recall a single instance of doubt being expressed by any one as to the direct encouragement and suasory power of the master. The student thought it a piece of good luck to be thrown in Knox's way, and proudly valued any prize or honourable distinction won in his class. Hundreds of those who thronged the benches of Old Surgeons' Hall still live to speak in rapturous terms of the " great teacher," and in the rank and file of these are to be found men of high distinction in the practice of their art, in zoology and natural history, in the walks of literature and general science.

Large space would be required to enable me to name the distinguished " Knoxites," and to allude specially to some and not to all would involve me in a delicate task. Among those who lent ear to Knox's first course of lectures were two youths who have since risen to the height of their selected calling, and as they are admirable representatives of his school in zoology and surgery, I may be permitted without bias to name them. One was Richard Owen, of Lancaster, who truly received zoological inspiration from " lectures the most brilliant ever delivered on anatomy," and to-day speaks of

---

[1] I may be pardoned for using this simile, drawn from observation in the treatment of cholera, and a striking case of successful transfusion after puerperal hæmorrhage—a case which my deeply-lamented friend Sir J. Y. Simpson used to cite as the most satisfactory example of the kind in British obstetric medicine.

Knox's influence in prompting him to visit the Jardin des Plantes, and seek the teachings of the French *savans*. Any words of mine regarding Professor Owen would be but a faint echo of the verdict of Europe at large; nor is it necessary to dwell upon the " Lothian lad," William Fergusson, who owed nearly all to Knox, and now occupies so proud a surgical position in the metropolis. How many others there are of great and distinctive merit in Edinburgh, in Glasgow, and throughout Scotland; whilst from Cumberland to Cornwall, and in the large towns of England ; in Ireland, the United States, British America and British Colonies ; everywhere the majority of medicals who were educated previous to 1842, and who have reached superior positions, were " Knoxites." The provincial medical schools, the Queen's Colleges of Ireland, had men of the same order to represent their anatomy, physiology, and surgery at starting ; whilst numbers of leading men in the public services owed their advance to the influence of their great anatomical teacher. Many are gone who held up the " Knox light " to the advantage of their times ; but others remain in whom their master's spirit has kindled a true love for science. Among those whom I remember to have called forth the Doctor's hopes are Professors J. H. Bennett and George E. Day ; Dr. Boyd, of London ; Dr. Adams, of Glasgow ; Mr. R. T. Lightfoot ; Dr. Kelburne King, of Hull, &c. British anatomy and surgery owes no little to Knox's methods, and his inoculation of the minds of thousands whom he educated for every walk of professional life. Professor Goodsir's letter (Anatom. Memoirs, vol. i. p. 142), to his old master on this very subject, in 1854, might be cited, but abundant evidence exists throughout the country in support of this opinion.

A pause in the narrative would have been more consonant with my feelings than noting those who occupied Knox's benches, the noting which implies the recall to memory of dearly attached friends, and many noble sons of science gathered to the dust. Having enjoyed the closest intimacy of the men, how can I write without emotion of John Reid, of John and Harry Goodsir, of Edward Forbes, of Samuel Brown, among the chiefs of " the Brotherhood"? Who more distinguished in British physiology, in manly, honourable character, than Professor John Reid? Who more scientific than Professor John Goodsir, the true successor of Knox? Who offered more promise as a naturalist than the big-framed, bighearted Harry Goodsir? Who won the hearts of men more than Professor Edward Forbes? Who lighted anew the torch of philosophical chemistry in the spirit that guided Dr. Samuel Brown?[1] Sharing in the fame of their master were Hugh Falconer, one of the most genial of men and among the ablest of palæontologists ; the famous Perceval Barton Lord, who figured so nobly in India ; the clever chemist, R. Mortimer Glover, of Newcastle ; the gracious James Duncan ; the lively Archie Cockburn ; the excellent brothers George and Patrick

---

[1] I have elsewhere (Goodsir's Memoirs) spoken of these distinguished sons of science, and would willingly have said something of Falconer and P. B. Lord, R. M. Glover, and others named in the text ; but a suitable *in memoriam* would probably have extended this chapter beyond the wishes of my readers.

Newbigging. Of those personally unknown to myself, and belonging to a different path, were Lord Glenorchy, Sir George Sinclair, and greater than all others among the *literati* and strictly non-medical who assembled under the Knox roof, was the logician, Sir W. Hamilton, Bart., all of whom spoke in the highest terms of their anatomical teacher.

The name of Knox was like a sign of freemasonry ; and his Edinburgh associations often proved a bond of attachment to the veriest strangers in all parts of the world. By the camp-fires of Canada, under the Indian verandahs, in the tented field, on the heights of Balaclava, and wherever military or naval surgeons have congregated for forty years past ; hours of *ennui*, anxiety, and danger have been robbed of their trials, and even made cheery, by the introduction of the famed anatomist's name. If perchance one of the party could call up the visage, the style of elocution and mannerism of the teacher, the effects were exhilarating. "Another pipe, another story of the queer old soul," and with the revival of their students' days, surgeons forgot their pressing hardships, in reflecting on the world of the past enlivened by Knox. If anecdotes of the anatomist could stir the circulation of his pupils thousands of miles from home, the last *mot* or story, fresh from the mint of Old Surgeons' Hall, enlivened with treble force the dinner and supper parties of Edinburgh, of the medical class especially.

Time, it is said, occasionally makes sad havoc of personal reputation, and Knox was a melancholy instance of the truthfulness of this. If the tide of his prosperity

rose higher on the beach than any other anatomist of
the century, the ebb of his adversity receded to the utmost
verge of the sands, the very shoal. Like his great military
idol, he had had his Austerlitz, and now had come his
Moscow. Unsettled from 1842 to 1846, and moving to
and fro on both sides of the Tweed ; now living with an
old pupil, now searching for employment in London,
he was at length induced to give a few lectures on
the "Races of Men," in Newcastle-upon-Tyne, Manchester, &c. This peripatetic philosophizing made him
known to the general public, and helped his finances ;
but it was not exactly the position for a man of Knox's
calibre to occupy in England, that had its "Royal
Institution" and many chartered corporations under
whose wing he should have played a part equal to
the best-cultured minds of the day. His letters at
this period express disappointment, and no wonder.
Possessing the highest gifts of intellect, he obtained no
acknowledgment in the ranks of his own profession ; the
greatest teacher of anatomy could find no chair and no
lectureship in the mighty metropolis; and the Government, not knowing the meaning of the word science,
could not possibly see the merits of a man of genius.

CHAPTER XV.

Πολλὰ τὰ δεινά, κοὐδὲν ἀν-
θρώπου δεινότερον πέλει.

THE antiquity of Man, his geographical position and migrations, his capacities and beliefs, have engaged the thinking minds of every age; it is only in these latter days, however, that his true characteristics as a component part of the zoological chain have received due recognition at the hands of Science. Long prior to the reign of Queen Anne, or any other British queen, philosophers, as well as poets, had conceived the idea that "the proper study of mankind is Man;" but of what avail were poesy, theology, and the speculations of the schoolmen till Vesalius and his successors mapped out the human anatomy, and gave a philosophical direction to Biology?

Taking the biblical genesis as the text of man's natural history, there was but one genus—*Homo*, and but one species—*Homo* styled the *Sapiens;* and in accordance with the cry "Am I not a man and a brother?" men of every hue and dye were to be viewed as alike

partakers of the fee-simple of the earth. As long as
Science limited its prerogative to Mosaical traditions, the
legends of the Saints, and the doctrines of the infallible
Church, Adam and Eve were its anthropological idols,
and the wily-tongued serpent a miraculous conception—
nondescript and terribly wicked. This mythic credence,
or Eastern allegory, judged by the laws of ratiocination
and geological insight, could not possibly last. With
the growth of Western civilization questions naturally
arose as to Man being a single species, or if his first
genesis, "Eden's lovely pair," were black or white, brown
or red ; and how far his mental and moral nature were
reconcileable with his physical structure.

Looking upon the human family at large, it might well
be asked :—Were the Southern Islanders luxuriating
upon their enemies' warm vitals or an occasional relish
of " cold Missionary"— the Esquimaux peering out
from beneath his bearskin coverings like a timid
hedgehog, yet feeding with a forty-parson stomachic
power, on whale blubber—the black-ebony African in
his nude, chewing the sugar-cane—the countless families
of deep olive, sooty, and ochre-red, grandly feathered and
tattooed, some with noses rung like a Durham ox, others
with lower lips fashioned like egg-cups, or seeking
beauty in paint, mutilation, and deformity, fetish worshippers and other animalized anthropoids :—were all
these sprung from the loves of Adam and Eve, and were
they to be held of the same stock as Socrates, Galileo,
and Newton ? Many and ludicrous were the attempts
to solve these and other questions pertaining to Man's
position, but to no effect till Johann Friedrich Blumen-

bach's dissertation, "*De Generis Humani Varietate Nativa*," was read at Göttingen in the autumn of 1775. A few months prior to Blumenbach, John Hunter,[1] an Edinburgh graduate, selected for his thesis the Varieties of Man ; so that Edinburgh and Göttingen made the first advance to ethnology. As the Scoto-Britannicus proceeded no further in the work, the German got the field to himself, and maintained it beyond his professorial jubilee. Blumenbach's labours formed the text-book of Cuvier, Lawrence, Pritchard, Nott and Gliddon, Latham, Waitz, Morton, Pickering, and others.

Anthropology may now be said to be in a promising way : accredited facts and a stricter observation and analysis of humanity in well-trodden fields are being accumulated, and, what is of more import, are freely discussed and interpreted on scientific grounds alone.

Knox, as a youth, was greatly influenced by the stirring events of the Napoleonic epoch. Pressed forwards by the tide of human thought that swept away so many of the effete formulas of the eighteenth century, Knox came to view the passing events of his adolescence as having a more lasting influence than popular passion concentrated upon a revolutionary storm and a national conflict. The spirit of the Old Gaul, though springing from a single city, the capital, it is true, had been sufficient not only to upset the

---

[1] This John Hunter has by some continental authors been mistaken for the great surgeon, comparative anatomist, and founder of the museum of the Royal College of Surgeons, London. The former had a very ephemeral fame, whilst the philosophic labours of the latter placed him in the very front rank of medical discovery, and there he will stand as the historical John Hunter.

oldest dynasty in the world, but to make Europe stand
aghast at the dazzling blaze of French aggression. Well
versed as Knox was in historic lore, and the progress
of modern polity and civilization, nothing in past times
appeared to him so strange as the impetuous force of
the Celtic wave rushing from the banks of the Seine
across the Alps, spreading over the southern plains of
Europe, and even traversing the " Great Sea " to the
land of the Pharaohs and the Solomons.   Then arose
the opposing forces, the marchings and countermarchings
of the Allies from Madrid to Moscow, and all directed
to crush the Corsican phenomenon at the head of his
Celtic tribes.   Why should the French become so for-
midable at the close of the eighteenth century, that
they could tear State treaties to rags, set alliances at
defiance, and make havoc in Europe ?   Some other
source than geographical position, mere numbers, or
cunning diplomacy, ruled events ; and Knox sought
for the *rationale* in the blood of the race.   It was the
Celt who had broken loose from his Bourbon chains,
and, fired by the old spirit, military and marauding,
had carried the revolutionary torch from Alp to Alp,
from city to city, till the tocsin of war resounded
through Europe.   The "*Marseillaise*" with its " *Citoyens
aux armes,*" the *bonnet rouge*, and " Goddess of Liberty "
idols were but the thermidor efflorescence of French
glory ; the loftier and more ambitious design of carrying
the tricolor triumphantly to the ends of the earth lay
in the sap of the race—the blood of the Gallic Celt.

As proving an early penchant for the study of Man,
Knox, immediately after graduating in 1814, visited

the Highlands of Scotland for the purpose of observing the Caledonian Celt at home. In the military hospitals of Brussels, crowded with Waterloo victims, he studied the "Pruss" and "Frank," the Sclavonic, the Basques, and other waifs and strays of the rank and file engaged at Mont St. Jean. In Africa, at the Cape, he had more specific data for observation.

Knox sought to give a new direction to the study of Race. In the first place, he wished to have a faithful record of Man's normal structures, his osteology, nervous system, &c., then the deviations, rudimentary, excessive, or abnormal, so as to make the history of the physical man as complete as possible : this, he maintained, could only be done by competent persons, thoroughly educated for the work by a knowledge of comparative anatomy as well as the human. He aimed at a knowledge of Man in all his entirety— geographical, historical, and physical. Being debarred from taking part in the greater inquiry that involved much travel and years of devotion, he occupied himself mainly with the history of Man, as far as that history bore upon the rise and fall of nationalities in the present century. The questions involved in this pursuit than which nothing could well be more deeply interesting to both governments and peoples, were so adroitly entered upon by Knox that in time he gained the distinction of having made them very much his own.

He argued for the strictly scientific path of inquiry in studying Man, and through all his varied relations, savage, social, or intellectual ; and this entirely apart from all preconceived Mosaical and Aristotelian notions.

U

He saw in the coalescence, the dynastic growth and "solidarity of peoples," a manifestation of the blood affinities of Race. The historical patriotism and conservation of public feeling or a national life were to be found with those of unmixed blood; indeed, he looked upon the homogeneity of Race as the only reliable basis of a well-founded nationality. Race was the instrument in Napoleon's marvellous rise; it was not less the cause of his disastrous fall. With differences of race came diversity of thought, contentions, and war; and no rule, however autocratic, could long maintain the *status quo* against such discordance and blood temper. Espionage, prisons, and the scaffold might serve for a time, but would not kill the hydra-headed power that demanded government in sympathy with racial predilections.

In offering a synopsis of the history of his own epoch, Race *quoad* the polity of Europe formed the main basis of his argument. He saw the operations of Race upon the wheel of Fortune all over the world's area, and as clearly patent in the foreground of savagery as of civilization; he held that each political move in Central Europe revealed facts in support of his doctrines. Ten years before Knox lectured to any popular audiences on the subject I had been made partaker of his views on the history of races, and been much struck with their novelty and force; but what surprised me most was his bold asseveration of what he felt sure must come to pass in my time, if not in his own. He saw with the eye of the seer what was looming in the distance of Continental affairs, and unquestionably indicated the approach of the most stormy events in modern times; nay, more, he saw the fulfilment of his rashest prognostications. His prefiguring "the inevitable course of events" simulated the constancy of purpose that characterized the Roman Sybil, and, like her, he encountered a world of doubting and disbelieving Tarquins. The bold avowal of his sentiments implied the power to look into the seeds of time, whilst his prophetic warnings, fraught with interest, were at times as startling to his listeners as the "All hail" of the weird sisters on the blasted heath to Macbeth and Banquo. The actions of men, and the parts performed by the rulers and the ruled in Europe, were to Knox like a game of chess : here were kings and pawns on the board, and castles behind which were sheltered statecraft and priestcraft ; the knights might be military, diplomatic, or revolutionary, but ever sought to top over the pawns or to crush the people; and all the movements obtained direction from Race.

Happily for the character of Knox's "stars," and casting of the European horoscope, the dismemberment of the Austrian Empire, and the rise of the Italian Kingdom, that he had foreseen, are now patent facts ; and no better example need be cited of his clear insight into the future, his guide to which rested exclusively upon the likes and dislikes of Race. There was neither fancy nor guesswork in the Knox programme that pointed to a new interpretation of the world's history. His predictions had no alliance with the Keiths of the past, much less the Cummings of the present day, whose patchwork of Daniel, the Pope, and the Devil, with earthquakes to boot, are only suited to scare old women of both sexes.

Knox based his views of the coming time—earthly, be it
understood—upon the type and disposition of the actors
in the world's drama; and Race he held to be unchanged
and unchangeable. The stage, the orchestra, and the
scenic reliefs might vary with the fashion of the times—
the Consulate, the Commonwealth, or the *coups d'état* of
history—but the living forces would remain the same in
essence and manifestations: another drop of the curtain,
fresh buckram and hose, a loftier declamation, and the
moral epilogue was neither more nor less than Man
acting in accordance with the impulses of his race.

No one could converse with Knox without recognizing
the great space that man's nature filled in the schedule
of the anatomist's philosophy. Race would set aside
geographical position and boundaries, protocols, auto-
cracies, and the like; it overtopped restraints of every
kind, diplomatic or dynastical. Knox could not glance
at a cranium for the common descriptive anatomy
without speaking of its ethnological bearings; it was the
same with the external features and form of man generically and specifically. However much he might owe to
study and acquirements, Knox seemed to the manner
born to investigate distinctive anatomical characters:
even when walking along the streets, thronged with
men and women, he was always on the *qui vive* for
Race features. He could see at a glance what ordinary
men could hardly distinguish at their leisure; if his eye
was penetrative beyond most, his more gifted vision lay
within an alert and discriminative mind. Previous to
his time, little or nothing was heard about Race in the
medical schools: he changed all this by his Saturday's

lectures, and Race became as familiar as household words
to his students, through whom some of his novel ideas
became disseminated far and wide, both at home and
abroad. The terms "peoples," "nationalities," and the
like, used to constitute the staple vocabulary of writers,
without, however, any tangible groundwork or ideal
perception of the larger truths involved. Knox, travelling like a peripatetic from one great city to another,
helped to convey to the English mind a larger meaning
than hitherto existed of the history of peoples ; and this
he accomplished by holding up a mirror that reflected
not only the names and colours of humanity, but the
inherent virtues and vices—call them the distinctive
qualities—of Race. Though slow to admit any doctrine
not springing from its own loins, "Cockaigne" at last
came to recognize "there was something" in Knox's
arguments, and that his scientific texts might be
preached from ; even the *Times*, where few men would
look for any semblance of philosophy, began to write
of Race with as much pretension as any "old dog at
physiology."

He may have glanced at the plan of Daubenton,
founded on the structure of the head and on the relation which it bears to the trunk ; or the older plan
of Albert Dürer, who used a frontal, nasal, and maxillary line for his cranioscopic survey ; and the better
known facial lines of Camper as modes applied to
the discrimination of national crania as well as distinguishing them from the higher mammalia ; but beyond
a criticism of the weaker points in the doctrines of
Camper and his predecessors, Knox offered no further

elucidation of their views. The diversities in the osseous head of different nations, like of those of national countenance, were, according to Blumenbach,[1] reducible to five principal varieties. To this classification Knox objected, but he seemed less averse to Blumenbach's "vertical rule," deduced from observing crania from behind the vertex, having their cheek-bones placed in the same horizontal line, arranged in a series : this "vertical rule" claimed attention very markedly when the head of a Georgian woman, distinguished by the symmetry and beauty of all its parts, was placed between the cranium of a Tungoose from the north-east of Asia, and that of a negress from the coast of Guinea. As "the facial angle" led Camper to propose three varieties of Man—Caucasian, Mongolian, and Ethiopian —Blumenbach obtained *inter alia* the same notions from his "vertical rule ; "—the superadded American and Malayan holding middle places between the Caucasian and Mongolian, and the Caucasian and Ethiopian. Alexander Walker, a distinguished anatomist, looked to the physical form and moral habit of man, and in

[1] There is a singular coincidence in the nature of the inquiries which engaged Knox and Blumenbach ; *e.g.* the Comparative Anatomy of the Eye, the *Ornithorhynchus Paradoxus ;* even beyond the biological field, as in medical and surgical practice, Knox ran in the Blumenbach groove when he discussed the frequency of hernia, &c.

Both Blumenbach and Knox had the art of calling things by their right names, and of not sparing the rod when pseudo-science and charlatanism deserved it. In speaking of the Sloth, Blumenbach said the animal could never be brought to move both feet at the same time. "When it goes, it moves first one foot, stops, and sighs. Ah ! it could not have been in the universal menagerie of Mount Ararat, because it lives in Brazil only; if it had to come from Ararat to Brazil, it would not have been there yet."

some respects he claimed Knox's adhesion as better indications than those of Camper or Blumenbach.

From an early period in his career as an anatomical lecturer, he had pointed out the import of the study of Race, and, after 1834, had indoctrinated the majority of his friends with his more advanced views; it was in the year 1846 that he ventured to appear on a public platform to address a non-medical audience. In the language of the day, these lectures caused a sensation by their novelty, and led to much talk out of doors, and no small amount of controversy in the press. For the first time English mixed audiences listened to an original construction of human history, to the tracing of human character, individual, social, natural, to the all-pervading, unalterable physical characters of Race. In 1850 Dr. Knox published his lectures under the title "The Races of Men : a Philosophical Inquiry into the Influence of Race over the Destinies of Nations." A second edition was issued by Mr. Renshaw in 1862 : considering the nature of the work, its cleverness, originality, and the bold onslaught of the author on stereotyped prejudices, it should have sold in thousands.

Knox based his anthropological views on the physical structure of Man, or his zoological history. "Men are of various races; call them species, if you will; call them permanent varieties; it matters not. The fact, the simple fact, remains just as it was : men are of different races. Now, the object of these lectures is to show that in human history Race is everything." He believed that the mind of the Race, instinctive and reasoning, naturally differed in correspondence with the organization. He doubted if civilization had made much progress since the decline of the Roman Empire, and seemed disposed to think that Christianity was losing ground. Human history was not a chapter of accidents, "Race was everything, yet we know not the history of one race on the earth. All is conjecture, pretension, error, obscurity." He classified the history of Man with the history of the organic world, "as by the unity of organization Man is connected with all life—past, present, and to come. Other animals have but one history, their zoological; Man has two, the zoological and the intellectual." He objected to the philosophic formula of Blumenbach as being but an external-character naturalistic method of studying Man. To the Slavonian or to the South and Middle German, to Goethe, Oken, Von Martius, and a host of others, he attributed a truer theory of nature based on Transcendental Anatomy.

In his first lecture he astonished his hearers by saying that the Celtic race does not, and never could be made to comprehend the meaning of the word "liberty"—an opinion deduced from past history—1791, 1815, and 1830—and which received ample confirmation by the events of 1848 and 1851. On each of these occasions supreme power was in the hands of the Celtic French, but to no avail. To-day France is under a Napoleon and arbitrary power. Knox was specially strong, if not dogmatic, on the character of the Celt— his "furious fanaticism, love of war and disorder, hatred for order and patient industry, and no accumulative habits," and as clinching the contrast between the

Saxon and the Celt, from personal character and feeling, said : " As a Saxon, I abhor all dynasties, monarchies, and bayonet governments, but this latter seems to be the only one suitable for the Celtic man."

In matters pertaining to the history of Man he was not sparing in his criticism of universities, colleges, and schools, to whom the world owed "the perpetuation of error, and of neatly-formuled untruths : " he had as little sympathy with the "trashy, popular physiologies " that would attribute the dulness and phlegm of the Dutch to their living amongst marshes, or the vigorous calf of the Frenchwoman's leg to there being no side pavements in Paris—opinions that had been advanced by Andrew Combe and Sir Charles Bell.

He held that as regards individual existence, time is a short span ; a few centuries, or a few thousand years, more or less : this is all a man can grasp, and for that period, at least, organic forms seem not to have changed. " So far back as history goes, the species of animals, as we call them, have not changed ; the races of men have been absolutely the same." Again, he says : " Look more narrowly into the races of men, and you will find them to be subject to diseases peculiar to each ; that the very essence of their language is distinct, their civilization also, if they have any." Two questions, he thought, remained beyond human inquiry :—First, the origin of life on the globe ; secondly, the secondary laws which create out of primitive forms, the past, the present, and the future organic worlds. Wishing to confine his remarks to Man merely as a material being, the most perfect, no doubt, that exists, Knox concluded his introductory chapter as follows:—" In woman's form I see the perfection of Nature's works; the absolutely perfect, the beautiful, the highest manifestation of abstract life, clothed in a physical form, adapted to the corresponding minds of her race and species."

In his lecture on the " History of the Saxon and Scandinavian Race," Knox's satire is manifested against ingenious priests, Jesuits, and subtle casuists, from St. Cyril downwards to Dr. Buckland of the nineteenth century, and the framers of treaties, protocols, and alliances. " The Scandinavian or Saxon," wrote Knox, who wished to avoid the words " German " and " Teuton," as liable to *equivoque*, " was early in Greece, say 3,500 years ago. This race still exists in Switzerland, forming its Protestant portion ; whilst in Greece it contributed mainly, no doubt, to the formation of the noblest of all men— the statesmen, poets, sculptors, mathematicians, metaphysicians, historians of ancient Greece." He attributed to the Saxon inordinate self-esteem, love of independence, which makes him dislike the proximity of a neighbour, hatred for dynasties and governments, and considered him democratic by nature, indeed the only democrat on earth who comprehended the meaning of the word "liberty." Of the origin of the Saxon race, and not less its English portion, he was by no means clear, yet he quoted Livy as to their physical character; *e.g.* fair hair, blue eyes, fine complexion, " not a well-made or proportioned race, falling off most in the limbs ; the torso being large, vast, and disproportioned." The Saxon was not suited to America

and Australia, and a *real native* permanent race of pure
Saxon he held to be a dream which never could be
realized. Here is his description of the Saxon:—
" Thoughtful, plodding, industrious beyond all other
races, a lover of labour for labour's sake, he cares not
its amount if it be but profitable; large-handed, mechanical, a lover of order, of punctuality in business,
of neatness and cleanliness." Again: " This genius is
wholly applicative, for he invents nothing. In the fine
arts, and in music, taste cannot go lower;" but they
delight in " prize-fights, bull-baiting with dogs, sparring
matches, rowing, horse-racing, gymnastics."

In his " History of the Celtic Race" he maintained
that whether French, Irish, Scottish, or Welsh, the
Celt was always the same, unaltered and unalterable.
Civilization and education may modify, religious formula
is the result of Race; morals, actions, feelings, &c.,
flow from physical structure. Long prior to Cæsar's
time the Celtic race had overflowed its barriers, crossing
the Alps, sacking Rome, invading Greece, and plunder-
ing Delphi. From Brennus to Napoleon, the war-cry
of the Celtic race was, " To the Alps—to the Rhine."
War is the game of the Celt. Herein is the forte of
his physical and moral character; in stature and weight,
as a race, inferior to the Saxon; limbs muscular
and vigorous; torso and arms seldom attaining any
very large development—hence the extreme rarity of
athletæ; hands broad; fingers squared at the points;
step elastic and springy; in muscular energy and
rapidity of action surpassing all other European races.
His natural weapon is the sword. Jealous on the point

of honour, his self-respect is extreme ; admitting of no
practical jokes ; an admirer of beauty of colour and of
form, and a liberal patron of the fine arts.   The musical
ear of the race is tolerably good ;   in literature and
science he follows method and order; in the ordinary
affairs of life he despises order, economy, cleanliness ;
regular labour he holds in contempt.   Irascible, warm-
hearted, full of deep sympathies, dreamers on the past,
uncertain, treacherous, gallant, and brave.

In discussing the physiological questions—Do races
ever amalgamate ?   What are the obstacles to a race
changing its original locality ?—he answered the first
query by a direct negative, and pointed to Spanish
America, also to Ireland, where the Celt and Saxon hate
each other.   Contrary to current Evangelical opinions,
he held that Protestantism did not alter the Celt, and
that the Presbyterian Caledonian Celt had the same
faults as his Papal brother across the water; that Christianity had little or no influence over human affairs,
further than a State engine serving political purposes.
His second query took him back to the Phœnician,
Greek, and Coptic colonies; but what was of more import
to modern history, he had poor hopes of John Bull's
future as a denizen of North America, instancing the
changes going on in the United States man, and his
different appearance from the European.   The ladies
early lose their teeth ; in both sexes the adipose cellular
cushion interposed between the skin and the aponeu-
rosis and muscles disappears, or at least loses its adipose
portion ; the muscles become stringy and show themselves ; the tendons appear on the surface, &c.   The

French Celt he maintained would never become a colonist in Algeria, and that he did not thrive in Corsica.

In his second lecture, embracing the physiological laws regulating human life, he pointed with triumph to Guizot and Metternich among the converts flocking to his standard, and admitting "that 'race,' as well as 'democracy,' or socialism, or bands of peripatetic demagogues, or evil spirits,[1] may have had something to do with the history of nations, and more especially with the last revolutions in Europe." Mere climate could not by any process of time form a new race ; the Bosjeman could not be convertible into an Amakoso Caffre or Saxon Hollander. Any change in structure or colour can at once be traced to intermarriage, but he did not believe that the new product arising from intermarriage, or a mixed race, would stand its ground : " 1. By reason of the innate dislike of race to race, preventing a renewal of such intermarriage ; 2. Because the descendants will of necessity fall back upon the stronger race, and all traces, or nearly so, of the weaker race must in time be obliterated."

Knox looked upon human history as but of yesterday compared with the period through which the globe has rolled in space, "through which life has undergone its ever succeeding developments ; yet Man, up to the earliest recorded time, did not differ materially from what he is now ; that there were races then as now ; that neither over them, nor over the living world around, has climate or external circumstances effected any serious

[1] Metternich had spoken of "evil spirits," and Lord John Russell of " peripatetic demagogues," in their explanation of the events of 1848.

changes, produced any new species, any new groups of animal or vegetable life, any new varieties of mankind."

Looking at the two sides of St. George's Channel, where two nations equally civilized and favoured by climate had lived for hundreds of years almost *cæteris paribus*, and finding one nation respecting, the other despising the law ; " the one Protestant and tolerant, the other Catholic, fanatical, and persecuting ;" Knox could not believe that distinctions so wide were the result of accidental circumstances, or that the British and French could be " spoken of in the abstract as the branches of one great family, of some ideal Indo-Germanic stock, of some fabulous Caucasian family, who would never have differed had no seas divided them."

His description of the gipsy on the southern borders of Scotland, the intermarriage of the gipsy woman with the Saxon, and all the speculations expressed as to the nature of this wandering tribe, are set forth in Knox's usual style.

The Coptic, Jewish, and Phœnician races, of course come under his cognizance ; but it cannot be said that he throws any light upon them. Of the history of the Coptic, the ancient or modern Egyptian, Knox, like hundreds of others who have preceded him, offers nothing tangible or satisfactory ; he has his hypothesis, around which he weaves a large amount of weft, more coloured than substantial. The best German minds have been devoted to Egyptology, and the French helped a little in the same direction ; but the ethnological history of Egypt, of surpassing interest to mankind, as yet remains untold.

And this is all the more curious, as of the fertile and inhabited lands of the earth, Egypt is held by latest observers to be of the most recent geological formation. Human history extends only to the Egyptian dynasties, a kind of evidence not to be overlooked in showing that Man has had his most ancient resting-place by the banks of the Nile ; how long antecedent to the building of the Pyramids, and the enjoyment of life's luxuries, physical and æsthetic, will ever remain beyond all record. If grounds for speculation daily arise as to the past and present history of Man, they come with more marked force to the mind absorbed in the study of the ruins of the Pharaohs and their predecessors—in the Temple of Columns at Karnac, or in the dark caverns of the Tombs of the Kings on the heights above the plains of Thebes.

Knox was facetious upon the Jews, whom he looked upon as composed of more than one race—Coptic, Chaldean, and Phœnician—and his opinions gave rise to much newspaper discussion at Manchester, the great emporium for both Jews and Gentiles. He would not admit of the true Jew ever marrying with the Saxon or any other people, so that the elopement of Jessica with Lorenzo from old Shylock's house was a Shakesperian fancy, without the slightest ethnological support. Yet Knox might have allowed with Lancelot Gobbo—

> " There will come a Christian by,
> Will be worth a Jewess' eye."

He had no belief in the conversion of the Jews, and if his description of their race be at all correct, they are hardly worth the pains. It was his solemn conviction "that a real Jew would never alter, for nature alters not, and therefore conversion was impossible.[1] As for their being a dispersed race, they were so in Cicero's time, and hundreds of years before the taking and destruction of Jerusalem by Vespasian." "The question always returns," says Knox, "why were they a dispersed race, and why are they now a dispersed race? No sane person doubts their power to seize Judæa if they thought fit. One of their capitalists might actually buy it from the present Turkish Government."

His "Remarks on the Jewish and Coptic Chronology" imply no belief in the generally accepted views on this subject: the Coptic and Mosaic records were not trustworthy; their authors, like the Chinese, Hindoos, and others, wishing to appear the earliest in history, sought to identify themselves with the great creative power.

Knox's description of the Jew seems to have been drawn from Amsterdam, and Shoreditch, London. Oriental travel, it need hardly be said, would have profited him more. Could he, on an early spring morning, have observed the "Jewish household outside

[1] Having made personal inquiries in the Judæan stronghold of "converted Jews," where English sympathies have been strongly enlisted, and where, more wonderful to say, Scotch money has been most incautiously spent on the same "cursed tribe," I have no reason to doubt Knox's opinions. The fact of so rare a phenomenon as a converted Jew, even at an Exeter Hall May meeting, might make the sanguine Christian pause before he throws away his money on Hebrews. The so-called "converts" presented to my notice in Palestine (and they could be counted on the fingers) had none of the features of the "unmistakeable Jew;" they appeared of a spurious breed; probably Knox would have classified them with the Coptic division, with whom they ranked for cunning.

the gates of the city of David," inhaling the incense-breathing morn, and gathering the wild roses of Sharon, he would have enjoyed another sight, imposing of itself, and more truly characteristic of the race. There the patriarch and his spouse realize the ancient type ; there the daughters of Jerusalem, robed in the purity of brides possibly waiting for the bridegroom's coming, present the regular fine chiselled features, the bland and bewitching eyes, the exquisite bust and Medicean Venus form, gushing in feminine attributes and attractiveness. Of Syrian women, who are, as far as my observations go, among the fairest on earth, the young Jewess budding into womanhood is the cream of joy and loveliness. A "Sabbath morning" in the Ghetto of Rome, or a few hours any day of the week on the bridge connecting Stamboul proper with Pera (Constantinople), along which the nations of the earth seem to pass to and fro, revealing the best and worst of their kind, would also have modified Knox's picture of the Jew's physiognomy.

" The Dark Races of Men " occupy upwards of 100 pages of Knox's work. He was disposed to think that there must be a physical and psychological inferiority in the dark races generally, as since the earliest times they had been the slaves of their fairer brethren.[1] He describes the exterior of the dark man, his physical characteristics, the non-amalgamation of the Saxon

---

[1] The late lamented Dr. James Hunt, founder and president of the Anthropological Society, read papers on the Negro's place in Nature, to the British Association, which he afterwards published in the *Anthropological Review.* His views coincided with those of Knox, and perhaps are more amplified in detail than his coadjutor the anatomist's.

X

with the dark race, the threatened extermination of the
race by the organized hypocrisy of the said Saxon ;
here and there interspersing his anthropological views
with remarks upon governments, missionary schemes,
and the like.   Looking upon the black man as differing
from the white man "in everything as much as in colour,
he is no more a white man than an ass is a horse or
zebra."   He has much to say about the Chinese, and
the praise bestowed upon the race by Humboldt and
Schlegel : the latter thought them highly civilized,
and instanced their canals, bridges, &c. ; but, writes
Knox, "this is a great error ; the beaver, the bee, and
the wasp and ant would, in this case, be civilized ; the
hillock of the African termites is a more remarkable
labour, comparatively, than the pyramids to Man ; Man
builds, cuts canals, makes roads, instinctively, exactly
like an animal; these are no proofs of intellect or pure
reason ; each race builds after its own kind. The Saxon
is not disposed to build; the ancient Copts, Phœnicians,
and Greeks were, on the other hand, remarkably so, and
builders *par excellence*."   The doom of the dark race was
sealed; nothing but the tropics could save him from the
sword of the Celt, and the conventions, treaties, and
law of the Saxon.

Knox seems to have overlooked the fact of English
colonists carrying with them to unknown lands more
than the sabre and rifle, the law and the prophets ;
namely, alcohol, smallpox, and other forms of physical
disease and distemper.   Whisky and other social evils
are the accompaniments of modern Christianity ; they
are the latest emblems or croppings out of civilization,

and assuredly they are the most potent agents of all in civilizing the aborigines *off* the face of the earth. How effectually they have done their work in the present century may be gathered from the history of every British foreign possession. Look at Tasmania, with its 7,000 aborigines in 1803, sabred and Christianized by the English till not a single individual is left! For several years back there had been but one black representative of a population that under ordinary increase should have reached 20,000; and he, known as "Lanney,"[1] or "King Billy," the very last of his tribe, died early in the year 1869. It was the same with the Botany Bay blacks, who, in little more than sixty years after the occupation of their lands by the Anglo-Saxon, became extinct.[2]

[1] There has been a colonial fight over "Lanney's" dead body. The Colonial Secretary had promised Lanney's head to the Tasmanian Royal Society, while Dr. Crowther wished to send the entire skeleton to the College of Surgeons, London. The old days of body-snatching, or rather mutilation, have been revived at the antipodes. Some one ran off with the cranium, and Dr. Stokell, surgeon to the hospital, made sure of the hands and feet; hence it would appear that "Lanney" dead is a greater bone of contention to the doctors than "Lanney" alive, seeking salvation, was to the missionaries.

[2] A body of benevolent Christians, many years ago, determined to evangelize the Botany Bay blacks, and told off a band of missionaries for the purpose. Behold, there was but one of the aborigines left!—a dark "grinning Diogenes," who used to crawl out of his tub to beg coppers of the passers-by; he was called "Rickety Dick," and died in 1840.

CHAPTER XVI.

RACES OF MEN.

PROFESSOR TIEDEMANN noticed the great size of some African skulls in Knox's museum, and was disposed to question the opinions proclaimed by the historian Gibbon as to the inferiority of the Negro. Knox thought there must be a physical, and consequently a psychological inferiority in the dark races, not depending altogether on deficiency in the size of the brain *en masse*, but rather perhaps on specific characters in the quality of the brain itself. In all discussions as to the respective merits of brain-power he saw that the quality of the brain structure—be it firm, fibrous, with more or less of grey matter—should be fully considered. An instance of the import of such inquiry was shown to the Royal Society of Edinburgh by the late Sir W. Hamilton, Professor of Logic, already spoken of as a pupil of Knox's, when he was contravening the doctrines of the phrenologists. He had two noteworthy skulls upon which to found his comparisons: one was that of a Malay robber and cut-throat, who ended by murdering his wife and getting hanged for his villany; the other was the skull of George Buchanan, the Scottish historian, preserved in the museum of the University of Edinburgh. One skull was presumably a bad specimen of a nation reckoned bad; the other a very good instance of a nation reckoned good. The calibre-compasses were applied and bump after bump measured; and after balancing all in accordance with a phrenological survey, the *Malay* was declared to transcend in goodness the *Buchanan* example by such-and-such a cipher of inches. Thomas Carlyle, from whom I partly quote, might well say to Sir William the next time he met him: " Malay cut-throat *versus* Buchanan: explain me that; till then I say nothing."

Knox's seventh lecture on the History of the Celtic Race abounds with interesting matter. His pictures of the French, Hibernian, and Caledonian Celt are drawn to the life; their character is summed up in the brevity of epigrams; and as you read his description you walk the streets of Paris with *Monsieur*, or you sit by the hut fire or on the potato-heap with the children of Connemara, or stand on the coast of Dornoch from which the Caledonian Celt departs with the exclamation " We'll maybe return to Lochaber no more." Knox had but a poor opinion[1] of the Celtic race compared

[1] Dr. R. Druitt read some passages of Knox's work to the late Lord Lyndhurst, whose "aliens in blood, in language, and religion" speech to the House of Lords had been severely handled by the O'Connellite party and the press. In Knox's description of the Celt the ex-Lord Chancellor found consolation to his wounded feelings. Both Lord and Lady Lyndhurst wished their estimable medical friend, Dr. Druitt, to express to Dr. Knox the delight they had in perusing "The Races of Men," and their wish to see the work freely circulated in the best English society.

with the Germans, whose general characters occupied another chapter.

" As early as 1820–21 I became convinced that the elements of mind to which the German owes his vast reputation as the most philosophical of all men, the most abstract in reasoning, the most metaphysical, the most original, and, in a word, the most transcendental,—the element of mind which produced Kant, and Goethe, &c., is not, cannot be Saxon—cannot be Scandinavian."

Withdrawing a part of his praise from " the Saxon, or North German," he bestowed it upon the Central German race, a darker and a differently shaped race ; and to them and the pure Sclavonic race belong German litera-ture, science, and art.   He calls the Sclavonic " a noble race, the most intellectual probably of all."   Inferior in external form or *physique*, short in stature, and of dark hair and complexion, they are superior to the Saxon and Celtic races in their taste for music, architecture, and the fine arts generally.   Knox evidently augured great things from the Sclavonic race—eighty millions in number, under the despotism of three dynasties—Haps-burg, Brandenburg, and the Muscovite—demanding a political unity and only in need of a leader.   After asking the amalgamation theorists and others to look at Central Europe, its state in 1815, its condition now, Knox goes on : " The Sclavonian wants a leader ; so does the South German ; so does the true Saxon or North German.   They are quite sensible that at present, though broken into fragments, the day may come when Nature must again assert her rights in spite of treaties and protocols, partitions and adjustments.   The balance of power in Europe must ultimately rest, not with families, but with races : the question of European civilization must repose on the same basis."

In his brief sketch of the Sarmatian race he seems to have imbibed the Napoleonic dogma of either a Cossack or a Republican Europe—the balance of opinion weighing towards the dominance of the Muscovite power, to be exercised through the Sclavonian as the nearest path to the gates of Constantinople. He had no sympathy with the Russ, low in the scale of humanity and low in morals.

No chapter of the "Fragment," as he chose to call his volume on the "Races of Men," will be read with greater interest than the one headed "Question of Dominancy:—England : her Constitution and Colonies : —Nationalities." He viewed the present Norman government of England as antagonistic to her presumed Saxon population : that the land of Ireland and of Caledonian Scotland was in the hands of the hereditary descendants of the Norman, and that England was daily following the same steps. When Sheffield was agitating for "financial reform," Knox advised the reformers to look at the land question—not forgetting, by the way, to call the "Church rampant, Norman, bloated with wealth—corrupt beyond imagination, and a population priest-ridden." As the Saxons are democrats, nothing will ever satisfy them but self-government, and no Government can long hold a Saxon colony. The really momentous question for England as *a nation* is the presence of three sections of the Celtic race still on the soil : the Irish Celt is the most to be dreaded.

His concluding lecture embraced : " Ancient Greece—
The Fine Arts—The Perfect and the Beautiful—Relations
of Philosophy to ' the Perfect and the Beautiful ' —
Theory of Species, or Individualism—Theory of Unity,
or Universalism—Application of the Laws of Transcendental Anatomy to the Past, the Present, and the Future
of the Organic World—Unity and Variety." Having
such texts as these, Knox might well preach one of
his largest and most telling discourses. Let the
reader imagine a chapter in Knox's best style on the
Homeric ballad, the Parthenon, the Apollo and Venus,
Athenian Philosophy and Philosophers, the picturesque
banks of the Koonap, the human form divine and
especially beautiful women, embryology and cyto-
genesis, the Goethian and Sclavonic ideas in contrast
to Paley and the Bridgewater Treatise schools, history
and logic, error and Transcendentalism, glances at the
earth's history from the muddy waters holding the
Megatherium to these latter days in human history,
with its *demo* and other *ocracies*, its theologies:—fully
realizing *de omnibus et quibusdam aliis !*

In an appendix, he treats of the " Origin, Civilization,
and Extinction of the Dark Races of Man," and " The
Antagonism of Man to Nature's Works." To " the
Bridgewater school, the sturdy utilitarian, the dogmatic
Jew," he left " the jesuitical task of discovering in physical
and moral suffering a benefit and a pleasure." Looking
to " mental and bodily diseases, pestilence and famine,
wars of opinion ! war to the knife ! &c." he held Man's
fate to be " severer than that of the lower animals : they
have no aristocracy, no priests, no kings ; they are

spared this triple curse; nor can a dark and fearful future be depicted on their brains, in terms so strong as to make them believe that millions of invisible beings walk the lower regions of the atmosphere, wholly occupied in leading them to destruction." His notes are as enlivening as his text, and nothing more need be said.

A second edition of "The Races of Men" appeared in January 1862; it differed from the first only in having attached to it a supplement, consisting of four chapters: 1. "An Inquiry into the Laws of Human Hybridité;" 2. "On some Ancient Forms of Civilization;" 3. "Africa, its Past, Present, and probable Future;" 4. "The Present Phasis of Ethnology."

After quoting largely from Livy, as to the history of the Gauls, and Paul Broca's definition—"a hybrid is a living being, the product of a mixture of two species more or less remote"—Knox seems to agree with Buffon, Voltaire, and Cuvier, "that species have not altered since the earliest historic times. Confining himself to human *hybridité*, he asks: "Is it true that all the races of mankind intermingle freely with each other, giving rise to a fertile progeny? Look over the world as it now exists, and say where such a hybrid exists; for to prove that all races mingle freely with each other, it must be shown, not only that this is so, but that there results a self-supporting progeny, characterized by all its newly acquired moral and physical properties, without recourse being had to either of the primitive races. Now this has never happened either in respect of dogs or men—the two genera which have been chiefly appealed to in this inquiry." He believed that from the earliest historic times mankind were already divided into a certain number of races, perfectly distinct. In reference to the Biblical theory of the origin of the Negro race, he quoted M. Broca's clear refutation of that theory from the Hebrew writings themselves, but doubted if it would "put a stop to the infamous hypothesis which had been engrafted on the Book of Genesis by modern divines." As the law of living beings was obviously that every living being should bring forth after *its* own kind, Knox was of opinion that the various species of animals, Man included, have never varied, are immutable, unchangeable, if not eternal; that as they are now, so were they when Man first commenced to engrave on stone or record on parchment what he saw in the external world." He would not sanction the idea of a human hybrid being permanently fruitful, and *inter alia* appealed to the hybrid produced between the male European and female Australian as seeming altogether sterile from the first: in this view he would appear to be supported by M. Pouchat.

"The races of man," writes Knox, " differ from each other, and have done so from the earliest historic period, as proved—

" 1. By their external characters, which have never altered during the last six thousand years.

" 2. By anatomical differences in structure.

" 3. By the infertility of the hybrid product, originating in the intermingling of two races.

" 4. By historic evidence which shows that no distinct hybrid race can be shown to exist anywhere."

Again he says : " Though of distinct species, all the races of men belong to the same natural family, the embryo of each species containing within itself the rudiments of all the others. The human family stands profoundly apart from all others, implying that in the great chain of beings constituting Nature's plan, some natural family filling up the link has disappeared.

In concluding his chapter on Human Hybridité, he states that " the mingled races of Europe are not hybrids; the Basque remains distinct from the population of Old Gaul, and the Sclaves retain everywhere the peculiarities of their race. The 'old Pruss' is still distinct from the Scandinavians, Sclavonians, and Teutons who groan under his abhorred rule. . . Of all countries Italy is the one which ought to have proved, by its population, the substitution of a hybrid for a pure race. Nothing of the kind exists. The sterility of hybrids is the check which Nature employs for the preservation of her primitive forms of life. There is a *consanguinité*, no doubt, in all that lives ; for life, being a property inherent in matter, must at its origin have been one ; but this *consanguinité* does not extend to or exclude specialities. It goes no farther than their *genera*, and most commonly not so far."

In his brief notice of " Some Ancient Forms of Civilization," he discusses the " origin of Art," and then goes on to "the Arab race," whose history he traces in his usual graphic way. With Mahomet as their leader, they conquered a great part of the civilized world, and had they not been checked by Charles Martel, Knox fancied, the Koran might now have been

taught at Oxford and Cambridge as "the Book" which
must supersede all others. He seized the chance of
showing how the history of the Arab brings out the
questions of the future of intrusive races into continents
of which they are not the aboriginals and the influence
exercised over the invading race by coming in contact
with those of a higher or lower civilization. " Brought
in contact with many races, they adopted the inventions
of none. The Koran was the tomb of truth in science,
literature, and art. Though conquerors of many races,
they gave origin to no hybrid race. They attempted
settlements or colonies on three continents, and failed.
Nature gave them desert Arabia as their home, and
there only do they thrive."

His views of " Africa, its Past, Present, and probable
Future," are stated with great boldness, and, whether
altogether or only partially correct, are worthy the
attention of both the politician and philanthropist. As
a sojourner in Southern Africa, he claimed the privilege
of writing from personal observation, and a long life's
interest in all matters pertaining to the history of an
important English colony. There is, as indeed prevails
everywhere in Knox's writings, much reflection, both
in form and statement, and large notice of the Celt
and Saxon, in their relations to the Negro and other
races.

" The present phasis of Ethnology" afforded him the
opportunity of speaking more directly of his own endea-
vours to indoctrinate the English mind with a knowledge
of Race from an original point of view. Before 1848, not
a thought was bestowed upon Race by the English press.

He accused the *Times* of plagiarizing all his ideas without the slightest acknowledgment.[1]

In surveying the affairs of Europe, the progress of the Italian question, and the breaking up in part of the Austrian Empire, Knox had reasons to congratulate himself, for in a few short years there had been a fulfilment of the most important of his predictions. Those who felt disposed to laugh in 1846 at Knox's theories of Race, were surprised at the historical endorsement they obtained in 1860. The idea of supporting ethnological propositions by the testimony of ancient monuments seems to have occurred to Knox long prior to Messrs. Nott and Gliddon, in proof of which he referred to M. Milne-Edwards, the French physiologist, and M. Thierry, the historian.

No well-educated person could look at the "Irish difficulty" of British statesmen, the conflicting interests on the banks of the Rhine and the Danube, or the larger field of American politics, without acknowledging the significance of the anthropological views enunciated by Knox. Reasoning from geographical and philological data, as much as from the individual being, Man, the ethnologist was led to an ideal grouping of the families or races. This was but a conventional assumption or

---

1 In a characteristic preface to his work, Knox said : "Physiologists will dispute with me the great laws I have endeavoured to substitute for the effete commonplace of the schools ; geologists will think me hasty ; theologians—but here I stop ; a reply shall not be wanting. As to the hack compilers, their course is simple : they will first deny the doctrine to be true ; when this becomes clearly untenable they will deny that it is new ; and they will finish by engrossing the whole in their next compilations, omitting carefully the name of the author."

mode of treating a noble theme; it had no claim to be viewed as a zoological classification. Moreover, it failed to convey any truth that could be made applicable to the solution of many problems affecting humanity. Knox saw the inadequacy of a mere formula wanting in scientific purpose, and offering no explanation of the mighty events clustered around the growth of the first French Empire, much less the disturbing influences at work during his own more peaceful epoch. Blumenbach and his successors did not foresee the threatening storms which burst over Europe in 1791, in 1830, and in 1848; and they failed to comprehend the proximate cause of the varied revolutions of the century. What was the science of Man worth, if it rested content with the mere lineaments of form, the colour of the skin, and the outward life of a people? Each generation will rise higher in the belief that the proper study of mankind belongs to the philosophic anatomist who could marshal the data around him, and grasp the psychological criteria (or evidence) along with the *physique* of Race. It was idle to expect any indications of value, much less reliable data, from political economists, military chiefs, and diplomatists, who looked to intrigues in the administrative bureaux and the game of hazard in the hostile field for the *status quo* of nationalities. Man *per se* had no significance to governments beyond the "heavy battalion" work or as load to the dice, one throw of which might decide an autocracy or a constitutional monarchy for the joy or hate of peoples. Previous to Knox, writers on ethnology had made no advance to solve the circumstances affecting Italy and Germany after the Congress of Vienna (1815), and, like thousands of others totally unconcerned with the history of Race, looked upon Austria as one of the strongest and best-disciplined powers in Europe. Nay, the sun had to set on the bloody field of Sadowa (1866) before the self-opinionated diplomats could see the position of the House of Hapsburg.

Blumenbach's writings had not reached the core of anthropology, or Metternich, the fitting instrument of Austrian tyranny, would hardly have talked of Italy as a "geographical expression." Had Knox's views been understood on the Continent in 1849, the Austrian's boast of Novara would have been tempered by the probable contingency of a Solferino, or the more applicable instance of Garibaldi's campaign and success from the Sicilian coast at Marsala to the banks of the Volturno.

Knox aimed at the pith and marrow of the question at issue, or the blood of the Race : there he saw the true history of Man, his struggles and his aspirations ; one set of men praying for a king—Saul and the prophets ; another demanding a republic, but all governed by a natural impulse that would prevail sooner or later against the edicts of Councils or military despotisms. Peace prevailed in a community consisting of one race only, and there public sentiment was respected ; on the other hand, empires like Austria, composed of many and diverse ethnological elements, must in the course of time go apart, or succumb to greater and more lasting disintegrations.

To attain the veritable of Race, the physical structure, the actions and demeanour of the man, and his adaptation to peace or war, the industrial or fine arts had first to be grasped; in short, the *physique* in its entirety, and the man in his ethical, intellectual, and social relations. Then the brain power, the capabilities of the people as reflected in their literature and science, their penchants for home or colonization, their moral sentiments, national traits, historical manifestations, naturally completed the groundwork of the study of the anthropologist. This was pretty much the mode pursued by Knox in reading Man's position and place in the great Cosmos. He cared little for the Natural History classifications met with in acknowledged authors; he looked for the marked traits or attributes of a people, those basial elements, the genius, the temperament, and the instincts of Race. In the analogy of true or structural elements among a body of men, in their common adhesion to matters of polity and observance, in their unanimity of sentiment and healthy fraternization—call it patriotic or, as in some, communistic—were to be found the faithful indications of Race. It could only be by examining the physical, artistic, educational, and historical developments of Man that you could hope to comprehend the individual species and his congeners. A common error prevails in speaking of peoples living under one dynasty as being a distinct race or nationality—forgetting that dynasties are family arrangements where *might* prevails over *right*, and quite regardless of the wishes of the governed. The Hungarians, Slavs, Croats, &c., under the ban of Austria, are oft designated Austrians : even Ministers and the House of Commons talk in this way. Though ethnologists and men of thought knew otherwise, it fell particularly to Knox to put the matter more broadly and intelligibly before his country-men. He did a good part in showing up the fallacy of imperial rule being viewed as pertinent to the character of the people under its control. Austria, just instanced, has reaped bitter experience and as yet untold humiliation from its ignorance, or self-will, and its total abnegation of the rights of her people to be ruled according to their natural instincts.

In the application of his knowledge of Race to past and present history, he hoped also for enlightenment as to the future history of Man, particularly in Europe. No one can question that he succeeded in demon-strating from a new base line the construction of a larger survey than had ever been taken of Man's history as deduced from Race. The age had hardly been edu-cated to the belief of history being dependent on the blood and temper and natural proclivities of Man. The undying influence or inevitable tendencies of Race con-stituted the Knox text, and no text was ever better handled; it was the Alpha and Omega of numerous disquisitions; it always turned up afresh like the ever-changing aspect of the sea's surface, influenced or not by tide or zephyr. If assertion and dogma appeared to prevail in the advocacy of the new theory, did the earnest appeals to history made by Knox not show his profound conviction of the soundness of the doctrines he sought to establish? Neither force nor reiteration of statement would ever found a theory, but Knox, it may be fairly said, enunciated truths from data open to the scrutiny of all men, and as patent as current history

Y

itself. Allowing for slight trespass to the right and left of his argument, or beyond the logical verities, his theories, so novel and instructive, deserved greater attention than was awarded them. They would have been of large value to the Cabinets of the Great Powers since the advent of the nineteenth century; and could they have been acted upon at the Congresses of Vienna[1] and Verona, assembled to solder the broken fragments of kingdoms and duchies left by Napoleon *le Grand*, there would have been less dissimulation and fraud, and vastly less protocolling and check-mating during these latter days of European history. Moreover, many of the rankling sores of the body politic, the inheritance of "Constitutional mongers" of "the Holy Alliance" sort, which might have been healed if honest races had got their own, were subjected to constant irritation, till at length the ichor of discontent prevailed over the bonds of Metternich, and revolutions disturbed the whole Continent.

Look at the present disquietude abroad; it was also predicted by Knox, who, though dead seven years, seems yet to speak from the tomb. Whilst living, he fulfilled too strongly the adage applied to the

---

[1] Talleyrand never believed in the permanency of the balance of power established by the Congress of Vienna. He saw there would be a tendency on the part of the Germans to unity, and he argued that one of the Great Powers of the Confederation would spring up, and that Power could not be Austria, composed as she was of distinct and conflicting elements, which prevented her from being united at home, or capable of acting effectually abroad. This arch-diplomatist understood the influence of Race in history, and could, in 1837, foresee what came to pass in 1866, the victory of Prussia in her struggle with Austria for predominance in Germany.

fate of prophets,—the commercial and legislative publics
having their Delphic oracles in the Stock Exchange and
Ministerial portfolios—for why should the salt of the
earth countenance an English ethnologist basing his
views of nationalities on Race? Moreover, Europe had its
saviour in "the man" of the *coup d'état*, and why more
saviours than one for one epoch? "*Quosque tandem*," &c.

The correctness of Knox's views as to indigenous
races holding their own against their conquerors is well
instanced in Algeria. The French got possession of
Algiers in 1830, and meant to establish an important
colony and to make it a paying concern; the produce of
its southern climate, the fruits and condiments, were to
contribute to the markets of Paris and the luxuries of
the aristocracy. Administrations, governorships, and
military training for 100,000 troops—Zouaves and Spahis
to don the semi-oriental costume—Imperial visits and
mighty complacency to the tribes once led by Abd-el-
Kader, were part of the scheme; and, to crown all,
the "oldest son of the Church" fraternized with the
Mahometan banners and complimented the green-
turbaned Ulemas, and all for the glory of France! What
is the result of nearly forty years of Viceroyalty, aided
by scores of thousands of bayonets? The colony of
Algiers contains only 220,000 Frenchmen, and these are
so dissatisfied that great numbers meditate change of
quarters. On the 17th October, 1868, some of the best
agricultural class sold their stock and land and emigrated
to Brazil; and a thousand others were prepared to follow.
This fact is highly significant; as Cobbett would have
said, "the straw is moving," and the French rat may

have to yield his forty years' foraging to the *native* or
true Algerine animal.

He saw the futility of Missions, and oft described the
charlatanism of such schemes.   Christian Missions to the
followers of Islam! To benefit or destroy ? Mahometanism has *its* book, that does not require to be elaborated
by millions of sermons.   Mahometanism is peaceful,
sober, and virtuous.   Can this be said of the denizens
of British cities ?   If light weights and measures, food
adulterations and poisonings, baby-farming, limited lia-
bilities, Overends and Gurneys, commercial Quakerisms,
social evils, divorce courts, church squabblings, and
endless modes of deceit be desirable to propagate
abroad, then Christian England, as a perennial fertilizer
of such commodities, has a great mission before her.
Perhaps the heathen may prefer his *status quo* and a
respectful distance from Exeter Hall indoctrination.

Knox differed greatly from some of our modern writers
whose ingenuity enables them to explain everything in
the history of Englishmen, from the paint and tattoo of
their aboriginal life, be it that of the Druid, the cannibal,
or the holocaust, down to the Victorian crinolines and
chignons.   Such gifted persons speak in *ex cathedrâ*
fashion, and as often without trustworthy data.   The
pages of Cæsar are quoted as if the Roman had been a
learned authority on the varieties of man ; even Huxley,
as if forgetting the inductive philosophy and the patent
facts under his own cognizance, binds himself to Cæsar.
Now, considering the reputed origin of the Britisher—
Taranis-worshippers, Celtic tribes, Romans, Jutes, Angles,
Danes and Norsemen, *et cetera ;* then the mythic and

the traditional blending with the semi-historical and fanciful record,—Knox might well have doubts as to the component parts of what is styled " the English Race." Neither anatomically nor metaphysically can they be readily understood ; on the other hand, the Irish Celt need not be confounded with the so-called Teuton, whatever locality be fixed upon within the four seas for observation.

If Defoe, in his wrath against the Stuarts, said that Englishmen were the mud of races, Knox hesitated not in his leisure to call them a mongrel crew. Emerson thought there was an anthology of temperaments suiting the sky and soil of England, and he compared them to the varieties of pear-trees suited or unsuited to the soil of the orchard in which they are planted. In our discussions (Knox and self) as to the Norman invasion by 20,000 European vagabonds, Knox was highly diverting at the taste of the hour for the pride of descent from men who showed their merits on their shields— the wolf, the swine, the jackal, and snake being fitting emblems of their human characters and tendencies. If, as Alfieri said, " the crimes of Italy were the proof of the superiority of the stock," he may have borrowed this paradox from the founders of the English House of Lords, who refer the ornaments of their birth to the Norse piratical crews and the Norman free-lances ; men of whom the best that can be said is, that they were *chevaliers d'industrie*, having in their trail the scum of Europe.

The questions affecting man's hybridity so frequently engaging Knox's mind, also the permanence or decay

of the fresh products from the admixture of races, bid
fair to be solved in the course of time, and that time
not so very far distant. The United States of America,
now traversed by a line of railway from sea-board
to sea-board, its mighty commerce and mightier ag-
gressiveness, its growing population that daily receives
accessions from almost every quarter of the globe—a
flow tide of peoples without an ebb, and these peoples
the very motley of creation—would appear to offer the
elements upon which the types (if such a term is ad-
missible) of hybridity will one day be revealed in
unmistakeable colours. Look to the past and present
history of the States ; its wild Indian or parent stock,
the English Puritans and their slaves, the run of British
immigration since the peace of 1815, the great exodus
of the Irish Celt in 1846 and onwards to the "land of
freedom," the tide of Germans, Scandinavians, French,
Chinese, Japanese, and Mexicans ; and all marshalled
under the "stars and stripes," and working for the
almighty dollar and the continuance of their species,
pure or collateral. Analyse its millions—its European,
its Asiatic, and its African graftings upon the original
stock. Such a conglomerate the world never saw before
of white and brown, olive and black humanities, and all
free to roam in polyandrous or polygamous fashion.
The Vale of the Mississippi will indeed beat all creation;
for where does history reveal such gathering or assimila-
ting of peoples, such association of interests, and such
consanguinity ; to say nothing of the outer forces
directing the commerce and agriculture, and not less the
politics, the ethics, and the beliefs of New America ? As

"miscegenation" is one of the grand topics of "women's platforms" in the States, and the fair girls of the New Agapemone period stand forth as abettors of coloured connubial unions for the millennium of spinsterhood; hybridity is not only going ahead, but advancing to Niagara and far beyond.

Who is to divine from the aspect and tendency of the present times what will come to pass before the dial points to the year 2000 A.D. ? Let the mind reflect on the basis of the new Genesis in the broad expanse of the far West,—the Agapemone of the "mighty creation" in all its colours, types, and forms. Fancy John Chinaman seduced from kith and kin and yoked to Widow Malone, "ochone, ochone;" Cornelius O'Dowd mingling his pure Phœnician blood with the dark pigments of an odorous African ; the black-ebony "Pompey" and "Cæsar," so much alike in white chokers and blue coats and yellow pants, leading two fair-complexioned girls from "fifth avenue," Philadelphia, to the altar, or portals, if you will, of miscegenation ; "Tomahawka" forsaking his back-woods, war-whoops, and savagery to espouse a philanthropic Quakeress,—the pure white and drab of art setting off the red brown of nature's nude, and creating æsthetic thoughts in the wedding guests as to the pretty hybrids of the future; the big raw-boned Scotchman dividing his basin of brose with a dwarfish squaw from the Polar regions ; the Dutch Boer tripping it to the lively guitar of his hot-blooded Mexican spouse ; and lastly, the Anglo-American of 300 years' growth, Puritan, Quaker, Prelatic, or Papal, looking on and hardly knowing whether to join hands with the coy Welsh maid of

Wesleyan piety, or the voluptuous girl of Cadiz, or the unadorned beauty of Japan.

Such assumptions are by no means exaggerated. Already the Mormonites from all lands rush to the arms of Brigham Young, the prophet of Utah, and everywhere communities of "holy brothers," and holier sisters, spiritual wives, Perfectionists, and other orders of the mutual love sort, are being founded under circumstances most alluring and sensual: such promise in their way to emulate the concubinage of David and the Israelites, or the warmer Egyptians, to say nothing of the loves of "burning Sappho" and the heydays of voluptuousness at Baiæ! If in our good Protestant and monogamous times he be a wise child that knoweth his own father, what chance will there be for wisdom itself, when New America realizes to the full the tide and free admixture of peoples, to proclaim even the race of 'the individual man, much less his special genesis?

As if driven along by the impetuosity of his ideas, and the relish for saying startling things in a startling way, Knox was apt to break the thread of his discourse in sundry entertaining modes. "Sailing orders" with Knox were but a general manifesto of his good intentions; for being his own Jupiter and Æolus to boot, he would now enjoy an hour of the gentle zephyr—the delicate irony; then have a turn of the stormy blast or strongly denunciatory; indeed, nothing could be more curious and diversified than the records of his log-book. "The Fragment" is exceedingly characteristic of its author, his vices and his virtues. His discursiveness and repetitions are vastly too common ; even the pictorial part, the woodcuts, are made to do duty over and over again, and for what purpose the said deponent knoweth not. His definition of species and their varieties is not always precise, and there is an occasional hiatus in the argument ; also a rash statement and a rasher inference. Writing *currente calamo* and very much as he used to address an audience, he advanced his first thoughts with the same authority as he should have advocated a well-digested opinion. His style is happily the very antipodes of that in vogue in medical literature ; it is exceedingly pointed and racy, and thoroughly fulfils the Knox desideratum of hitting the right nail on the head and driving it home. His love of epigram and greater love of satire often merited rebuke, for in this latter respect his injudiciousness cropped out pretty freely. Some of his historical statements were loosely set forth ; and it may be said of " The Fragment" generally, that it wanted revision at other hands than the author's. But, giving all prominence to these blemishes, who can read a page of the book without pleasure and profit and singular delight ? The suggestiveness of his remarks, the graphic narrative, and the raciness of style, are Knox's own ; then the scenic-like pictures he presents pass before your eyes with all the novelty of a lively panorama to infantile minds. In your general admiration you overlook the lines of incongruity, the deficient perspective, the too-heightened colours, or too-glossy varnish of the artist ; because the general effect of his pictures is so grandly suggestive.

" The Fragment : or, Sketches of the Races of Men,"

can hardly fail to obtain a place in history ; and when it comes to be read by the light of another century, by which time human prejudices, now very much on the wane, will no longer affect a free expression of thought on all matters affecting the social and religious position of our species, it is more than probable that Robert Knox will have accorded to his memory a higher praise than his contemporaries willingly conceded to him during life. General consent has awarded him an exalted platform as an anatomist, and he was undoubtedly the greatest teacher of his day, but posterity will probably figure him as the chief anthropologist of his epoch, and a pioneer of a philosophy that sought to recognize the true nature of Man, his instincts, his passions, his psychological leanings, and social influences.

CHAPTER XVII.

Congenital Deformity of Joints.—Contributions to Anatomy and Physiology in *Medical Gazette.*—Cervical Ribs.—Lectures on Physiology, &c.—Museums.—Potato Disease.—Agricultural Schemes.—Seeks Government employment.—Sphenoid Bone.—Fau's Anatomy.—Hip Joint, &c.

IN all that related to fact and observation in reference to or in illustration of science, Knox was scrupulous to a degree that nothing but the truth should be emitted. In describing the results of his own investigations, he was ever anxious to keep prominently in view the tendency that preconceived notions or "idols of the mind" had in swaying inferences, or in disturbing the fair expressions of a fact. Speaking of an eminent anatomist, the author of a work on the arteries, and who had done much to illustrate the anatomy of the iris, but who from his peculiar bent of observation could see or describe nothing but blood-vessels, Knox referred to his own inquiries, by saying—"Here was a great difficulty; he could see nothing but *blood-vessels;* while I, gentlemen, I declare to you, had long the utmost difficulty in recognizing any organic structure but *nerves.*"

Though unable to vindicate Dr. Knox's behaviour towards his pupil and colleague Professor John Reid in 1841, I feel warranted in saying, and possibly repeating, that he always appeared solicitous to give honour to whom it was due, and a large meed of praise to deserving merit. Sir George Sinclair, in one of his letters to the anatomist, writes : " One of the most prominent features which characterized your prelections was the frankness, or rather the eagerness, with which you did justice to the *grand* discoveries and immortal writings of those who had preceded you in the career of scientific investigation." Sir George, who attended very regularly two winter and two summer courses of Knox's lectures, wrote from experience : " By your teaching you have succeeded in furnishing to your country many eminent and esteemed practitioners. You always contrived by the judicious exercise of genius to keep up the attention of your pupils, even when dwelling upon the least interesting branches of your course. No lecturer was, I believe, ever surrounded by a more attached or a more attentive audience."

He published a memoir "On Abrasion of the Diarthrodial Cartilages by Friction, and on their Atrophy from other causes," in the *London Medical Gazette*, November 4th and 11th, 1842. One of his propositions was, " that whatever alters materially and permanently the system of leverage natural to any joint, must, in the end, *rub* away, or destroy by *wasting*, or want of use, the cartilages and synovial tissue of that joint, and even the surfaces of the bones themselves, unless the injury were arrested by a timely eburnation of the bone; and that this effect might happen altogether independent of inflammation, ulceration," &c.

He gave an admirable description of the foot of the

child at the fourth or fifth year :—" Everything is taper, soft, gently traced; neither sinews nor veins nor bones are visible; the whole, in fact, is eminently beautiful, and in keeping with all those pleasing and graceful forms which render the child an object of gentle attraction even to the sternest natures of mankind." He was of opinion that the female foot, if finely formed, like that of the Venus, for example, retains in part " the infantile character associated in our minds with youth and health, grace, simplicity and truth, loveliness and confiding helplessness of the person."

He next adverted to the congenital deformity or peculiar dislocation of the great toe, or change in its direction from a straight line with the inner plane of the foot to that of an angle, more or less acute, with the metatarsal bone supporting it, until at last it produces a plaiting, as it is called, of the toes. This deformity he thought more common in the Saxon than the Celtic races; and seen " oftenest in large, raw-boned, ill-proportioned, tall persons—nature seemingly leaving in such persons the extremities unfinished." The deformity did not depend on tight shoes, as it exists among the poor who seldom wear shoes in Scotland, but on a congenital tendency.

He gave cases and drawings to illustrate his theory derived from some of the larger joints. An interesting paragraph in this paper refers to the rupture or dislocation of the bicipital tendon within the capsular ligaments of the shoulder-joint, and also brings out the case of Louis XV. described by Portal, and the success of the quack bone-setter in similar instances. Nor is he slow to defend the originality of his observations against

all comers—to wit, Professor Richard Partridge, who had
described a similar case to Knox, but omitted all mention of his "*earliest memoir* on the pathology of the
biceps tendon;" and who, "true to his class (Londoners),
was bound to strike out of his paper any view not of
London growth."

He remarks upon the interstitial absorption of the
neck of the thighbone, and cites cases related by Mr.
Geo. Gulliver,[1] "one of the most distinguished pathological observers of the present day," and whose memoirs
he held "to merit the deepest attention from all surgical
pathologists."

His "Contributions to Anatomy and Physiology" occupied several numbers of the *London Medical Gazette* from
Midsummer to Christmas 1842. His first contribution
(June 23rd) was entitled "Some Remarks on the Structure and Arrangement of the Spinal Arachnoid." Then
followed, "On some Varieties in Human Structure, with
Remarks on the doctrine of the Unity of Organization."
1. Osseous System—the Cranium. 2. The Humerus;
its supra-condyloid process; which was pretty nearly a
repetition of what appeared in 1841, already described
in page 294. 3. Osseous System; under which head he
describes the case of a young man of 25 years of age
with two episternal or presternal bones, occupying
precisely the position in which they were first noticed
by Beclard and Breschet, and Mr. King, of London. He

---

[1] Mr. Gulliver, F.R.S., so well known in the history of physiology
during the last thirty years, writes in very flattering terms of Dr. Knox's
abilities as a lecturer and man of science. He attended Knox during part
of a winter session.

doubted M. Breschet's opinion as to these presternal bones representing the rudiments of a cervical rib of which the vertebral portion is very usually found in connection with the seventh cervical vertebra. Knox had never seen but one instance of these bones. He held it to be more philosophic to suppose them rudimentary "than to adopt the Bridgewater and Guy's Hospital physiology,[1] which argues that every animal is made for itself alone, stands alone, and has nothing to do with any other, and that the individual organs of man and animals are to be explained by a physiology whose highest stretch of generalization is to represent the *mamma* of the human female as having been purposely created double, that the accidental loss of one, by milk abscess or otherwise, might occasion no interruption to their function! Profound philosophy! but proving, at the same time, to how little purpose Mr. John Hunter lived and laboured, and bequeathed to Britain his immortal museum, seeing that into the educational institutions of his adopted city he failed to introduce a single spark of his philosophy."

Under "Muscular System" he described the *musculus-hepatico-diaphragmaticus*, and the *scalenus anticus* divided into two portions, betwixt which the subclavian artery passed across the rib, which arrangement was found in the subject with the episternal bones.

In future numbers he discussed the "Variety in the Form of the Human Pelvis and its component parts, and the Transcendental and other Physiological Laws as applicable to the Pelvis and its Varieties." He stated

---

[1] Knox here gave a reference to Sir A. Cooper on the *Mammæ* and Bridgewater Treatises, *passim*.

that he had examined the pelvis of five women of different ages who died soon after delivery, and found in all of them a relaxation of the articulations of the pelvis to a greater or lesser extent, so that he was disposed to look upon it as a regular and healthy process. In September his contributions were—

1. "Obliteration of the Cavity of the Tunica Vaginalis Testis in middle and aged persons."

2. "On a Congenital Deformity of the Head and Neck of the Femur."

3. "Observations on the Muscle of the Lachrymal Sac, or Tensor-tarsi."

4. "A Reply to M. Malgaigne's memoir, entitled ' Recherches sur la Fréquence des Hernies selon les Sexes, les Ages, et rélativement à la Population.' "

On November 3, 1843, his memoir on "the Cervical Ribs in Man" appeared. After noting that M. Hunauld, in 1740, had the merit of discovering the nucleus of bone anterior to the transverse process of the seventh cervical vertebra, "so frequently present, so varied in its form, and which is, in fact, a rudimentary cervical rib," he instanced his own observations, illustrated by numerous drawings. "The pedicle or footstalk of the transverse process of the seventh cervical vertebra may, and probably always does, comprise the following elements : 1. A germ for the posterior arch. 2. One for the anterior. 3. A short nucleus for the articular surface. 4. A separate and distinct germ for the rib. These different germs are developed in a great variety of ways. Sometimes the rib extends to the sternum," as Hunauld reports to have seen ; " more frequently it stops short, and terminates by a rounded free extremity, or unites with the first true rib ; sometimes it is very short and rudimentary, but still distinct from the anterior root of the transverse process ; at other times so intimately united with it that there is no distinguishing between them. Lastly, the rib may be wanting altogether, and so may the anterior root of the process ; or this latter may be wanting, and then the rib seems to take its place by completing the foramen : it was that misled Hunauld." He looked upon the anterior roots of the transverse process of the seventh cervical vertebra as resembling the dorsal processes, and wished the attention of anatomists to this view.

In his second memoir, Nov. 10, 1843, he described more minutely the anatomical preparations illustrating the cervical ribs. He also described the cervical vertebræ of the Aï (Three-toed Sloth—*Bradypus Tridactylus*, Linné), and instead of wishing to alter the nomenclature of the human osteology, on account of the eighth and ninth vertebræ of the Three-toed Sloth being supposed to be dorsal vertebræ, he preferred the theory of M. De Blainville, "which, by arranging the cervical vertebræ into three or more groups, admits of an increase or decrease in their number, without the violation of any other well-established philosophic theory."

In his concluding paper (Nov. 17) he divided the seven cervical vertebræ of Man into three groups. In the 1st and 2nd groups, the first, second, third, fourth, fifth, and sixth vertebræ were alike in both Man and the Aï; whilst the 3rd group showed the seventh cervical vertebra of Man opposed to the seventh, eighth, and ninth of the Aï.

" That the transverse processes present probably in all the vertebræ a double root presenting various stages of development.

" That the anterior roots of the transverse processes contain the elements of at least two structures, viz. a process which in the intermediate cervical vertebræ, extending outwards, unites with the posterior root, and so forms the foramen for the vertebral artery ; and a shorter or stronger part, which ultimately becomes the *facet* for the articulation of another element; that is, the head of the ribs." He looked upon the seventh cervical vertebra as combining the characters of both regions, viz. cervical and dorsal.

As regards the genus *Bradypus*, the eighth and ninth vertebræ he considered to be analogous to the seventh in Man, carrying ribs more rudimentary than in Man, being limited in their development to the tubercle and a portion of the body, whereas in Man the cervical ribs had a head and neck, tubercle, and body complete. Those who wish for a more complete history of the Cervical Ribs should consult a memoir by Professor Wenzel Grüber, of St. Petersburg, published last year.

In the same *Medical Gazette*, vol. xxxiii. (Session 1843–44), he published six essays " On Hermaphroditism," which were professedly reprints of papers he had communicated to the Royal Society of Edinburgh in 1827 and 1828. Also five contributions on the *Corpus Luteum*, in which his brother takes part. His observations on the anatomy of the Inguinal Canal, p. 536 of volume just cited, tend to confirm the accuracy of Mr. Guthrie's dissections.

At the end of the Session 1843–44, the students of the Edinburgh Veterinary College presented Dr. Knox with a handsome gold medal "as a token of their gratitude for his long-continued kindness in affording them free access to his valuable lectures on Human Anatomy and Physiology; and for the unremitting interest he had uniformly manifested in advancing and advocating veterinary science." The written testimonial was on parchment, to which the signatures of the students were affixed.

Dr. Knox's "Lectures on Physiological Anatomy, the Special Physiology of Man, and on the Anatomy of Tissues, Morbid and Healthy," appeared in the *Medical Times*, vol. xii., extending from April 5 to July 12, 1845. These lectures sometimes bear out their title of anatomical, physiological, and pathological essays, and contain much of value to the student of medicine; but divergences into other paths are far from being uncommon, and the fine arts and "pictorial anatomy" teachers now and then come in for a sly hit. Here is a reference to music :—"To thousands, nay, to millions, the Norwegian airs of Rule Britannia, the Duke of York's March, and God save the Queen, appear to be musical ; they fancy them even grand and beautiful ; but what is passing strange, they really imagine them to contain a good deal of music in their composition. Now, those having really a musical ear, and who feel that the frightful noise made by an 'orchestra and the whole

strength of the house,' in performing (so they call it)
one of these 'coarsest of all successions of simple
sounds' (for airs we can scarcely call them), is, in point
of fact, not music, are not bound to alter their
opinions merely because a race destitute, as a race,
of a musical ear fancy such things to be musical;
neither is there a necessity for those possessing a
sound eye and taste for beauty in high art, being
obliged to give way to the opinions of those not gifted
with such feelings" (p. 21).

His fourth lecture contains a number of measurements
of the cranium, including the face, of individuals of all
nations.   His notions as to bulk of brain being the
measure of ability and power and genius are expressed
thus :—" The largest-headed men of my own acquaintance have been town councillors and jobbers about
public offices—men of energy no doubt, calculating men,
unscrupulous, dishonest, but destitute of genius or elevated
thoughts ; a small-headed vain man is usually selected
as chairman.   This class must, I think, also include all
statesmen who are found competent to hold office, the
least inkling of honesty of purpose being a total and
absolute disqualification " (p. 56).

His fifth lecture contains further measurements,—"the
absolute height of the cranium and face when placed on
a horizontal surface, from the base to the vertex."   The
table would indicate that the Scotch head " possesses an
elevation of probably a quarter of an inch over that of
the Hindoo head; an important difference, no doubt, and
yet scarcely adequate to the explaining why a handful
of adventurers, whose doings have at times been suffi-

ciently clumsy, should be able to hold in the most abject slavery a hundred millions of their darker brethren" (p. 75). Other measurements of the cranium, and a description of the osseous component parts, afford him opportunities of blending physiological and pathological comments, and these are not altogether without interest.

His two last lectures, "On the Supposed Advantages of a knowledge of Anatomy to an Artist," are highly characteristic of his historical survey, from Da Vinci to Haydon and Sir C. Bell, and to the great damage of many reputations and of persons who had long been cited as authorities on English art, and on theories of beauty. Mr. Haydon's lectures are severely handled. Haydon had written, "Industry will improve mediocrity, but will never elevate mediocrity to power." Upon this Knox adds : " By power is of course here meant *genius;* for as to elevation to real power, why, mediocrity is your only chance ; it secures your entrance into good society, a *fauteuil* at the council table of all Royal Societies and Academies. In town councils it secures the mayoralty for its possessor, in universities it is the only sure passport to a chair " (p. 266).

His paper on the Nostrils of the Horse, published in the *Veterinary Record,* is copied in p. 287 of the *Medical Times,* vol. xii.

In December 1845 he attended a meeting of the Birmingham Pathological Society, and explained the advantages of modelling specimens of pathological anatomy according to the plan of Dr. Felix Thibert. Some time afterwards the Doctor was engaged in

Thibert's Museum (when established in London), showing from wax models the more instructive parts of the
human anatomy to popular audiences.   However profitable the pay, the engagement must have been of the
most irksome nature to a man of Knox's capacity.

Two lectures by Knox on "Anatomical Museums,
their Objects and Present Condition," appeared in the
Medical Times, July 18 and 25, 1846.   They contain
much sensible advice, which is all the more valuable
as coming from a man of thorough experience in the
formation and direction of museums.   In 1820, the
College of Surgeons of Edinburgh, according to Knox,
contained from 200 to 300 preparations put up in a
fashion entirely antiquated and useless.   Though the
first and second Monros had made a collection of physiological, pathological, and zoological specimens, the
first scientific or Comparative Anatomy Museum in
Scotland was made by Dr. Barclay.   In 1821, not a
single skeleton of a fish was to be found in the Hunterian Museum, Lincoln's Inn Fields, London.

Like many other men, practical or theoretical,
agricultural and scientific, Dr. Knox had *his* words on
the potato disease of 1845–46 (*Medical Times*, Jan. 3,
1846).   The theory he propounded was, that " organic
changes, dependent on atmospheric causes, had exposed
the tubers to an attack of a parasitic fungus, destroying
its substance, and unfitting it for the food of either man
or beast."

In February 1846, Knox was gratified by a letter
received from Professor Robert Harrison, of Dublin, who,
after examining the works of Cuvier, Carus, and others,

gave Knox the credit of having been the first to discover
and make known the peculiar air-bag in the Emeu.   In
the tenth volume of Meckel's Comparative Anatomy
the structure is alluded to, but by no means accurately
described ; and whilst Knox's name is mentioned, Professor Harrison considered that Meckel had not shown
" the credit and respect due to the discoverer of such a
very anomalous structure."

In the autumn of 1846, Knox was in London seeking
a Government appointment.   He tried both Lord John
Russell and Earl Grey for employment in a survey
of Africa, and though his claims were supported by
the Marquis of Breadalbane and Sir George Sinclair,
he met with no success.   Knox's scientific attainments
were of too high an order for the Whig mind to understand ; moreover, nepotism and party ruled official life.
Knox was not a Border Elliot or a Highland Campbell,
or he would have been made to fit any vacancy in
the State.

Writing from Birmingham (Dec. 9, 1846), where his
lectures on Race had been so well received, Knox condemned the rush to the press so marked in London,
and then called Goodsir's attention to the "immense
dissections" made by his brother and himself, which had
not been published.   The opportunity was now come
for Edinburgh as a school regaining its position, as De
Blainville had proposed to him (Knox) to translate his
works with additional remarks; all his own drawings for
illustrating the series would be done in Paris.   As Sir J.
McGregor and others were favourable to the scheme, he
hoped Goodsir would join him in issuing a quarterly

fasciculus on the Vertebrata. Nothing came of this proposal.[1]

Knox's mind was fertile in resources, and no department of knowledge escaped his attention. About Christmas (1847), when residing for a short time in Clarke Street, Edinburgh, he submitted to Mr. David Milne, of York Place, a proposal to establish " an Agricultural School or College, within the walls of which should be taught the sciences bearing on Agriculture, and in particular the sciences of Chemistry, Vegetable Physiology, Veterinary Medicine, and Geology." Mr. Milne replied in very pleasant terms, remarking, *inter alia :* " It is a bold conception, and the execution of it might well fire the ambition of a patriot. . . . I believe there is now sufficient intelligence in the country to see the importance of an institution which proposes to promote the art of Agriculture by the lever power of science."

In the autumn (August of 1847), Knox wrote Lord Lincoln, then Commissioner of Woods and Forests, respecting South Africa and its applicability to an extensive scheme of colonization. His Lordship expressed himself greatly obliged by the interesting details furnished him, but made no further reference to Knox's application. Twenty-five years before he addressed "the State officials," he had advocated such colonization, and dwelt much on the advantages of Africa to English phthisical patients and others as a sanatorium.

In the summer of 1848, Knox began a series of Lectures on the Races of Men, in the *Medical Times.*

[1] See Goodsir's Anatom. Memoirs, vol. i. p. 142.

They appeared from week to week, and constituted twenty-four in all. As in 1846 he had publicly foretold the coming approach of that great struggle between the dominant races for supremacy that burst over Europe after the days of February 1848, the flight of Louis Philippe, and Austria's Metternich, he was proud to revert to the accuracy of his prophecy. He pointed out with special self-satisfaction the views he had held as to Austria having no existence as a nation, and hardly a habitation or a name, and that Germany had still to be formed, limited, and consolidated. It need hardly be said that these lectures were worked up for his " Races of Men."

Dr. Knox never had an abnormal structure submitted to his examination without being able to throw some light upon its nature. In the apparently most ambiguous instances he was sure to ferret out some fact that would lead to a further *éclaircissement.* The originality of his observations and the breadth of his generalizations were frequently proved. When he found the sphenoid bone particularly small in size, and a distinct narrowness of the base of the cranium, he argued that there was a relation between the development of the sphenoid and the activity of the cerebral functions. So far-fetched an hypothesis excited the laughter and ridicule of the hard matter-of-fact kind of persons, who asked, " What next?" Later observations, however, especially those of Virchow, confirmed Knox's views, and showed that the size of the bone has much to do with the configuration of the head, and, necessarily, its capacity for containing nervous matter—the fatuous and insane having but a small sphenoid compared with the man of intelligence. Though Knox had publicly spoken of the great import of the sphenoid as far back as 1834, it was 1848 before he published anything on the subject. His paper on the "Importance of the Sphenoid Bone, and its due development in Man," appeared in the London *Medical Times* for July 1848. In a previous number of this periodical he had described an adult cranium of a fatuous person in whom there was nothing amiss but the incomplete development of the sphenoid—it being no larger than in a boy of ten or twelve years of age. He got Mr. Hallett, Professor Goodsir's demonstrator, to make measurements of the sphenoid in different races of men, and of different ages : eighty measurements were taken.

Virchow, in his Treatise on the Development of the Base of the Skull (Berlin, 1857), drew special attention to the early ossification of the sphenoid as affecting the formation of the skull, or, as he termed it, "strongly shortening the base." This condition he noted along with the deep fossæ of the nose and prognathous face met with in the Cretin, thus corroborating the views expressed by Knox upwards of twenty years previously. The plates given by Virchow to illustrate the ossification of the three embryonic portions of the sphenoid are very conclusive in character.

In his "Library of Illustrated Standard Scientific Works," Hippolyte Baillière published "Fau's Anatomy of the External Forms of Man," for the use of artists, edited with additions by Dr. Knox, 1849, 8vo. text, and an Atlas of 28 plates 4to. plain and coloured. Both text and illustrations were admirably done, and if English artists cared to study the science of form, they had it faithfully set before them in Fau edited by Knox. The Appendix, constituting one-third of the entire text of 313 pages, is from Knox's pen; it embraces his observations,—(1) "On the Elgin Marbles;" (2) "Egyptian Gallery—Coptic Race;" (3) "The Antique Statues of Greece compared with the Living Model—the Athlete of Ancient and of Modern Times;" (4) "An Analysis of the Beautiful in Form;" (5) "The History of Artistic Anatomy, and its utility to the Artist;" (6, and finally), "On the *Ecorchée*, or Plastic Anatomical Figures of the Schools—on the Dead and Living Anatomy." In these six chapters Knox gives a fair abstract of his views of Anatomy *quoad* Art; and perhaps few men in England were better entitled to advance an opinion on the relations of the human form to true art than himself. He had his ideal of the beautiful, like all men who have written on the subject, and whether that ideal be right or wrong in its construction, it is worthy of study as emanating from a man thoroughly conversant with all the data upon which an artistic theory can legitimately be based. He showed that the anatomy of the schools was not properly the anatomy for the artist; and that the success of Da Vinci, Michael Angelo, and Raphael in representing the human form, rested more upon the study of the model than dissections.

In the *Medical Times* (June 28, 1851), he had some "Observations on Excision of the Pelvic Extremity of the Femur." He spoke of recommending the excision of the trochanter in a soldier of the 14th Regiment, then at Melsea Hospital (Hampshire), in 1816. It was not done, but the *post mortem* showed him to be right in his diagnosis. He cited other cases, as if claiming priority in the suggestion of the operation of excision of parts of the femur, and of the trochanter in particular. He wrote in high terms of Mr. Fergusson's operations upon the hip, and the suggestive pathological questions pertaining to them. From other and quite independent sources there are good grounds for believing that Knox was the first surgeon to recommend excision of the head of the femur in this country.

Dr. Knox in 1853, or thereabouts, either purposed lecturing on or publishing "The Descriptive and Surgical Anatomy of the Fasciæ and Aponeuroses of the Human Body." His notes from cases in the surgical practice of Liston and Syme, now before me, would imply publication, but on the next page is the following:—
"Lecture 1st.—Of the general Cellular Envelope of the Body. The methods of teaching anatomy, whether by oral instruction or by published treatises, have all more or less this disadvantage; they do not, nor can they be expected to describe and group together the organs, such as those I am about to speak of, in a way at once practical and philosophical; minutely accurate in detail, yet neglecting not those large views first taught by Bichat and confirmed by all subsequent anatomists; supporting each important fact of detail by a reference to the practice of ancient or of modern surgeons;— alike instructive, whether successful or unsuccessful; judicious, though bold; timid, yet mischievous, scholastic, or empirical." He then argued that rational practice in surgery at least must be, or ought to be, based on

minute accurate descriptive anatomy ; and in the hope of supplying what seemed to him wanting in respect of the anatomy of some parts of man, he had selected the fasciæ and aponeuroses for his description.

Another memoir he purposed writing was "On the Laws regulating Human Production, Mortality, and Increase. By an Anatomist." A few pages were written out, but in too fragmentary a form to be noticed here.

In October 1853 he gave the introductory lecture to the Royal Free Hospital School of Medicine, and was said to have made an impression upon his audience. He alluded to the circumstances which had borne down upon his Edinburgh career, and showed the gravity of the anatomist's position in England previous to the year 1830.

CHAPTER XVIII.

THOSE who wish to see Knox in his own humour,
jaunty, free, egotistical, and happy, should read his
"Great Artists and Great Anatomists: a Biographical
and Philosophical Study," 8vo. (Van Voorst, London,
1852). It was said that the boldness if not heterodoxical
flavour of some of the author's statements alarmed one
or more of the London publishers. However this may
have been, John Van Voorst, with his usual public
spirit, issued the work, and it is one that should be
read by every man who can relish an intellectual treat,
whether interested or not in art and anatomy. The
biography and philosophy of the work remind you of
his "Races of Men;" and both volumes should be regarded as rare specimens of "high art" in literature—
painted by a knowing hand, whose brush permits of
no cobweb and gossamer, and no mazy perspective.
The English reader of to-day would appear to relish a
different style of art than Knox's—the "high falukin"
of the Beales and Bradlaugh "spouters," or the Braddon

"Brummagem ware"—so much the worse for public taste and morals to boot.

Along with the central figures of Cuvier, Geoffroy St. Hilaire, Da Vinci, Angelo, and Raphael, are grouped men of every age and clime, and fragmentary remarks of the most varied description. No man of the diviner sort in history is passed by, and each portrait done by the limner Knox is surrounded by the art, the literature, and the science of the epoch in which the genius lived. His canvas is like one of John Breughel's big copper sheets, where human figures blend with landscape, and animals, and flowers, and insects, testifying even to the whole "creation": oddly enough, a further comparison could be instituted between the anatomist in his showy attire and the decorative person of the artist known as "Velvet Breughel." In reading the "Great Artists and Great Anatomists," you are now side by side with the *savans* of the Institute; now listening to Napoleon under the shadow of the Pyramids of Egypt; now with Linnæus in his wanderings; now examining *"Les Ossemens Fossiles,"* or made spectators of the Shakespearian drama; and so on. Men of every type, with all their passions and prejudices, and all the varied cosmopolitan phases of life, are presented on the Knox panel with a fair share of the Breughel colouring. In one page you are *vis-à-vis* with Laplace and Arago, in another, among the pedants of Oxford and the cliques of London. The curtain rises upon "La Belle France" carrying her sons of genius in *Io triumphe* fashion, whilst the master minds of England are retiring from sight—being frowned down by the theologians of

Exeter Hall and the "nobodies" of a British Parliament. Nature's transitions of organic life are not more varied in time and circumstance than Knox's narrative; more-ever, the racy style, the pointed satire, the sweeping generalizations, all add to the charm of the book.

In January 1852, Knox, who was then applying for an appointment in the British Museum, was advised by his excellent friend Mr. Murray, of Great Stuart Street, Edinburgh, to be cautious how he spoke of the management of the Museum or those holding office. "You will make enemies who may do you infinite mischief, and not the less because all you say against them is true." Turning to another subject, and also a letter he had received from Knox, he writes: "The affairs at the Cape are getting worse and worse. You are too true a prophet; for all you have told me has completely come to pass. Your letter on that subject, with a little altera-tion, would make a good letter for the *Times.*"

"A Manual of Artistic Anatomy for the use of Sculp-tors, Painters, and Amateurs," by Dr. Knox, was published by Mr. Renshaw in 1852. The text was illustrated by numerous woodcuts designed by Dr. Westmacott. This manual contains a great deal of information set forth in Knox's best style: the third part of the volume is specially interesting, where the author dwells on the object and aim of art, and his analysis of beauty and his theory of the beautiful. He opposed the idea of poetry and music, the drama or the pantomime, belong-ing to the Fine Arts; nor did he show much more favour to architecture: with him sculpture alone is high art.

In the same year, at the instigation of his friend Mr. Renshaw, Knox wrote "A Manual of Human Anatomy, descriptive, general, and practical," illustrated by 200 engravings. In sending a copy of this well-got-up work to Professor Goodsir, and asking him to make it his text-book, he said that though he had always entertained a dislike to *Vade Mecums* and Manuals not written by anatomists, he was obliged to comply with the spirit of the age. After praising the printing, paper, and woodcuts, he spoke of "the text as the old story, the descriptive anatomy of Man, a kind of anatomy that few teachers here understand." In his preface, Knox calls it his latest work, and, *inter alia*, says : "For the medicine which appeals not to anatomy is empiricism, and the zoology not based thereon is not a science;" and of descriptive anatomy, "as the broad portal stone of that doorway by which all must enter who purpose exercising conscientiously the arts of medicine and surgery. Scarpa and Hunter, John Bell and Dupuytren entered by this gate." Professor Goodsir praised the manual very highly, and recommended it to his pupils.

Under the auspices of the same publisher, Dr. Knox translated Milne-Edwards's "Manual of Zoology," in 1855. A second edition appeared in 1863, edited by C. Carter Blake. Milne-Edwards's work, so popular in France, required but an English translator of Knox's breadth of mind to become as acceptable to British readers. Knox's additional observations enhanced the value of the volume, as many of these were strictly original and illustrative of his own zoological experience. Professor Goodsir wrote that it was "by far the best manual on the subject, and infinitely better than its numerous imitators." He and Professor Allman, also Mr. Sedgwick, of Cambridge, made it their text-book, and, if I am rightly informed, Oxford and other examining boards adopted the manual.

Referring to the *status quo* of England and the Continent in 1853, Knox writes : " Strange revolutions are taking place in the world, which still moves in *a circle*, for in my younger days I remember precisely similar war and other cries ;—Invasion—Buonaparte—our Altars and Hearths—Church and State! To me it is perfectly amusing to hear the same thing repeated after nearly half a century. It is much the same in medicine : I used to read the journals until I found them stuffed with matters discussed thirty years ago and more, and now brought forward as something new." He alludes to some dissections engaging him, and adds : " So you see that I am still the same as when you first saw me, full of life, mad after the discovery of the unknown in science, and as respects these matters as regardless of the diggings and the diggers as if they were situated in the moon. It is the first time, I believe, in human history that mere *brute labour* is to take the ascendant of all other qualifications."

About this time, Knox issued a prospectus announcing the publication, on the 1st of October, of " Researches, Anatomical, Physiological, and Pathological,"—to be completed in four parts. The work was to be " published by the Messrs. Longman, in the style and of the size of Lardner's Encyclopædia, and by subscription." He assigned good reasons for collecting all the memoirs he had contributed to the different societies, and making the medical public aware of his "theories and opinions;" but I cannot learn that anything was done to fulfil the promise of the prospectus, upon one page of which the titles of no less than forty-five papers are recorded. The absence of subscribers' names, it may presumed, stood in the way of accomplishing it. Nor was this to be wondered at in England, when, as Liebig wrote to Faraday, "works of a practical tendency alone awaken attraction, while the 'purely scientific,' which possess far greater merit, are almost unknown; yet the latter are the proper and true source from which the others flow."

In May 1854, Robert, the son of Dr. Knox, died of heart-disease in Edinburgh. It was a great blow to the father, from which he did not recover for months. The young man was exceedingly like the Doctor in looks and manners, and promised well in point of ability and conduct.

In 1854, Messrs. Routledge and Sons published a shilling volume for Knox—"Fish and Fishing in the Lone Glens of Scotland; with a History of the Propagation, Growth, and Metamorphoses of the Salmon." The edition was soon disposed of, as every angler of the Tweed and its tributaries, the lairds of the "lone glens," as well as the lads of "Gala water," had their copy of Knox on Fishing. If there was not so much to learn of Izaak Walton's craft from its pages, the reader could count upon the science of the anatomist, his description of British fishes, their characteristics—external, dental, and osteological—and many useful hints besides; to say nothing of the picturesque landscapes, the funny maxims and moral reflections.   His old pupil, Dr. Robert M. Glover, said he read the book with exquisite delight, and felt as if "the green leaves rustled in the song, and the streams murmured pleasantly with all their waters." The book revived some old friendships, and got Knox invitations from "fishing folk" in every district of Scotland, none of which could he avail himself of. Yet he wrote for the dweller in towns, who " instinctively feels that, ceasing to be a man as nature made him, he is becoming a citizen—a cit! Abhorred word! I would rather dwell, as I once did, amidst the wild and now desolate dells of the Anatolo, leading at the base of the beauteous Boschberg the life of the wandering Caffre, than listlessly pace London's idle busy streets, with nothing to look at but miles of hideous brick walls, with holes in them called doors and windows.   Odious commonplace! You mask humanity, and mar the better part of human nature."

In the *Lancet* of November 19th, 1853, Knox has some remarks on " The Cholera Fly."   Attention having been called to the coincidence of swarms of flies and the advent of Asiatic cholera, Knox spoke of his experience in 1831–32, and his visits to Fisherrow, a few miles east of Edinburgh, of a lady calling his attention to a number of dead flies of a peculiar form and colour, with yellow stripes on the abdominal region, and numerous minute opaque particles evidently discharged by the flies ; that a person in bravado took a quantity of this deposited matter, which brought on an attack of cholera.   In reference to an appearance seen by hundreds, and which was much talked of at the time, Knox and his brother, whilst fishing in the Annan and examining the banks of the Solway, " saw in the extreme distance, as if hovering over the town of Dumfries, a vast cloud in motion : it extended from earth to heaven, and resembled a cloud of flies." The cholera reached Dumfries that day, and did not leave the town till it decimated its population of 15,000 inhabitants !

In the *Lancet* of November 4th, 1854, " Xavier Bichat, his Life and Labours: a Biographical and Philosophical Study," contained an exceedingly characteristic essay of Knox's, in which Bichat stands surrounded by the political and dynastic associations of the French Revolution; Bourbonic and Hapsburg discouragement of science; medical teaching, and the like, or rather the unlike. He looked upon the history of anatomy as wrapt up in Bichat. He stated that anatomy was a haphazard sort of study in 1810, when he began it, and that it was not much better in 1825, when he gave his first course of lectures on Descriptive Anatomy. He traced Bichat's history as a child of the Revolution ; his precocious intellect, when at the age of twenty-eight he wrote his essay, "*Sur la Vie et la Mort*," and all the salient points of his remarkable career. " It was by the force of genius, instinctive, profound, that, arriving at certain generalizations, he found a new era—the era of facts : he taught the scientific world to speak and think as he did. If he did not succeed in laying a true basis for biology, it must be remembered that the laws of life transcend, in seeming complexity at least, the laws of inert matter : in living bodies all is mystery—their origin, persistence, extinction. He failed where Hunter failed ; he attempted *physiologie*

positive, but it would not do.   Is Cuvier's merit the less
that he could not explain the successive zoologies which
have appeared on the globe but by the clumsy inter-
position of a succession of miracles?"   Knox boasted
that he introduced Bichat's teaching of anatomy into
Britain.   Comparing Bichat with Cuvier, Knox said,
"Cuvier spoke to mankind, but it was Bichat's fate and
misfortune to limit his researches to one animal: that
animal, it is true, was Man, great and all-powerful only
in his own conceit."

His remarks "On the Aztecque and Bosjesman children now being exhibited in London, and of the Races
to which they are presumed to belong," appeared in the
Lancet, April 15, 1855.   Taking the figures which Cas-
tenada—the Mexican employed by Dupuis, the Spaniard,
when exploring the ruined cities of Central America in
1805–8—copied from the bas-reliefs of Palenque, Knox
saw the closest resemblance between these and the
Aztecque children, and believed that he saw an identity
of race.   Considering the remoteness of the period when
these bas-reliefs and paintings were figured on the ruined
temples of the cities of Guatemala, he sought support to
his views in what he called the law of " interrupted
descent," which he thus explained :—" A race of men
or animals may be so reduced as to be thought extinct ;
still some remain, and such as do are of course the direct
descendants of an ancient race.   Or the race may be
quite extinct in that locality, and should individuals
appear, having an identity of features and form with
the ancient, such a phenomenon is explicable only on
the physiological law of interrupted descent."   As negro

blood once introduced into a family will reappear after some hundreds of years without any new infusion, the same with the Jew and Gipsy." He believed there was Jewish blood in the Aztecque children, and thought the primitive races of men might be detected in the features of the inhabitants of localities where a mixed population predominates.

In another article upon the Aztecques, he alluded to the supra-condyloid foramen and webbed toes and fingers, and maintained "that the human family as it exists is one quite apart from the highest four-handed animals." Again : " Some men are born to grow up with webbed fingers and toes, and others with the median nerve and humeral artery and bone of the arm arranged as in the cat and tiger. Do these deformations prove an approach to the lower animals—of an affiliation with a lower class of animals ? Not in the least ; they are merely characteristics of 'retrograde development ;' for, failing in the development of a specified zoological form, Nature produces another, but it does not follow, nor indeed is it true, that all such developments are necessarily the affiliation of a natural family with the one next in serial unity."

At no time could Knox perceive any *serial* affiliation between the human family and the highest apes existing. " I do not mean by this that Man stands apart from the living world, and that a gap exists in Nature's works. But what I mean is this, that the *seeming* gap must not be offered as proof that such really exists. Apes are not convertible into men, and for this simple reason, they do not belong to the same natural family."

He followed out these speculations still further in his " Introduction to Inquiries into the Philosophy of Zoology," in the *Lancet* for June 1855. Should fossil Man be discovered, Knox thought that his relations to the present or living world would be the same as the extinct Solidungula and Carnivora to the living— *generically* identical, *specifically* distinct. " For who, by examining merely the skeleton of the Hottentot, could have re-constructed, had the race been extinct, that singular specimen of humanity ? I go further: were the Jew extinct, no zoologist that ever lived could have re-discovered in the cranium and skeleton those unaltered and unalterable features of a race the most remarkable perhaps on the globe."

He believed that the existing species of men belonged strictly to one great natural family ; that the species are separated from each other by anatomical and natural history characteristics, as wide as those marking species in any natural family ; but would not admit of Man's affiliation with the highest Quadrumana, nor *vice versâ*.

His " Contributions to the Philosophy of Zoology," extending over June, July, August, and September, bore more especially on the natural history of Man, and afforded him abundance of texts from which he might preach *suo more*. Here is a specimen of his style and thoughts :—" In every embryo of every species we have *the possible* of all forms appertaining to that family at least. The destruction, then, by geological or other phenomena, of all the species, saving one, of any natural family, would not necessarily extinguish that family,

since in the embryo of the remaining species there
exist the elements for the re-appearance, perhaps
under modified forms, of all the extinct species. As
of fishes, so of Man : one natural family—one embryonic
form, equal to the production of all species in accordance with the essential conditions of existence in time
and space."

Among other crude opinions hazarded by Knox, one
related to the Jews, whom he thought were becoming
extinct, as "their children cannot be reared even in
Jerusalem."

He dwelt largely upon dentition, and Natural History
character, and in writing of the Salmonidæ, *inter alia*,
expressed himself thus :—"The living zoological world,
as it now exists and has existed, is a self-created, self-
creating world, ever alive, never decaying, never old.
Life is coeval with the globe."

Knox remarked upon Goethe's idea of "the germ of
any animal being the germ of every other." "This is
the highest generalization. It connects the living and
extinct world into one great self-created chain ; it connects it with the physical history of the globe itself—
formed by a word, developing in its history an idea—that
idea the universal and the eternal. Physically speaking,
it means the development of the eternal germs of life
in time and space, agreeably to laws inherent in their
nature ; the material form they assume is the combined
result of these laws, and of the external circumstances in
which they are placed."

He communicated several papers to the *Lancet* in
1856, and commenced in January with what promised to

be a series of " Contributions to Surgical Anatomy and
Operative Surgery." His second paper (May 17) was
more a history of cases derived from various sources, civil
and military, both at home and abroad. In his third
(July 19), he recounted instances of bad operative surgery,
and urged the advantage of anatomy. On August 30th,
September 6th and 13th, he wrote " On Organic Harmonies : Anatomical Co-relations of Methods of Zoology
and Palæontology." He reverted to the opinions
he had expressed in 1830 to the Royal Society of
Edinburgh, and which controverted Cuvier's ideas that
there exist certain anatomical co-relations which, when
once detected in one animal, furnish a law applicable to
all. Knox wished to show that he never mistook the
method by direct observation for any laws of co-relation
or organic harmonies admitting of any *à priori* reasoning. In his third chapter on this subject, he condemned
F. Cuvier for omitting to notice in his work on the
Cetacea, both his (Knox's) papers on the Dugong and
Cetacea. In opposition to Baron Cuvier, Knox had
shown that the Dugong did not belong to the
Cetacea. He felt the littleness of F. Cuvier the more
that, like John Hunter, he (Knox) had spent much labour
and time, and hundreds of pounds sterling, in the dissecting of the Cetacea.

The war with Russia and the siege of Sebastopol
roused Knox's patriotism to fever heat ; the military
ardour of his adolescence was revived in his " sixties ; "
and from time to time he addressed himself to the
heads of departments in the War Office and Admiralty.
The dire antagonism of the Saxon to the Sarmatian or

Russ was as strongly manifested by Knox as by any
subject of her Majesty's ; and at length he became
desirous of serving his country either as physician in the
Crimea or staff-surgeon. His application to the Government was backed by Lord Murray, of Edinburgh, in a
note to Lord Panmure. He was sixty-three years of age,
yet as active as ever ; so that his friend Mr. (now Sir
Wm.) Fergusson had no hesitation in stating in his letter
to Knox : "You seem to me as full of energy as ever,
and I need hardly say that your intellectual powers
seem equal to any of those former efforts which in early
days made you *dux* of the High School of Edinburgh,
and the first teacher of anatomy in Europe." Mr.
Coulson and numerous friends spoke to the same effect
on Knox's behalf, but those in power were too prone
to nepotism and "taking care of Dowd" to heed the
application of a man of genius like Knox. Considering
the class of medicals sent out to the Crimea to aid the
strictly military staff, it said but little for those in the
sunshine of office that so distinguished a man as Knox
should be left out in the cold. His age, it might be
supposed, could hardly be an object with a sexagenarian
Administration at home and Peninsular Generals in the
field forty years after Waterloo, and these Generals red-
tapists of the reddest dye ! Lots of civilians, and some
of them not worth their rations, had been appointed,
yet Knox, the teacher of thousands, and of those too
who held high place in the Crimea, could not be accepted !
He had military experience, had been present in two
campaigns in Caffraria, and in many dangerous *com-
mandos*, and was the sole surgeon in charge of posts

forming the left division of the African frontier for nearly three years. All these recommendations went for nothing ; such was the mode adopted by British Secretaries of State to make the Crimean struggle the most disastrous to our prestige and honour the world had ever witnessed.

He had correspondents in the Crimean Army, and was well posted on all the movements of the besieging force. He knew the hardships to which his professional brethren were exposed, the faulty commissariat, and all the evils of the situation ; and used his pen pretty freely to show up the errors of the Government in the *Morning Advertiser* and other newspapers. He also addressed himself frequently to the Secretary of War and Sir James Graham at the Admiralty, giving various suggestions well worthy the consideration of those in power.

He had communicated his views on the needful reforms to be instituted in the Crimea to render our army healthy and efficient, to his old pupil, Sir George Sinclair, who replied, *inter alia :* " I have read with very lively interest your recent remarks on the state of matters in high places with respect to the public provisions for medical and chirurgical aid, in connection with the army and navy, and it appears to me that the gratitude of the country is due to you for pointing out so plainly the defects which it would be most important and most opportune to rectify or to remove. If the distinguished men who have it in their power to bring you forward in some public capacity, as superintendent of a professional department, or as an instructor, on a great scale, of the surgeons and anatomists of a future age, they would, in my opinion, reflect great honour upon their own discernment, afford high gratification to your numerous pupils, and make a grateful though tardy reparation for past slights and shortcomings to one who has most truly rendered good service to the State by training up so many men of eminence in the most useful of all departments—Medicine."

On the 22nd of September, 1856, the Academy of Sciences of the French Institute received from Dr. Knox in manuscript an essay entitled " *Travaux sur l'Adaptation focale de l'Œil*," and appointed a Commission consisting of MM. Quatrefages and Claude Bernard to examine the said essay.

On the 18th October, 1856, Dr. Knox was appointed Pathological Anatomist to the Cancer Hospital at Brompton. "The committee of the Hospital, impressed with the benefit likely to accrue to the Hospital by Knox's eminent name and talent, deemed themselves personally obliged by his acceptance of office."

In the *Lancet* of May 1857, Knox wrote a letter to Isodore Geoffroy (St. Hilaire), member of the Institute, on " The Food Question in France," in which he strongly condemned the use of horseflesh. He maintained that the use of such food would argue an unwholesome condition of the social positions of a nation. On the Scythian desert, the Mongol, the Calmuck, or the Tartar were horseflesh eaters ; and so were the African yellow or Bosjesman races ; but the savage Caffre and not overnice Negro never touched horseflesh. He had tasted the flesh of the wild horse, and pronounced it carrion.

He advised France to improve her breeds of cattle and sheep, and to imitate the English feeding of both ruminants. He did not like the French artificial mode of rearing fish practised at Thuringen. " Look to Africa," was his counsel to France, not without some sly hints as to the inroads of the Saxon Boer from the extreme south being met by the Gaul.

On August 23 (*Lancet*) appeared his " New Theory of Race"—Celt *versus* Saxon. Dr. McElheran had read a memoir to the New York Academy of Medicine, in which he claimed for the Celtic race predominance in America. This idea being in opposition to Knox's views, he replied to his former pupil, and in a very characteristic way. Dr. McElheran had called "the carnivorous Saxon" the " outer rind of humanity :" this was enough to call forth the Anatomist.

Dr. Knox communicated no less than eight papers to the *Zoologist* during the years 1855 1856, and 1857. " Some Observations on the Salmo Estuarius, or Estuary Trout," appeared in vol. xiii. p. 4,662 (1855). He described the estuary trout taken at the mouth of the Nith where it joins the Solway, and in the Tyne in East Lothian, as being a foot in length generally, and feeding on small shrimps. He distinguished this trout from the true salmon found in the same net, the food of which salmon consisted of the eggs, or remains of eggs, of the Echinodermata ; and from the sea-trout, or *Salmo fario*, living on the sand-eel and small herring; and from the common river trout and parr, which had been feeding abundantly on flies, cod-bait, &c. As food for man the estuary trout was excellent; the flesh is of a pink colour, and quite equal to the finest river trout of England and the celebrated Lochleven trout. He showed the specific characters of the said trout, external and internal, and formulized the dentition.

In the same paper he described the law of *edentulation* (loss of teeth) as regards the vomerine teeth in the Salmonidæ ; also the natural family of the Salmonidæ, and of the different trouts caught in Scotland. He used the dentar formula of M. Valenciennes as his guide in the description ; admitting, however, that it was a partial law applicable to some continental species, but inapplicable to the great family of the Salmonidæ as they now exist in the creations of the globe.

His paper "On the Food of certain Gregarious Fishes" (*loc. cit.* p. 4,709), which had been read to the Linnean Society in 1854 (*Proc. Linn. Soc.*, No. lx. p. 354), supports the views he had originally made known to the Royal Society of Edinburgh on the salmon, vendace, herring, &c. discussed in Chap. X. of this work.

His " Inquiries into the Philosophy of Zoology (*loc. cit.* p. 4,792) led him to discuss the views of M. Valenciennes (*Histoire Naturelle de Poissons*), particularly as to the dentition of the Salmonidæ, to which he was opposed. He gave measurements of three distinct families, and the arrangement of their dentition. He believed the colouration of the Salmonidæ obeyed fixed laws. He discussed the proportions of the Salmonidæ as compared with each other and the generic animal, and continued : " Species are only real in so far as regards Man's observing powers : they seem to form no part of Nature's scheme or plan, which obviously fills up all gaps, leaving

no link deficient in the chain. . . . Unless we are prepared to adopt the doctrines of chance, there can exist
only one creative idea, and consequently one creation.
The theological doctrine of Socrates, worked into a
system by Philo-Judæus and his followers of 'the
final cause' school, applies merely to simple mechanical
laws of obvious significance and application : it has
nothing to do with the great laws of life, the laws of
formation and deformation, the laws of unity of the
organization in all that ever lived ; the law of serial
unity, which makes the living and past organic worlds
one, and not many."

In his essay "On the Growth of the Salmon from
the Egg to the Adult" (*loc. cit.* p. 4,792), he speaks of his
own observations, and those of Hutchinson of Carlisle
in 1782, of his contemporaries, Andrew Young of
Invershin, and Shaw of Drumlanrig, of the great
Willoughby in 1686, and other authorities.

His "Contributions to the Philosophy of Zoology"
(*loc. cit.* p. 4,837) are but a text for advocating the
transcendental in anatomy ; nor is there much to be
learned from "The present Condition of the Salmon
Question considered Physiologically" (vol. xiv. p. 4,985:
1856); or "Some Remarks on the Skeleton of the Head
of the *Urus Scoticus*, or White Ox, obtained from the
park of Cadzow, the property of the Duke of Hamilton"
(vol. xv. p. 5,417 : 1857.)

He had a long article on "Zoology, its present Phasis
and future Prospects" (*Zoologist*, vol. xv. pp. 5,473-5,502:
1857), which afforded him the opportunity of speaking
his mind on various matters affecting zoological study

and pursuits. He accused the *parti-prêtre* of having degraded science in England ; the same existed in France, but was swept away by the French Revolution. " With us on the favoured side of the Channel, *sot* George succeeded *idiot* George ; the English mandarins, with whom, of course, was the English *parti-prêtre*, successfully resisted the claims of man to be free ; the progress of science, especially of zoological science, was successfully resisted. . . . Gibbon's name could only be mentioned in a whisper, and to speak of Voltaire otherwise than to vituperate, was sure to entail on the speaker or writer a torrent of abuse."

He admitted that all this had changed. The paper is a capital example of Knox's pictorial, disquisitional, and discursive writing, embracing the *Historia Animalium* and the latest of the Cumming prophecies done up in high sarcastic method. He held that "sound zoological science never existed in England ; that it vacillated between the extreme of utter scepticism and the most slavish of doctrines, the theory of final causes. . . . . Continental scientific men look on with wonder, and ascribe it to the climate, and to the temper of the islanders : a hypocrisy which has been called ' organized,' but which must mean ' organic,' has no doubt something to do with it. The question resolves itself into this— Is life an inherent quality of matter from the beginning, an essential to it, and requiring but certain circumstances to call it forth ? This is a simple enough proposition, perfectly intelligible, and in every way probable ; so soon as it has been demonstrated it will take its place in science—but not till then."

B B

He gave Buffon the credit of the theory of primitive worlds, and to Voltaire the expression that had been applied to the physical world,—"the laws of deformation are as constant as the laws of formation."

In the endeavour to obtain a clue to the whole of Knox's writings, I visited the shop of H. Baillière in Regent Street (June 1869), and from a remark made to me a few hours previously, was induced to inquire if Knox had ever written on the Social Evil; the reply, as I expected, was in the negative. Seeing the urgency of my request, the obliging foreman handed me the only volume ever published by H. Baillière on this subject. Opening three pages at random, I unhesitatingly declared Knox to be the writer of the bracketed portions of the volume entitled "The Greatest of our Social Evils: Prostitution, as it now exists in London, Liverpool, Manchester, Glasgow, Edinburgh, and Dublin: an Inquiry into the Cause and Means of Reformation, based on statistical documents. By a Physician." (London: Baillière, 1857.) The "Physician's" style could be none other than Knox's, and documents are now in my possession to prove the accuracy of my first conjecture. The work is based on Léon Faucher's "*Études sur l'Angleterre,*" and Dr. Richelot's "*La Prostitution en Angleterre,*" and Parent Duchâtelet's "*De la Prostitution dans la Ville de Paris.*" The subject could hardly be to Knox's liking, but being cast on the literary world for his bread and butter, he had, at Mr. Baillière's suggestion, undertaken to translate and extend the labours of the French authors given above, and to introduce along with his own observations the opinions of accredited

English authors. Knox's own portion is not the least interesting part of the work, as containing statistical and other information on population, manners, emigration, tendencies of race, historical criticism, and the like. Among other curious statements in the book, Knox attributes a great deal to fortune-telling as a cause of prostitution.

"Immorality and libertinage," wrote Knox, "belong to all countries and to all times; nor would it be easy to determine under what forms of society, under what kinds of government, under what systems of religious belief, immorality, using the term in its widest acceptation, has most prevailed. Rigid Presbyterianism and Sabbath worship avail nothing towards mitigating the evil; they clothe it simply with the garb of hypocrisy, and driving it from the open streets, force it into the domicile. . . Society will and must, sooner or later, have recourse to a system of control; that control in free countries can only be exercised over the more daring and profligate, who, throwing aside the ties of family, the respect for society, self-respect as well, and that modesty which, when natural, exalts woman above all price, chooses to set up for herself and on her own account, without a partner of the other sex, a traffic which, although sanctioned and legalized by some nations who, I believe, claim to be Christian, society will not tolerate in her when it assumes this independent form. Against this open prostitution, society, in general, claims a right of control; in England it has hitherto been merely denounced. The time is sure to come when society must adopt more active measures against

the growing evil. But before attempting this, might it
not be advisable to employ with more energy the
existing modes of repression which continental writers
admit and prove have never, in the United Kingdom,
been fairly brought to bear against this the greatest
of Social Evils ? "

In an appendix he quotes St. Augustine, who looked
upon bad women "as a natural constituent and essential part of the order of human affairs as instituted by
Providence, as contributing to the sum total of human
happiness, and as a natural arrangement not admitting
of correction by human means." Whilst the Saint
pointed out the infamy of the whole class of prostitutes
and panders, he continued :—" *Aufer meretrices de rebus
humanis, turbaveris omnia libidinibus : constitue ma-
tronarum loco, labe ac dedecore dehonestaveris ;* " thus
he held prostitutes to be part and parcel of the great
Providential arrangements.

Since Knox wrote, the question has absorbed a large
share of attention, and the "Contagious Diseases Act"
would imply a determination on the part of the Government to meet the worst features of the Social Evil.
To-day (April 1870), some of our leading politicians
and divines, spinsters young and old, wives as well as
matrons, are in the field discussing a dirty subject : the
Westminster Review has also reviewed the whole question at length. If, as has been conjectured, 56,000
persons of the productive class in London alone are
annually more or less incapacitated from profitable
labour by this malady of the sexes, and that from the
same cause our army loses in the course of a year six

days' service of the whole force, it seems high time for a people's Parliament to interfere. The question is one of extreme gravity to the nation at large, and not likely to be settled by aproned ecclesiastics, spinsters of a certain age, and matrons seeking publicity at the cost of delicacy of feeling. Where is the shade of Mrs. Ellis, and where are the model "Women of England" in these days of grace?

CHAPTER XIX.

IN 1857 Dr. Knox issued his brief work, "Man, his
Structure and Physiology; popularly explained and
demonstrated, with eight moveable dissected coloured
plates, and five woodcuts" (Baillière, London). This
work was quite elementary in design, yet meant to be
educational : he held, that without a knowledge of the
facts and deductions it contained the general student
could make no sound progress in zoology, and the
professional student would become an unsafe practitioner, and the palæontologist a mere dreamer. The
dissected coloured plates remind me of the work of
Dr. Alexander Ramsay, a lecturer on anatomy in
Edinburgh early in the century; where, probably for
the first time in Britain, this kind of illustration was
adopted. This little volume added nothing to Knox's
fame ; it fell short in value of the " Popular Physiology"
of his distinguished pupil Dr. Perceval B. Lord—issued
by J. W. Parker twenty years previously. Considering

their size, the plates convey a great deal of information; and here and there in the text are Knox's characteristic touches. He held that Man stood apart from all other natural families, that between him and the highest of the Apes or *Simiæ* there is a gulf, even as regards structure, which renders wholly inappropriate the fashionable term of "anthropomorphous apes." It is curious to observe M. Pruner Bey travelling over the the same ground—"*Société d'Anthropologie.*" An abstract of his paper appears in the *Cosmos* of May 28, 1870.

From time to time Knox reverted to his "old hobbies" in Natural History. The Cetacea, upon which he had written so ably, seem to have engaged his attention to his last days. In the autumn of 1857 he inquired of Professor Goodsir as to the exact arrangement of the cervical vertebræ in the true whales, and referred him to his own preparation of the "young *Mysticetus*" for examination; as he was wishful to see if Eschricht and G. M. Van Beneden, who had lately published a memoir in the Bulletin of the Royal Academy of Brussels, were right in their views. Van Beneden held that in *true whales* the cervical vertebræ at every age form one mass, never showing even in the fœtus any traces of division into district bones, or cartilages, as the case may be. The anatomical facts furnished by the young *Mysticetus*, afforded, as Goodsir observed,[1] no support to the views of G. M. Van Beneden; so the conclusion arrived at by Knox was, that the actual number of

---

[1] Professor Goodsir's letter is in my hands; but as a copy appears in the *Proceedings of the Linnean Society*, London, vol. iii. 1858, pp. 63–76, it is unnecessary to quote it here.

cervical vertebræ in the *Mysticetus*, as in most other mammals, is seven.

Knox's last "Contributions to the Anatomy and Natural History of the Cetacea" were read to the Linnean Society, October 6, 1857. He spoke first of the Dolphins, and secondly of the Balæna Whales. In this paper he held that the number of vertebræ comprising the vertebral column exclusive of the cephalic, should determine the species of the Cetacea. He gave a tabular view of the number of vertebræ determined by himself and others; thus his own were—*Mysticetus borealis*, Greenland, 48; Great Northern Rorqual, 65; Lesser Rorqual, 48; *Delphinus Delphis*, 65; *Delphinus Phocæna*, 65. He wished to divide the Cetacea into whales with whalebones, and whales with teeth. Those with whalebone have rudimentary teeth in both jaws in the fœtal state. In certain species of *Delphinus* the vertebral column is composed of 61 vertebræ, in others of 65, in others of 66, in others of 81, in others of 90.

Speaking of the Balæna Whales, he refers to the Queensferry instance (February 1834), and that the number of vertebræ in the Balænopterous whale was 48, while the Rorqual *giganteus* had 65, and held the difference to be specific. In this whale he saw a canal in the centre of the spinal marrow. The nerves of the lung and stomach terminated in loops. The arterial plexus surrounding the spinal marrow and extending into the chest was an intercostal artery that never gave off any branches, but continued of the same calibre throughout, making innumerable flexuosities or turnings.

Writing from Colchester (no date), where he had been

lecturing, to his nephew in Edinburgh, and enclosing post-office orders for the maintenance of his family there, he remarks : "You cannot think what pleasure I have in making you all comfortable. I do believe that were it not for this pleasure I would not take the trouble to take another meal ; for I am tired of the world, its humbug and commonplace. . . . The morning is, as usual, misty, cold, rainy, dark; and I hear the east winds singing mournfully through the crevices of my bed-room. Let us fly to finer climates, where we may at least see the sun."

In a letter from Guildford : "Do not forget to make all round you comfortable. Mary (his eldest daughter), I suppose, manages chiefly; let bonny Bre and Bob have some pocket-money for sweets." Again : "I wish you were all here in London, but I know you are all comfortable and happy" in Edinburgh.

On various anatomical questions, human and comparative, Knox was consulted by both lay and clerical correspondents throughout Britain. Captain Basil Hall, who had been discussing the anatomical arrangements of the tiger's claw with Knox, makes an allusion to his own *penchant* for science, and in a way that had nearly cost him dear :—"I once entered a lion's den (old Nero's), and while I was sitting on his back, thought it a good occasion to lecture on this favourite fancy of mine. But the monarch of the woods, not having the love of science in his royal breast, gave such an infernal growl that it lives in my recollection to this hour."

In January 1859, Dr. E. Zimmerman junior asked Knox for information of his "late colleague, Dr. Vesalius, a native of Brussels, who died at Zante in 1564:" in justification of his question he appealed to Knox on the ground of his "well-known and well-merited position in the literary world."

When opportunity offered, he took care to ventilate his views on Race and Acclimation in the *Lancet* and other medical journals. He did not believe that the widespread Roman colonies succeeded to any great extent in altering or modifying the character of the original races of the conquered countries. "None of them ever became Roman or Italian, properly so called ; the intrusive race, in fact, after a few centuries, disappeared, and the population regained its primitive type or character—a process of depuration hastened, in all probability, by the circumstance that the Italian youth alone emigrated to foreign lands, intermarrying with the races amongst whom his lot was cast."

"The question of acclimation, which to many may seem a merely theoretical and philosophical question, is, on the contrary, to Britain, one of the most pressing nature, and eminently practical. On its solution depends the existence of what some are pleased to call "the Colonial Empire of Britain."

"The opinion gains ground that after some centuries the fate of all intrusive races is to die out, whether the land of their adoption be within or without the tropics, unless their numbers be fed by continual immigration from the parent stock. But be this as it may, the question which interests Britain at the present moment is, the maintenance of armies of Europeans in such a state of efficiency in her colonies as to render unnecessary the employment of natives, enlisted amongst the aborigines of the land thus held by military occupation. The revolt in India presents on a gigantic scale all the dangers of such a policy as the disciplining and arming races of men wholly and for ever antagonists to our own : whilst the same process—namely, the calling the peaceful labourer and merchant of European descent from vocations on which all civilization ultimately rests—must assuredly end in the speedy disjunction of these colonies from the mother country. Events productive of the same results, though springing from a different cause, lost to Britain the greatest colonial empire the world ever saw—the United States of America. To hold distant countries in any kind of subjection to Britain, her armies must be composed simply of the natives of Britain, born and educated in the land of their forefathers, proud of their nationality and of their European birth and education. . . . Armies are ever healthiest on the move—an observation which is true in more senses than one ; and on this theory, supported as it is by innumerable facts, we ground our belief in the possibility of maintaining the armies of England in a healthy condition all over the world, simply by judicious and welltimed frequent transference from one climate to another. . . . Are we to have another expedition to China on the model of the Crimean ? If any reasonable fears be entertained on this head—and numerous precedents warrant the reasonableness of such apprehensions—then the nation cannot too soon insist on the formation of a *Conseil de Santé des Armées,* to see to the due administration of a portion of the twelve millions

sterling which the country has voted for the maintenance of the power and dignity of England at home
and abroad."

Under the name of "A Traveller," he wrote " Contributions to the Natural History of Man," in the *London
Illustrated Magazine*, in 1854 or thereabouts. The
magazine was conducted by Richard Brinsley Knowles.
In his first chapter, headed " The American Race—the
Aztecques," he objected to the word Caucasian, as there
was not a shadow of proof that the European races
originated in the mountain country of the Caucasus ;
that the term had risen into an unexpected and un-
merited celebrity in consequence of its adoption by a
modern novelist, Disraeli ; adding, as if to swamp the
rosewater duchess-creative M.P. for Bucks, " that the
theories of the vulgar are the cast-off speculations of
philosophy." He speaks in another passage of Blumenbach's mantle being " new, glossy, shining, and
substantial," but that Pritchard wore it threadbare, so
that "none but an enlightened Quarterly Reviewer
could venture to call it a mantle at all. Not so the
bold and chivalrous author of ' Tancred ' and of
' Coningsby.' True to *his race*, he picks up the worn-
out, threadbare rag, and *declares* it to be a sound
and excellent garment—'as good as new.' And now,
patched with scraps and bits of Literature and Science
—curiosities in their way, no doubt—here we have it
palmed on the world as a new garment. With its
renovation and restoration, it has got a new name : it
is now called ' the Caucasian theory ' ! "

In another article he treats of " the Earthmen tribe

of the Bosjesman and Hottentot races of Southern Africa," and upon this subject, as upon all others of African growth, he fulfils the remark of the Roman poet from whom he quotes—

" Africa semper aliquod novi offert,"

interspersing his remarks on the *physique* of the different humanities with the grand scenes before him—Nature in all her wondrous beauty and variety.

Knox was made Honorary Fellow of the Ethnological Society of London, "the highest honour the Society had in its power to bestow," said the secretary, during the session 1860–61, along with Von Baer, Boucher de Perthes, Nott, Renan, and other *savans.* On March 6, 1861, he read a paper " On the Collection of Human Crania and other Human Bones preserved in the Crypt of the Church at Hythe, Kent ; " and on the 19th of the same month his observations " On some Ancient Forms of Civilization."

Excepting the president, Crauford, and the indefatigable secretary, Dr. James Hunt, few men took so active a part in the service of the Ethnological Society as Knox did at this period of its history. The Society showed its approval of his marked interest by electing him " honorary curator" of its museum on the 20th May, 1862.

In the spring months of 1861, it will be remembered that Du Chaillu was " the lion " of the London Geographical Society : in Knox's opinion the Frenchman was also in the hands of a clique. In speaking of Du Chaillu, he reverted to some intercourse he had had

with the greater traveller Dr. Livingstone, and of
Dr. L.'s expressions of regret to him that he had not
read "The Races of Men" and studied the history of
Man more than he had done; and further, that he had
not placed his manuscripts in Dr. Andrew Smith's and
Knox's hands: "as it was," said Knox, " Livingstone's
book was unreadable, but it suited the Geographical
and the Missionary bodies." I should have had some
doubts as to the propriety of quoting Knox's statements upon Dr. Livingstone and the Geographical
Society, had not corroborative evidence come within
my knowledge only a few months ago, in Edinburgh
(December 1869). No one need be told that the great
traveller's book was imperfect in many matters pertaining to science, and that it could not well be
compared with works of a similar nature published by
French and German authors.

To the *Empire*, apparently a weekly Radical print,
Knox contributed several articles, chiefly political or
condemnatory of the Sanitary Commissioners. "A
Plea for the Thames" was a hard hit at the "Sewage
Agitators," the Board of Health, Commissioners of
Works, &c.; and his article on the "Sanitary Movement" of the following week is still more characteristic
of his slashing style, as the following quotations will
prove :—

" The surplus population, and what to do with it, has ever been a
favourite subject of speculation with the metaphysician and the statistician.
Already, in the fourth or fifth century, St. Cyprian, looking around him
at the profusion of human life in Northern Africa, where now there are
not half a dozen persons to the square mile—to those places, now desert,
where Carthage once poured its thousands and thousands of armed men—

St. Cyprian defended the establishment of monastic institutions on the ground that the earth (meaning a few miles around his diocese) was over-populated ! Malthus followed to the same tune, but the good man, also a kind of monk, however, really believed in what he wrote. Not so the priest, St. Cyprian ; his white lies were his own invention, intended to delude mankind, and lead them into deep and damnable error. About ten years ago Lord Derby tried the stale and oft-repeated trick ! As Colonial Secretary, he showed by statistics that in the wide colonial domains of that queendom on which the sun never sets, there was not a spot whereon a labourer could reside with the smallest hopes of bettering himself ! And yet this man enjoys the confidence of England !

" Such are statistics in the hands of the *talented* and *unscrupulous.* St. Cyprian, in the fifth century, asserted the world to be over-populated. Lord Derby, in the nineteenth, did the same. The excuse for the Saint was his profound ignorance ; the British lord could have no such excuse. . . . . Holiness is a great gain to bishops and priests, no doubt still more to the governing body ; it is also an engine of great power when cleverly handled by a Sabbatarian nobleman, as a Shaftesbury, Ebrington, or Gros-venor. It is not the first time that men of this stamp have succeeded by its means in trampling out the very intellect and soul of a nation of free men. Free men ! what nation can be called free, governed by such laws, and trampled on by such men ! But the Sabbatarian host, having 'made common cause with God,' act in His name, and at times irresistibly."

He had commenced a memoir " On the Laws regulating Human Production, Mortality, and Increase," and it was his intention to arrange his matter under three heads: " 1. Man's productive powers, and the laws which seem to regulate them. 2. The laws of his mortality or annihilation. 3. His increase."

Another idea of Knox's was to re-edit Alexander Walker's work, " Intermarriage ; or the Influence of Physical Laws over Health, Beauty, Intellect, Deformity, Disease, Insanity ; " with "numerous notes and additional observations." Several fragmentary notes which he had made on intermarriage would imply that he meant to carry out his plan.

As Secretary to the Ethnological Society of London, and afterwards President of the Anthropological Society, Dr. James Hunt[1] had frequent communications with Knox, both personally and by letter. The following excerpts from his notes to Dr. Hunt may interest the reader. Writing in August 1860, Knox observes as to the *Hatchet question*, flint-headed arrows, &c. as being the precursors of bronze, iron, and steel: " I confess to you that I doubt the theory. It depended on the race, the locality, and the exigency; they do not imply in themselves a great antiquity: nothing of the sort appears in the Homeric Ballad, in the Tombs of Karnac [Thebes?], nor on the Obelisks." In a postscript referring to Race, he adds: " I observe in a critique on Gervinus's work on the history of the past half-century, in a late number of the *Saturday Review*, that Gervinus had adopted to the full the views I took many years ago of the causes leading to the demoralization and breaking up of the so-called Spanish Republics of America; he ascribes it to the hybridity of the people. The reviewer was bound in justice to me to have said that Gervinus had merely adopted my views, but he does not say so."

Referring again to Spain (Dec. 1860), he asks: " Did you see Don Pacheco's candid speech to the Cortes?

---

[1] Dr. Hunt, the indefatigable anthropologist, who founded and for some years ably directed the London Anthropological Society, is now beyond my thanks. His attendance at the Exeter meeting of the British Association, and his zeal for the science he so diligently espoused, obliging considerable exertion during intensely hot weather, proved too much for his delicate constitution. He was suddenly seized with cerebral symptoms, which proved fatal in a few days, at his residence, Ore House, Hastings.

He confesses that the Spanish race in Mexico are reduced to 8,000 ! that the half-breeds are worthless, &c. ; but was not all this foretold nearly twenty years ago in the Fragment on the Races of Men ? "

One of the pleasures of the New Year of 1861 to Knox was his being unanimously elected Foreign Corresponding Member of the Anthropological Society of Paris : moreover, as the learned secretary, M. Broca, informed him in a very kind and handsome letter, he was the first foreigner who had obtained the honour.

On the 18th January he wrote : " How the present state of Europe proves my theory of Race ! Look at Ireland and Austria. The *Times* of this morning admits that the theory has always been acted upon by Louis Napoleon, and that it will break up Austria and Mexico when the present mongrel race will die out in about a hundred years !"

He stated in his letters of this period that he was busy collecting facts " On the Antiquity of Man on the globe, the grandest of all scientific inquiries." Every now and then he hit the " parsons " very hard, and probably they merited it. Thus he writes : " I do not wonder at priests and Governments not liking ethnologists ; the hard matter-of-fact statements lately brought forward make short work with the Utopias of Church and State."

Knox had been criticised for speaking too freely of our relations to the coloured races of India, and for his un-English feeling ; and on seeing the *Times* in the same vein, he asked Dr. Hunt if he had seen Russell's remarks on the conduct of the English to the coloured races of India, and continued : " When you next hear of my un-English feelings on these matters, you can point to the much stronger language of Dr. Russell and the *Times*. But the truth is, the clergy do not like the inquiry into Race, and so they get up any objection against its advocates. They assert that I disparage their efforts at Christianizing Africa ! What do they think of the Christianity of Virginia and Georgia, and of the doings of the English in India ? "

In reference to Darwin and his opponents, Knox in May 1861 wrote : " A serious onslaught has been made on Darwin by Mr. Sedgwick at Cambridge ; also by Dr. Clarke, both great men, the former especially ; but priests in holy orders. That is enough. I continue of the same opinion in respect to Darwin's work, namely, it leaves the question precisely where it was left by Goethe, Oken, and Geoffroy St. Hilaire."

Some of his ethnological inquiries and observations read, or intended to be read, to the Ethnological Society were published after his death by Dr. James Hunt in the *Anthropological Review*, vol. i. 1863 :—1. " Inquiry into the Influence of Climate and of Hybridity over Man," pp. 246–263. 2. " On the Application of the Anatomical Method to the Discrimination of Species," pp. 263–270 (copied from the *Medical Times* and *Gazette*, March 14th, 1863) ; and 3. " On the Deformations of the Human Cranium, supposed to be produced by Mechanical Means."

The meetings of the Geographical Society used to amuse him greatly. Under Sir Roderick he witnessed from time to time the " lightness " of the proceedings and gaiety of the assembled, the dilettanteism of science if not buttered and sweetened, the "grand exhibitions" with Chaillu and the gorilla to boot, and other lions and lionesses, as the case might be, in pants or petticoats. Nothing diverted him more than the appearance of a negro "black massa" pitted against the white man, and prompted by Dr. Hodgkin, the Quaker, for the fight. The negro, in defence of his own order and their possible liking to "cold missionary," cited history, and talked of British cannibals. "Now," said Knox, "the story of the cannibalism of the natives near Glasgow rests on the very questionable authority of Saint Jerome. I would not *have believed the Saint on his oath, nor any other saint.*"

Full of literary projects, Knox was preparing an essay "On the Origin of the Arts," which he intended to make his best memoir, and to present it to the Academy of Belles Lettres in Paris. "Deep reflection on the subject has convinced me," says Knox, "that the question is really an ethnological one." Probably he would have gone along with Mr. Fergusson (History of Modern Architecture), who stated that the true glory of the Celt in Europe is his artistic eminence. The same ideas crossed my mind when writing the first pages of the "Life of Watson, the Sculptor," in 1865 and if my memory aids me, Mr. Ruskin has given expression to similar opinions.

In 1861 he was "maturing some new views on the functions of the brain." It would have been gratifying to find in his writings any indication of the nature of his thoughts on a method so deeply interesting to the physiologist, and upon which he had bestowed so much attention. He had previously admitted that there were not sufficient facts to attempt, with any success, a classification of the races of men.

Towards his last days he contemplated publishing a large work in two volumes, with the title, " Contributions to the Scientific and Educational History of my Times." It is greatly to be regretted that he did not live to carry out such a work.

A more fertile pen than Knox's was seldom if ever wielded, and its scope was far from limited—indeed much too general, for with greater concentrativeness on his part greater results might have been obtained. Unfortunately, his pen was too often driven by the necessities of life, and occasionally in a direction but little consonant to its master's feelings, and therefore less likely to contribute to his scientific reputation. It was all the more painful to reflect on such opposing circumstances, as no man had fewer wants or less regard for filthy lucre; whilst his heart was hourly linked with an intense regard for the advancement of professional knowledge. One day in the office of his friend Mr. Renshaw, Knox said with great energy and manifestation: " I would rather be the discoverer of one fact in science, than have a fortune bestowed upon me." Here he spoke most truly and advisedly as to the principles which had guided him through life.

Knox had no regard for the English Universities ; and he used to cite Lord Palmerston's remark to the House of Commons, namely, that all he ever learned was in the University of Edinburgh, under Dugald Stewart ; that during the first year he was there he was busily engaged in *unlearning* all that he had acquired at Cambridge. Knox believed that the members of the Ethnological Society "who stood up for English Universities never were there, and probably were not aware that these institutions are strictly theological institutions based on the edicts of Pope Boniface."

He frequently gave popular lectures on Race, Civilization, the Origin of the Arts, Leonardo da Vinci, and other notabilities in history. When lecturing at Hendon, near London, on Race, he showed some skulls in support of his views. When he spoke of the crania of the lower orders of civilization, where space for brain was wanting, he compared such to persons who go to Oxford to chop theology and logic for five years. He of course ignored the Mosaic record *quoad* Man.

·His visits to Southampton as a lecturer proved too much for a lady in the neighbourhood, who became enamoured of his person and cleverness, and evidently looked forward to marriage with the weird anatomist. Cupid won the spinster entirely; Knox had had experience, and *knew* the byways of womanhood. Maria was comely, and comfortable in means; Robert, however, had passed beyond his sixtieth summer. In this, as in too many cases, true love did not run smoothly; at any rate nothing came of the promised conquest of our hero.

In his latter years Dr. Knox took to practice in the Hackney district, and, marvellous to say, did a great deal in the obstetrical department. Let the old pupils of Knox picture their teacher trying to fill the his-

torical page, tracing the growth of the Egyptian dynasties and the formation of the Assyrian marbles,
and recording in graphic line the progress of race
and civilization, whilst his ears were dinned by the
voluble Mrs. Gamp and puerperal groans. Whoever
employed Knox professionally, liked him exceedingly.
Ladies in expectation would "expect" *too soon*, that
they might secure the services of the delightful doctor
in good time, and not unfrequently they would not
tolerate his leaving for days after the event. Having
his papers by him and every home comfort, he had
the pleasure of complying with the wishes of his friends.
He was kind to the poor, and prescribed gratuitously,
and often found them food and luxuries ; then, he used
to say, he was the happiest of practitioners.

He lectured at various public institutions, in and
around London, frequently, and at some of the large
towns, *e.g.* Sheffield, Southampton, &c. His style of
lecturing was so novel and captivating, that many
who scarcely sanctioned his doctrines and flings at
the ecclesiastics, attended him for a treat. Others
were so pleased that, though strangers to him, they
asked if he would come and dine, and stay all night.
Invitations of this kind were frequently offered to
him, nay, were extended far beyond all reasonable
limit ; so that Knox might literally have lived with
private friends, and found a comfortable home in
every district in London. "Hang up your hat in
the hall, Dr. Knox; call for what you want; we dine
at six ; our evenings and Sundays are entirely at
your disposal, and above all we shall be delighted

to have you here!" Such were the character of his invitations, and the modes adopted to get hold of the conversationalist Knox, the best of story-tellers, and the most sympathizing of mortals.

In the last year of his life his pen seems to have been as active as ever in controverting the errors of others, and in the advocacy of his own opinions. Professor Schaaffhausen, in a communication made to the Society of the Lower Rhine, holding its meetings at Bonn, in March 1862, endeavoured to show that there was a continual increase in the rate of the pulsations of the heart from morning to evening. In the London *Medical Times and Gazette* of May 31, Knox goes over his old ground, and cites Dr. Guy, Dr. Graves, and M. Quetelet, as supporting the views first expressed by him in 1814, and oft confirmed since; and naturally expresses his surprise at the German's unacquaintance with his theories of the differential pulse.

On August 2, 1862 (*loc. cit.*), he had "Some Remarks on the Formation of Membranous Cysts in the Interior of the Urinary Bladder." This paper shows his marvellous retentive memory even in his seventy-first year, his referring to cases treated by Liston in Edinburgh thirty years previously, and the pathological specimens in the Museum of the College of Surgeons.

Knox left heaps of manuscript written on small pieces of paper, and in the most perplexing manner on both sides of the sheet; and as if to make confusion more confused, he would occasionally carry on two subjects on the same sheet of paper: the

writing on one side being arranged vertically, and on
the other side longitudinally. Nothing could well be
more varied than his literary scope; and the same
might be said of his scientific walk. Descriptions of
varieties in the form, direction, and number of muscles,
also of arteries; in short, all the anomalous human
structures that he had met with in his Practical
Rooms during twenty years' observation were noted.
He looked to the "numerical anomalies of parts of
muscle" with as much nicety as he did to the points
of the osteogenesis, and with an eye to specific zoological features or type. In this department of inquiry he was followed by Goodsir; indeed, the scraps
of MS. lying before me recall the packages of the same
sort so lately turned over for the purpose of writing
Goodsir's biography : the like masses of waste paper,
emblems of waste labour and futile expenditure of brain
power.

The "threescore and ten of man's years" were felt
and acknowledged by Dr. Knox as having a true
meaning. His mind might seem as fertile and active
as ever; but the freshness of intellectual thought, the
acute perception, and the grander generalizations at
one time so apparent to the world of medicine had
become more or less impaired, and at all events
robbed of their gloss and attractiveness.

He talked with greater calmness of his contemporaries, and of the few, very few enemies 'that remained;
and seemed comforted in the possession of all that
nature required for the sustentation of his physical
man. He also expressed an affectionate regard for the

peaceful attitude of his latter days. Happily for him, his wants were few and easily supplied, now that the love of applause and the fiery ambition in life's fretful aim had quite passed away. His only son and survivor, and his attached friends in No. 9, Lambe Terrace, Hackney, sat around him, and listened with delight to his varied talk, his worldly experiences, his reviews of the different epochs of human opinion through which he had lived, and the part he had sustained amid a life of severe competition and contention. They were gratified above all other considerations to hear him express his satisfaction with what he had done in the cause of medical education and science, and to see his cheerful contentment in a sphere so little consonant with the heydays of his popularity and success. He went to bed surrounded by a household that never wearied of his talk; he rose to a simple meal which was to him as good as a feast; he then set to work with his pen and paper, and covered sheet after sheet with a flowing diction that no printer could keep pace with. If his mental energies seemed inexhaustible, his physical strength and walking powers were evidently on the decline. He complained of the enfeebled action of the heart, and his inability to ascend a staircase; he was fully aware of the approaching shadows of death; but this made no change in his conversation, and led to no religious manifestation.

In the autumn of 1862, he spoke of writing his life, and gave as a reason that he could explain the terrible events of 1828 better than any other person living, and further, that he would be able to prove his

entire innocence of all and everything pertaining to
the West Port atrocities.

He attended to his duties at the Cancer Hospital
on the 9th December, and came home tired and ex-
hausted.   After a glass or two of champagne he seemed
refreshed, and went to bed.   In a short time the noise
of laboured breathing was heard proceeding from his
room : he was found apoplectic, and with little or no
rallying of the powers of consciousness he continued
till his death on the 20th December, 1862.

As he had spoken of the heather and wild flowers
blooming in great beauty in Woking Cemetery, and
his wish to be interred there in some spot where the
sun might shine longest on the green sod above his
grave, his remains were deposited in accordance with
his desire, on the 29th December.   The funeral was
strictly private.

Sir William Fergusson is about to erect a suitable
memorial over the grave of his renowned teacher and
friend, to whom he owed so much.   It need hardly
be said that some sepulchral *in memoriam* is due
to the greatest anatomical lecturer ever heard in
Britain, the man of rare intellect, commanding eloquence, and genius.

CHAPTER XX.

SEVERAL newspapers noticed Dr. Knox's death. A leading article in the *Lancet* contained, *inter alia:* " His death was a shock to those friends and acquaintances who had seen him in tolerable health two or three weeks previously, but it was and is more especially felt by his few relatives and associates, who loved the old man for his most affectionate and cheerful disposition, for his promptitude in doing any kind action which could serve another, and for his high intellectual qualities. Like all of us, he had his faults ; but, as with most earnest men, those faults were superficial, and it is no abuse of language to say that a better-hearted man never existed. . . . He was a man, not to look at, but to converse with ; though no mere clothes-horse, such were his gifts of speech that his harmonious voice and earnest manner won the close attention of each listener. . . . His words always bore thinking of, and not uncommonly the more they were thought of the more was the speaker admired."

Dr. Druitt wrote the admirable notice of Knox in the *Medical Times* (Dec. 27, 1862). The following excerpts are quite to the purpose : " In gifts of speech he was unequalled. His voice bland and harmonious, his manner earnest and persuasive, his *facundia* —or by whatever other name we may call that seemingly inexhaustible flow of the choicest and most apposite language ; his clearness, his logical precision in speaking, and the enormous amount of information on all subjects connected with natural history and fine art, which flowed without effort from his lips, all conspired to make him justly a favourite with all who formed his acquaintance. . . . In spite of his savage Radicalism, and that during a part of his career he was not free from all blemish, he was, in private life, pre-eminently tender, friendly, and affectionate. . . . Fine art, its cultivation and estimation, were regarded by Dr. Knox like a lofty literature, a test of the true character of any race, of their power of appreciating truth, philosophy, and science. All mere *fashion*, all utility, perish from the face of the earth ! Those races only leave abiding memorials, who follow Nature and truth. Of course Dr. Knox loathed teleology, or the utility principle. . . . His grandest point is his incessant sarcasm at the blindness, the self-conceit, the utilitarian tendencies, the specious hypocrisies, the self-gratulation which is exhibited by us, who call ourselves the Anglo-Saxon race, and to a still greater degree by our unhappy relatives in America."

Dr. Knox was a member of several learned bodies or societies both at home and abroad. He appreciated the foreign distinctions which were conferred upon him as honorary tributes to his position in the scientific world : his British titles were of little or no value in his eyes.

Since the dawn of this century, when Geherner Hofrath Loder lectured at Jena on " Physical Anthropology," and sought to give a new direction to the study of man's nature by the application of a higher anatomy, no one had been more conspicuous than Knox in this special department of public teaching, or had done more to advance the study of Race within the medical circles, and among the educated classes of this country. The science of Man, as far as it is understood in Britain, owes much to the Doctor's advocacy of the question, or rather of one particular phase of Anthropology, and that of practical application to the national interests. Before his time the Races of Men were hardly heard of except in special works ; now the hebdomadal and daily press discuss Knox's theme with an ability that shows the growing strength of the doctrines he laid down, and at a time, too, when it was dangerous to speak of Man's genesis and position, except through the reflection of "*the* Book " and the interpretation of pulpit declaimers and other blowers of the soap-bubble sort in Science.

Dr. Knox possessed a happy versatility of genius that should have led to great results ; such endowment, it is true, occasionally proves as much a hindrance as a gain to scientific work requiring steady and thoughtful application. Caught by the sentiment of the hour, so tempting to men of his cast of mind, or striving to obtain fresh growths from one of his old leavens, a practice often betrayed, he showed himself less regardful of his programme and of the steps needful to initiate a theoretical doctine, or to establish a more apposite principle in biology. In the display of his abilities over a large range of literary and artistic observation, there was more of the instinctive dash than an earnestness of purpose. With greater precision, and a better-directed energy, his walk would have been higher and more commensurate with his rare intellectual gifts. He achieved much, it is true, and had a ray of concentrativeness fallen upon his work and been reflected on his page, he would have attained a higher eminence, and left a bolder inscription in the annals of British Anatomy and Physiology. Few men of this century had better brains, or held out greater promise of effecting right good work in science, than Robert Knox. It has been proved that his early years were exceedingly fruitful, and that anatomy in his hands derived a beneficial impetus, not only felt to-day in numerous medical schools of the kingdom, but likely to continue to be felt for generations to come. Who of the many distinguished teachers of anatomy gone before or culminating in Dr. John Barclay, have had such a noble following as the Owens, the Goodsirs, and others noticed in this volume?

Dr. Robert Knox laboured strenuously to educate academic youth as thinkers and workers in zoology; and succeeded in establishing a great school of anatomy.

His indoctrination will live ; indeed, he had the pleasure of seeing its fertile operations in the hands of Professor John Goodsir, who, during his twenty years' reign in the University of Edinburgh, must have taught upwards of 5,000 pupils, and very much on the Knox method of instruction. In the noble spirit that guided him through life, Goodsir gloried in his acknowledgment of the source of his own inspirations. Sir W. Fergusson, when so unfairly attacked by Professor Syme in November, 1856 (Vide *Lancet*), was also guided by the same grateful spirit, and publicly expressed the pride he had in having been associated with a teacher of such eminence as Knox— the greatest anatomist of his epoch.

A thousand regrets have accompanied my humble efforts to portray the historical Knox—regrets that his early promise was not sustained through his whole career. What might he not have been had the Fates been ordinarily propitious ! The Knox system of opinions, like the threads wrought by the Lachesis spindle, grew in junction and beauty, and bid fair to constitute a web of strength and durability, when the affair of 1828, the Black Atropos, came and impaired its integrity. It is possible that this might have been got over in time, had not the rivalry and personal enmity to which he was exposed proved too sadly disastrous. Relative to this hostility of feeling, it is curious to note Dr. Knox's dedication of his College of Surgeons "probationary essay " (1825) to Surgeon Wishart, of whom he speaks in high terms for his upright conduct towards his professional brethren, and as forming " a striking contrast with the unmanly, dishonourable, but too pre-

valent feeling which causes its possessor to sicken at
the mention of another's success, and stimulates him
to calumniate and detract from that reputation he cannot
hope to obtain."

His London life was in marked contrast with that
of Edinburgh, inasmuch as he had no class and no
platform ; whilst the *res angustæ domi* drove him from
the path of scientific inquiry and the higher aims of philosophy.   Forced contributions to medical and literary
journals or the daily press usurped the hours that should
have been devoted to the extension of biology, and to
the elevation of a name that might have proved a
British adornment to the progressive science of the
nineteenth century.   He had too much to do in the
currente calamo fashion ; indeed, from time to time, he
discharged the duties of a dozen " editorials."   He was
at home on the social, the sanitary, and the political
aspects of the day, the affairs anatomical and medico-
chirurgical, the Horse Guards, and Somerset House,
colonization and geographical discovery, priests and
petticoats, arts and artists, travel, natural history, and,
above all, Race. One day he figured as Spartacus writing
slashing articles for a Radical print, condemnatory of
parsons, politicians, and tuft-hunters—that was his *forte ;*
another day he was discoursing in the pages of the
Morning Advertiser, that odd representative of a dualistic
faith—beer and bigotry ; and though he did not write
for Licensed Victuallers or to please the Pharisee,
this must have been his foible.   In these instances the
guinea stamp prevailed o'er the man.   How far otherwise when he wrote for the Linnean Society, the

Zoologist, and the medical journals; there, science prevailed o'er the guinea, and Knox was then "a man
for a' that, and a' that."

No person had so many irons in the fire at once as
poor Knox. "A Dissertation on the Origin of the Arts"
—"A Critical Inquiry into the Nature of Beauty"—"On
the Intercalation of the present Living World with the
Fossil or Extinct," may be cited among the works he
had on hand and in progress towards completion ; and
only a few days before his death he had commenced
"A History of the African Travellers, Sparman, Le
Vaillant, Burchell, &c." One difficulty must have presented itself, that of finding publishers for works of this
kind, when the feeling of the day was by no means
favourably disposed towards the science and the varied
themes that he sought to expound. Perhaps the
world is much the same to-day that it was thousands of
years ago, when the most ancient literature of the Vedic-
Rig-Veda set forth—

> " How multifarious are the views which different men inspire !
> How various are the ends which men of various crafts desire !
> The leech a patient seeks ; the smith looks out for something cracked ;
> The priest seeks devotees, from whom he may his fees extract :"

yet who can believe in the successful competition of a
philosophic-mindedness like that of Knox, with the high
and low sensational, the bigamies and bastardies of the
fashionably current literature of these days of debase-
ment! What chance has true science, the science of life,
or the scrutiny of material forms, or the higher philosophy
of Man himself, with the mesmeric trance, the spiritual
" mediums," the calling of table-rapping spirits through

vile knaves "in the cellarage," the Exeter Hall intrusions into the councils of Providence, the "organized hypocrisies" of Disraeli Cabinets and Lothair-Caucasian myths, the hurdy-gurdies of art, and other go-rounds of the World's Vanity Fair ? The simple truth is, that the æsthetic aspirations, the broad science, the historic temperament and philosophic methods of Knox, came too soon upon the world's stage to be either understood or appreciated by the general public. His reasonings sounded of transcendentalism, whilst his talk breathed a doubting theism terribly incongruous with human creeds and low idealistic faiths. The anatomist was fifty years ahead of his time, hence his isolated position and the experience of neglect he sustained at the hands of Governments, chartered bodies, collegiate or corporate.

Dr. Knox may be said to have represented the intellectual qualities and the moral deficiencies of our nature. He made no religious declaration, and therefore belonged to no Church ; he nominally ranked with a large body of people designated "outsiders," or "Christians unattached." Well catechized in youth, as is the custom in Scotland, he knew the Bible intimately, and occasionally quoted it when wishing for an easy outlet to a pressing difficulty. Thus, in discussing the vital and chemical theories offered in explanation of the phenomena of respiration, none of which carried his entire conviction, he would cut the Gordian knot by saying— "But then, gentlemen, let us remember that HE breathed the breath of life into man's nostrils. How exquisite the sentiment !" All this was done with the gravity of an orthodox divine, and made a more profound impression upon his pupils than a long doctrinal sermon.

There were various speculations afloat as to his religious faith; and though this is a delicate subject to handle, especially if the man *sub judice* be charged with what the world in its wisdom calls heterodoxy, I hesitate not to disclose the whole truth known to me : half-truths only give rise to absurd innuendos and mysteriousness. In doing so, I shall but carry out his own wishes[1]—namely, to be known as he was on earth, and not as the "unco guid" of the Presbyterian Synods would have liked him to be. Knox, it need hardly be said, was as fully entitled to form his own religious belief as any man in broad Scotland. He had been brought up in the most rigid forms of the Christian faith, and had carefully studied all that pertained to its history, not uninfluenced, perhaps, by the example of his great ancestor, John Knox the Reformer ; he had been thrown among the paid advocates of the Churches, and *knew* the nature and merits of their advocacy, nowhere writ or upheld in the pages of the New Covenant: he noted the occupants of the chief seats of the synagogue, and the groups of feminine and emotional believers, yet the longer he lived the less he trusted to Sabbath respectabilities, and the proclamations of Zion from the housetops of a Mammon-built Church.

[1] A true Protestant in every walk of life, I hold that the world has nothing whatever to do with the beliefs of living men, if they choose to be reticent or non-demonstrative themselves. In these days of theological controversy, it is however of interest to know the opinions held by men of superior minds like Knox, particularly when the grave shelters them from the rancorous condemnation of would-be interpreters of Providence.

Some looked upon him as a Unitarian; if it were true, he then shared in the opinions held by Sir Isaac Newton,[1] John Milton, and John Locke, and a large and goodly company of noble names—the noblest, it may be said, in English history; opinions, too, endorsed by Channing and Emerson, and other leading minds of the United States of America, and by Herder and numerous noted Germans. Whilst he obviously sympathised with the fate of Servetus, and had no liking for the author of the rigid Calvinism that has tried many a young heart with its catechisms and unintelligible dogmas, he did not belong to the Unitarian school of thinkers.

He seemed to view all religious sects and denominations, from the Mummy-maker Egyptian down to the worshippers of the "Winking Virgin of Rimini" of these latter days, as much alike in character, having their origin in idolatrous credulity and ignorance. National Churches in his eyes were but part and parcel of the statecraft and priestcraft that crops out in every age and in every clime. In the fetichisms of the savage, the Dii Majores of the Greek and Roman, the Prophets of the Mahomedan, the Trinities of the Hindoo and Christian, he saw but the superstitious instincts of Man tamely submissive to artful schemers, whose purposes are best served by enslaving humanity and binding it down to the yoke of governmental and priestly tyrannies.

Without any outward religious manifestation, Knox was nevertheless a man of high reverence and belief.

[1] Some thirty years ago, when Newton's orthodoxy was being discussed, the impression I received was in favour of his being a pure Deist, rather than a Unitarian.

Walking out by the southern suburbs of Edinburgh and underneath the basaltic columns[1] of Arthur's Seat, his conversation would fall upon the constitution of the earth and the mighty physical changes it had undergone preparatory to its becoming the habitat of life ; the countless ages that had passed'; the insignificance of Man, though he would boast of his being the adorned capital in the temple of creation. He dwelt on Man's finiteness and inability, after tens of thousands of years' experience and increasing gain of knowledge, to fathom the mysteries of life—past, present, and future. In our sea-side rambles by the Firth of Forth, Knox, looking to the tidal wave falling at his feet, and wishing to interpret it in all its fulness of association, would become eloquent on the higher relations of Man towards his Creator. He expected the advent— far distant, it might be—of a clearer vision into the laws of the organic world, to enable "poor mortals" to grasp the grandeur of the great Creative scheme. Under a silence as serene as any "academic grove," and listening to Nature's music playing upon the pebbly beach, Knox would revert to the teachings of Socrates, and the greatness of a mind that could propound so bold and not less divine a sentiment as that pertaining to the "Unknown God." Though constant in his support of Aristotle's achievements in Natural History, and ready to uphold the prestige of

---

[1] Knox did not believe in such exaltations as Sir John Leslie, the natural philosopher, who forty years ago was afraid to pass underneath these columns, known as "Samson's Ribs," owing to his foolish credulity in the words of an old witch, who said that the said ribs would be sure to fall on the greatest philosopher of Scotland. Sir John owned this soft impeachment, and avoided the risk of fulfilling the old hag's prophecy—verily a safe one.

that noble work the *Historia Animalium*, Knox liked
to dwell upon the exalted genius of Socrates, who would
have but one God, and not a Trinity or Pantheon ; "the
Unknown God" rather than the many gods and god-
desses but *too well known* at Eleusis and elsewhere.
His views of Man, as part of the great organic scheme,
might be dogmatically asserted, as it has been by others
—"On earth there is nothing great but man : in man
there is nothing great but mind." But as the human
mind has never been able to comprehend the true God,
and is necessarily limited to the interpretation of His
works, Knox, with every respect for the declaration of
St. Paul on Mars' Hill, held by the philosophy of the
Greek sage, who would have raised an altar "To the
Unknown God;" upon which good men might con-
secrate good thoughts—the highest aim in religious
worship, and the best security for good works.

It would have been desirable to speak at greater
length of these conversations, so happily conceived and
so charmingly expressed ; but so many years have
elapsed since I listened to the anatomist, that I am
afraid they would lose much of their freshness and
interest in the narrative. In attempting to recall these
communings with Nature alongside so choice a companion, the man Knox himself, in deep earnestness,
pouring out enlightened talk with the fulness of a
libation offered to the gods, comes before me like a
living and veritable presence. Could his words be recorded they could only appear in formal lines wanting
altogether the brilliancy, the life, and the inspiration of
the speaker himself. He was "a being made of many

beings," and shone alike in every part of his multipled nature. You felt a genuine and immediate personal interest in his unflagging converse, and realized Words-worth's lines—

> " His gestures note,—and hark ! his tones of voice
> Are all vivacious as his mien and looks."

In his hours of communicativeness, and where more was meant than meets the eye, on matters of reve-lation, the Deistic feeling seemed to predominate in Knox's mind. His historical instances, the men whom he prized for their psychological gifts, their researches in science and philosophy, were reputed Deists ; *e.g.* Bayle, Voltaire, Hume, Condorcet, Goethe, Alexander von Humboldt, and Arago. Indeed, if the evidence of concurrent opinion be worth anything at all, Deism is the prevalent belief of all the leading minds in France, and probably of the Continent generally—the favoured Protestant Albion being by no means exempt. In confirmation of this view a late writer, as quoted by a London Episcopalian clergyman, states that " Rational-ism had made such progress in Germany that 10,000 volumes have been issued during this century denying the immortality of the soul."

If Knox ranked with those who preferred geological data to the traditions of Moses ; natural to revealed theology ; the laws of genesis to the doctrines of the "immaculate conception," the reader may rest assured that it must have been on a clear conviction that he founded his beliefs. Now, sincerity, as Sheridan said of virtue, is a fine thing, and ought to be respected in these days of unspeakable cant and hypocrisy. Unfortunately for the anatomist, living in the midst of a vaunting Protestantism called liberal and Christianized, his sincerity cost him very dear, as it had done thousands of others before and since his time. It was impolitic on his part, nay, adverse to all success in the world, to stand aloof from the Churches, whether established by law, or upheld by prophets of the Cumming and Tupper school. Perhaps in looking at these purely human inventions or institutions in all their professed integrity and orthodoxy to boot, he thought it better to take his stand with philosophers like Goethe and Humboldt than hang by the lawn sleeves and "holier than thou's" of the "self elect." Among the "eminently pious," Knox had no better repute than Goethe, who was talked of as a "Belial or corrupt spirit," whose dangerous character rested on a combination of genius and learning with demoniacal influence. The same charitable and Christian-like construction was put upon Knox, who, however much opposed to creeds, never dreamt of disturbing any man's faith. Knox was neither a Pericles nor an Anaxagoras, but he was as often arraigned before the gossiping tribunals of Edinburgh as if Lampon and other soothsaying sycophants of the Greek period had transmitted their malice from Lycabettus to Arthur's Seat.

"Under an Augustus or an Antonine, man was free to worship the deity of his choice or of his belief,—to practise whatever religious folly he preferred : throughout Europe, at the present time, to cease to be orthodox —to cease to conform—is to forfeit all or most of the privileges of citizenship." In penning these words in 1847, Knox had a home example of their truthfulness ; and many others less known to fame have suffered a similar ostracism.

The deeply meditating anatomist would rise to his own opinions, and with a rare courage believe and act independently of the prevailing sentiment ; to affect such a privilege he might have foreseen would not be held commensurate with the tone of British society. He may have hoped that the boasted civilization of the nineteenth century would, in time, come to recognize a true Protestantism, and that in shaking off the trammels of rudimental beliefs as persistent as paganism itself, the spirit of progressive thought would rise to a higher platform, and one broad enough to accept all men living honestly within the pale of their country's jurisdiction and the circle of approved morals. The history of our country was fraught with lessons calculated to teach him to be less credulous of either a charitable or a forgiving spirit in the world. Strong in his own individuality and the light that he possessed, he could not brook the restrictions imposed by men whose whole education was circumscribed by religious, and necessarily dogmatic, standards. Freedom of opinion in Knox was held to be egotism, waywardness, and wickedness.

" Oh that mine enemy would write a book!" and Knox might have added, "inscribe his name on the title-page;" but his opponents were more wily. It suited their tactics to deal in innuendos, suspicions, and the pious forms of sapping and undermining personal character, so prevalent in cathedral and Evangelical coteries. Not caring to

suit himself to the temper of the times, or to mollify
the rabidity evinced by Christians, he would hold
himself unshackled and unfettered ; and Edinburgh, not
liking this, first criticised, then censured, and finally
ostracized him from its high places of trust and distinction.

Knox lived to see great inroads made upon the old-
established Christian formulas and faiths, and considering what he himself had suffered, must have enjoyed a
hearty laugh on being told of his old friend the Zulu
accomplishing the conversion of a " Reverend Father in
God " from a belief in the inspiration of Moses, and,
oddly enough, by no greater argument than the simplest
rules of a Colenso arithmetic !

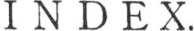

INDEX.

INDEX.

O.

"OINEROMATHIC SOCIETY," 133.
———————— Song, by Professor
Edward Forbes, 133.
Orang Outang, 218.
Origin of the Arts, 387.
Ornithorhynchus paradoxus, 25,
294.
Os femoris, fracture of, 208
Osteology, Comparative, De Blain-
ville's Lectures on, 216.
Owen, Professor, 165, 180, 281,
398.
Ox, the Wild, of Scotland, 209.

P.

PACHYDERMS, the Apodal, 165.
Painful Crepitation of the Radial
Extensor Muscles, 205.
Pancreas, Anatomy of the, 217.
Paré, Ambrose, 51.
Paterson, David, Knox's door-
keeper, 98.
Pathological Anatomist to the Can-
cer Hospital at Brompton, 365.
Paul Jones, the Pirate, 3.
Pericarditis, cases of, 19.
Philosophy of Anatomy, 243.
———————— of Zoology, 360.
Phoca Vitulina, Vasa Efferentia and
Afferentia in, 33; fossilized re-
mains of, 35.
Phocæna communis, 176–7.
Pictorial Anatomy School, 153–4.
Placental Tufts of Weber, by Knox,
219.
"Pocket Anatomist" exposed, 139.
Portrait of Dr. Knox, by Professor
Edward Forbes, 140.
Potato-disease, supposed cause of,
342.
Pulse, the Human, 7–8, 207–8, 391.
Pupils of Knox, numbers of, 130–4.
———— ———, the distinguished,
263, 281.

Q.

QUETELET, Professor, of Brussels,
207, 257.

R.

RACES of Men, chapters xv. and xvi.
———— Men, lectures on, 148.
———— Southern Africa, 24.
Radius, Fracture of, near Carpal
Extremity, 254.
Raphael, 52.
Rehearsal, a strange, by Knox,
134–6.
Reid, Professor John, 95, 133, 147,
157–8, 195. 208, 262–4, 282.
Reinhardt, Professor, 171.
Rennie, Professor, 189.
Religious opinions, chapter xx.
———— persecutions, 53.
Resurrectionists, 55, 60, 62, 65.
———— ————, stories of, 67–71,
103–4.
Resuscitation of the hanged, 49.
Rete mirabile in the Cranium, &c.
of the Cetacea, 170–1, 173–4.
Retzius, Professor, 180.
Robertson, Dr. Argyle, Edinburgh,
132.
Rorqual, the great, 166–70.
————, the small, 171.
Royal Society of Edinburgh, 36,
191–3, 270.
Royal Physical Society, Edinburgh,
5, 36, 248.
Royal College of Surgeons, Edin-
burgh, 37.
Royal Free Hospital, London, 349.
Ruysch, Frederick, 40, 52.

S.

SAINT JEROME doubted, 387.
Salmonidæ, growth of, chapter x.
Salmon Fisheries, Report on, 187–8.
Saxon Race, chapters xv. and xvi.
Scarpa, *Tabulæ Neurologicæ* of, 119.

THE END.

LONDON: R. CLAY, SONS, AND TAYLOR, PRINTERS, BREAD STREET HILL.